HEALING
AND
THE MIND

Also from Bill Moyers and Public Affairs Television

A WORLD OF IDEAS
A WORLD OF IDEAS II
JOSEPH CAMPBELL AND THE POWER OF MYTH
THE SECRET GOVERNMENT: THE CONSTITUTION IN CRISIS
REPORT FROM PHILADELPHIA: THE CONSTITUTIONAL CONVENTION OF 1787

HEALING
AND
THE MIND

BILL MOYERS

BETTY SUE FLOWERS, Editor
DAVID GRUBIN, Executive Editor
ELIZABETH MERYMAN-BRUNNER, Art Research

MAIN
STREET
BOOKS

DOUBLEDAY
New York   London   Toronto   Sydney   Auckland

A Main Street Book

PUBLISHED BY DOUBLEDAY

a division of Bantam Doubleday Dell Publishing Group, Inc.
1540 Broadway, New York, New York 10036

Main Street Books, Doubleday, and the portrayal of a building with
a tree are trademarks of Doubleday, a division of Bantam Doubleday
Dell Publishing Group, Inc.

Healing and the Mind was previously published in hardcover by
Doubleday, a division of Bantam Doubleday Dell Publishing Group,
Inc., in 1993. The Main Street Books edition is published by
arrangement with Doubleday.

"i thank you God for most this amazing" is reprinted from *Xaipe* by
E. E. Cummings, edited by George James Firmage, by permission of
Liveright Publishing Corporation. Copyright 1950 by E. E.
Cummings. Copyright © 1979, 1978, 1973 by Nancy T. Andrews.
Copyright © 1979, 1973 by George James Firmage.

Designed by Stanley S. Drate/Folio Graphics Co., Inc.

The Library of Congress has cataloged the Doubleday edition as
follows:

Moyers, Bill D.
    Healing and the mind / Bill Moyers; Betty Sue Flowers, editor;
David Grubin, executive editor.
        p.   cm.
    "A companion to Bill Moyers' public television series, "Healing
and the Mind"—Editor's note.
    Includes index.
    1. Healing—Psychological aspects.   2. Medicine and psychology.
3. Mind and body.   4. Psychophysiology.   5. Holistic medicine.
I. Flowers, Betty S.   II. Grubin, David.   III. Healing and the mind
(Television program)   IV. Title.
R726.5M69   1993
616'.001'9—dc20   92-31074
                                            CIP

ISBN 0-385-47687-6
Copyright © 1993 by Public Affairs Television, Inc., and David Grubin
Productions, Inc.
All Rights Reserved
Printed in the United States of America
First Main Street Books Edition: April 1995
10 9 8 7 6 5 4

THIS BOOK IS DEDICATED TO
my father, Henry Moyers, who loved this life despite his pain, and
to the men and women of the Fetzer Institute, whose mission is healing.

Bill Moyers would like to thank the following people for their work on the television series.

EXECUTIVE PRODUCER
David Grubin

EXECUTIVE EDITOR
Judith Davidson Moyers

PRODUCTION EXECUTIVES
Dana Fox
Judy Doctoroff O'Neill
Arthur White

PRODUCERS
Chana Gazit
David Grubin
Alice Markowitz
Pamela Mason Wagner

COPRODUCERS
Sam Sills
Kate Tapley

SEGMENT PRODUCER
Judith Towers Reemstma

ASSOCIATE PRODUCERS
Judy Epstein
Laura Jean Ozment
Rebecca Jo Wharton

PRODUCTION MANAGER AND
POSTPRODUCTION SUPERVISOR
Sally Roy

PRODUCTION COORDINATOR AND
POSTPRODUCTION COORDINATOR
Linda Patterson

CAMERA
Michael Chin
Mark Falstad
David Grubin

Bert Guthrie
Terry Hopkins
William B. McCullough
Allan Palmer
Frances Reid
Joel Shapiro
Gary Steele

SOUND
Francis X. Coakley
Stephen Longstreth
Michael Lonsdale
Roger Phenix

GAFFERS
Brent Lawson
Scott Ramsey
Mark Shankel
Dick Williams

ASSISTANT CAMERA
David Eubank
William B. McCullough
Rebekah Michaels
Hilary Morgan

EDITORS
Geof Bartz
Bob Eisenhardt
Larry Silk
David Steward

ASSISTANT EDITORS
Ann Collins
Nancy Beth Graydon
Melissa Neidich
Peter Stader
Patricia Streeton

SOUND EDITORS
Dan Edelstein
Ron Hershey
Melissa Neidich
Douglas Rossini

ASSISTANT SOUND EDITORS
Ann Collins
Lisa Prah
Elizabeth Rich

POSTPRODUCTION ASSISTANTS
Robert Featherstone
Adam Schenck

ADDITIONAL RESEARCH
David Gillis

MUSIC
Michael Bacon

SERIES OPEN
Maureen Selwood

COMPTROLLERS
Stacy Beatus
Jeannine Dominy
Diana Warner

EXECUTIVE ASSISTANTS
Claudia Odyniec
Deborah Rubenstein
Lee Taylor

PRODUCTION ASSISTANTS
Elizabeth Byard
Vivekan Don Flint
Brian Moore
Andrew Nugent-Head
Bill Nye

CONTENTS

III THE MIND/BODY CONNECTION

IV THE MYSTERY OF CHI

V WOUNDED HEALERS

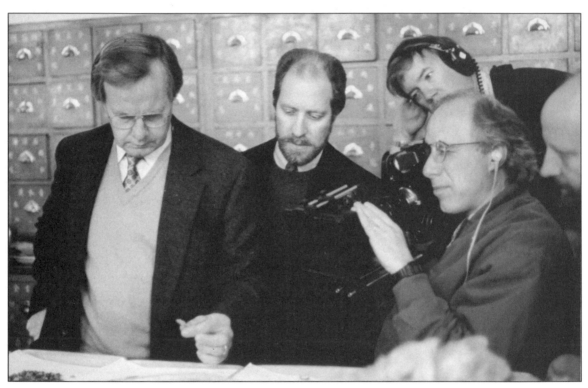

Bill Moyers and Dr. David Eisenberg are filmed on location in China by the team of David Grubin, soundman Roger Phenix, and lighting specialist Scott Ramsey.

INTRODUCTION

"Every education is a kind of inward journey."
—VACLAV HAVEL

I suppose I've always been interested in the relation of mind and body, growing up as I did in a culture that separated them distinctly. In science class we studied the material world, which we expected would someday be understood and predicted down to the last molecule. In philosophy we studied models of reality, based on the rational mind, that took no notice of conditions male and female, sick and well, rich and poor. And then in church we learned that we would someday take off this body as we might a suit of clothes and live as disembodied souls. Yet every day in this divided world of mind and body, our language betrayed the limitations of our categories. "Widow Brown must have died of a broken heart—she never got sick until after her husband was gone." My parents talked about our friend the grocer, who "worried himself sick," and my Uncle Carl believed that laughter could ease what ailed you long before Norman Cousins published his story about how he coped with serious illness by watching Marx Brothers movies and videos of *Candid Camera.*

Coincidentally, it was Norman Cousins who, many years after I left East Texas, helped me to put all this into perspective. We became friends in the 1960s, when I was a White House assistant and he, a famous editor and author, came down to Washington to advocate, passionately and puckishly, one or another of the humanitarian causes that commanded his enthusiasm. After I moved to New York, Norman and I sometimes met to continue our discussions of and debates over the state of the world. Then he fell gravely ill with a rare disease, and his extraordinary experiences as a patient became the subject of his best-selling book *Anatomy of an Illness.* When I needed help for loved ones in their own recovery, Norman was generous with his counsel, and our conversations moved from politics and world events to the subject of healing, to what he had learned and was still learning about emotions and health, laughter and medicine, mind and body. He became perhaps the country's best-known and most informed layman about these matters, approaching them, as another of his friends said, "with the discerning eye of a research scientist and the unabashed excitement of a child. He was a convert. He had a vision."

In 1980, Norman suffered a severe heart attack. Again he turned his harrowing recovery into a book, *The Healing Heart: Antidotes to Panic and Helplessness.* The University of California at Los Angeles invited him to become an adjunct professor of psychiatry and behavioral science, and until his death in 1990 he was the unofficial but enormously influential catalyst for the rapidly growing field of mind/body medicine. I went out in the mid-1980s to interview him for a television profile, and we talked late into the day about the innovative research being conducted by the UCLA faculty and other universities. "You have to treat this subject in a television series," he said. "Television's the new idiom, and this is the revolution that can really help people to understand their mind's power in healing. You must do a television series about it." I told him it would be difficult, in part because so many quacks were exploiting people's curiosity and yearning. Great expectations had been aroused in the 1970s, when people with cancer thought that mind/body interactions might work miracles, and those expectations had been cruelly dashed. The only way to approach the subject on television, I argued, was to acknowledge modesty, and television is not a modest medium. "But it has to be done one day," he said.

Norman's death quickened my resolve to act on his urging. So did the loss at that time of the person to whom this book is dedicated: my father. When my brother died in 1966, my father began a grieving process that lasted almost twenty-five years. For all that time he suffered from chronic, debilitating headaches. I took him to some of the country's major medical facilities, but no one could cure him of his pain. At one point during that ongoing search for help, a doctor tried to teach him that his headaches were somehow related to his grief. But my father persisted in treating his pain exclusively as a medical problem, and the headaches continued to torment him.

So there are many personal reasons for my interest in mind/body medicine. And there are journalistic reasons as well. In the past three years I found myself clipping more and more stories about new research and about the growing popularity of alternative medical practices among the general public. Doctors told me of patients increasingly seeking options that do not involve tests, drugs, and surgery. Shelf after shelf at the local bookstores filled with books on the subject. The Institute of Medicine at the National Academy of Sciences convened meetings on the extent to which stress and emotions may influence physical health. Experts in the fields of endocrinology, immunology, neuroscience, psychology, psychiatry, and epidemiology gathered to compare notes, findings, and doubts. Why is it, they wondered, that about 60 percent of outpatient visits to primary care physicians are related to stress or mind/body interactions? That perhaps one in five primary care visits are attributable "to major depressive anxiety disorders"? I read of one such meeting where a notable declared that "if this were a *medical* disorder that wasn't being diagnosed or treated, the situation would be regarded as scandalous." Meanwhile, Congress appropriated $2 million and the National Institutes of Health opened an Office for the Study of Unconventional Medical Practices, hoping to evaluate what truly works and to separate the quacks from the healers. Almost every week brought fresh reports of developments in a rapidly burgeoning field.

Then one day I met Robert Lehman. He had just become president of the Fetzer Institute and had resolved to make it the leader, through education and research, in expanding the development of health care approaches in which the mind, in all its dimensions, is applied to the health of the body. Ours was an instant kinship, providing the inspiration and impetus for the PBS series on which this book is based. Thanks to Rob's support, within a few months my longtime friend and collaborator, the filmmaker David Grubin, and I were beginning production on *Healing and the Mind*.

Two important questions shaped the series: How do thoughts and feelings influence health? How is healing related to the mind? We asked doctors in large public hospitals and small community clinics about healing and the mind in daily practice. We talked with people in stress reduction clinics and therapeutic support groups and learned about such techniques as meditation and self-regulation as well as about regimens of diet and exercise. We talked with scientists about mind/body research and about the fascinating new field of psychoneuroimmunology, which brings together psychologists, neurologists, and immunologists to explore mind/body connections. We traveled to China to experience a culture whose model of human health is so different from ours that my questions about the connection of mind and body could not be answered from within its frame of reference. When the regulation of chi, or vital energy, is the object of medicine, questions about mind and body make no sense.

The journey led us to a central question: What is health? When curing seems impossible, as in the case of terminal cancer, can we yet hope for "wholeness," the root of "healing"?

As usual with the exploration of complex subjects, there are more questions here than answers. And there are dangers, too. When I first proposed the series, one of my associates wrote an impassioned challenge to my intentions, for she feared that, "encouraged by the series, the desperately ill patient" might defy the physician, discard the medicine, stop the chemotherapy, and embrace an "alternative" treatment; or that the series might appear to support the kind of glib mind-over-matter thinking that makes people feel guilty about their illness. Her warning registered; the "Heal thyself!" message so implicit in some popular books promises more self-deception than self-healing.

I trust our work has avoided both dangers, first, by making clear that practically everything is still to be known about how the mind affects the body, and second, by emphasizing how much our Western medicine has to offer. Even in China, Western medicine exists alongside traditional Chinese medicine dating back thousands of years. We in the West do not have to give up our own proven resources in order to appropriate the best another culture has to offer; here may well be the crucible where East meets West to forge a new source of healing.

Exploration is the key. We have organized this book around the questions and answers we found during our journey, so that you, the reader, might join in our conversation. If the series and the book implicitly advocate anything, it is that the journey is worth making for what each of us might learn about this remarkable union of mind, body, and spirit that is the human being.

— BILL MOYERS

EDITOR'S NOTE

This book is a companion to Bill Moyers's public television series *Healing and the Mind*. Like most companions, it lives side by side with its partner but has its own individual life. In this case, the partner—the series—is full of action as well as the voices of many more people than can be represented here. How can the beautiful stroke of a Chinese calligrapher or the grace of a dying woman be embodied in this medium, which expresses the mind so much more effectively than the body?

And yet books have a place beside the fleeting images of the physical world we see on the screen. Here we can pause and contemplate what that calligrapher meant when he said, "When the mind is present in the heart, we call it happiness." Here we can read a poem by that dying woman and pause over the lines: "I can still see you gathered / — such an unlikely family— / and I know I can find / my way home." And here we can dwell much longer in the minds of the people Bill Moyers interviewed, for these pages give more of the conversation than is possible in the series. This book is also enriched by artwork which invites the reader's mind to wander freely between text and image, and beyond.

I'm grateful to David Grubin, the producer of *Healing and the Mind*, for all he contributed at every stage of this book. Judy Doctoroff O'Neill was also there at every step along the way, as was Judith Moyers. John Flowers, the editor's editor, offered helpful suggestions and encouragement. I also appreciate the practical support of Liz McAllister and Anthony Alofsin. Thanks to Elizabeth Meryman-Brunner, who found the images that enliven this book, and to Doubleday editor Bruce Tracy, who always managed to track me down in London for transatlantic copy-editing. I owe special gratitude to Chris Roberts, who deferred his Oxford education to spend a year working on this and other projects for Bill Moyers, and who, throughout a necessarily fast-paced process, was always gracious and helpful with just the right amount of urgency to allow us to make all the deadlines.

The vision and encouragement of Doubleday senior editor Jacqueline Kennedy Onassis is an important part of this and many other projects. She is one of my heroes, as is Bill Moyers, who continues "getting educated in public," as he once put it, for the benefit of us all.

—BETTY SUE FLOWERS
University of Texas at Austin

I

THE ART
OF HEALING

*"Remember to cure the patient as well
as the disease."*

—DR. ALVAN BARACH

Sirens wail through the night as ambulance after ambulance pulls up to the emergency room of Parkland Memorial Hospital, the public hospital in Dallas, Texas. The emergency area is so crowded that patients' beds line the hallways. Anyone who does not need immediate medical attention is sent to a packed waiting area. Men, women, and children sit silently, often in pain, waiting for hours to see a doctor. During the day more than 350 people may cram the waiting area of the outpatient clinic, until the line extends beyond the hospital door to the sidewalk. It is not unusual for some of these people, most of them poor, to wait ten or twelve hours to receive fifteen minutes of basic medical care. Like all public hospitals, Parkland is underfunded, overcrowded, and overwhelmed. Yet unlike most, it has resolved to change the way it practices medicine.

The man behind the change is Dr. Ron Anderson, Parkland's chief executive officer, a practicing internist and a Southern Baptist who has been influenced both by Native American wisdom about healing and by clinical experience demonstrating that patients benefit measurably when their medical treatment includes attention to their emotional needs.

Following Ron Anderson on his rounds with medical students, I listen as he stops at the bedside of an elderly woman suffering from chronic asthma. He asks the usual questions: "How did you sleep last night?" "Is the breathing getting any easier?" His next questions surprise the medical students: "Is your son looking for work?" "Is he still drinking?" "Tell us what happened right before the asthma attack." He explains to his puzzled students, "We know that anxiety aggravates many illnesses, especially chronic conditions like asthma. So we have to find out what may be causing her episodes of stress and help her find some way of coping with it. Otherwise, she will land in here again, and next time we might not be able to save her. We cannot just prescribe medication and walk away. That is medical neglect. We have to take the time to get to know her, how she lives, her values, what her social supports are. If we don't know that her son is her sole support and that he's out of work, we will be much less effective in dealing with her asthma."

Modern medicine, with all its extraordinary technology, has accomplished wonders, but Anderson believes that caring is also a powerful medicine. The most striking example of his emphasis can be seen in Parkland's neonatal intensive care unit. Like hospitals across the country, Parkland is dealing with a sharp increase in premature and low-birth-weight babies. The hospital employs the latest technology to keep those infants alive, but saving them, Anderson says, is not enough. Equally important is promoting the emotional connection between parent and child. Scientific research has shown that without human contact, a baby will wither and its normal development will be stunted. Babies need to be touched.

Cindy Wheeler is a neonatal nurse. I watch as she introduces Vanessa, a fifteen-year-old mother, to her premature son for the first time. In a room outside the intensive care unit, Vanessa scrubs her hands and arms. Cindy helps her put a sterilized gown over her clothing and then don a mask that covers her nose and mouth. They proceed through the double doors into a series of open rooms with row after row of high-tech medical machinery. In the middle of these islands of hardware is an incubator, a technological womb for Malcolm, Vanessa's tiny son. Protected by this space-age bubble, Malcolm looks more like a fetus than a baby. He is covered with tape and dotted with intravenous needles; tubes connect him to a series of monitors and machines. Cindy knows that Vanessa is frightened and wants to run away. She takes the mother's hand and in a gentle voice begins to tell her that it will be okay, that the baby needs her. She guides Vanessa's finger to Malcolm's miniature hand, whispering that all babies, no matter how old, will respond to the touch of a mother's hand by gripping her finger. The moment is crucial. Vanessa's tense ambivalence will either disappear or cause her to flee. The tiny hand closes around her middle finger. The mother smiles and closes her eyes. Her relief is palpable.

For many women like Vanessa, Cindy tells me, a baby is a status symbol, the first they can call their own. Their dream of a Gerber baby, a Barbie doll, is shattered when the child is born very small or critically ill. "Our mission," she says, "is to share our understanding of the loss they feel, and to help the mothers feel something positive from what otherwise can be a major disappointment and leave a deep psychological scar."

Many of the young mothers are from dysfunctional families. The hospital staff is often the closest they have come to having a nurturing family, and their experience in the neonatal unit is for some the first time they feel supported. To Cindy Wheeler and her colleagues, these teenage mothers are forced to make a decisive choice: to continue being controlled by their problems, or to take charge of their circumstances and, through caring, to make a difference. "Sometimes," says Cindy, "we get very angry at the mothers. A while ago, we saw mothers on drugs as a danger to their babies, and we kept them away from here. Just recently I became angry with a woman for taking drugs during her pregnancy. She was turning her baby into an addict. Her own baby! I wanted to slap her, but I controlled my anger. I told her that she should hold the baby because it was experiencing stress. Maybe it was the touch of that helpless child; whatever, the mother entered a drug rehabilitation program. And she's doing okay."

Listening to Cindy, I recall an essay by the physician and philosopher Lewis Thomas. Its point is that the dismay of being sick comes in part from the loss of close human contact; touch is medicine's real professional secret.

Far from Parkland, at Beth Israel Hospital in Boston, I hear similar opinions from Dr. Thomas Delbanco, an internist who has taken a sabbatical from his practice to head the Picker/Commonwealth Program for Patient-Centered Care. The issue of illness as a life crisis for patient and family, Delbanco says, has been given too little attention in the medical community. New studies are suggesting that patients who receive information and emotional support fare better on the average than those who do not. According to these studies, closer contact between physicians and patients can improve the chances of a good recovery.

Delbanco comes from a family of artists and plays the violin, an instrument whose uniqueness he compares to each individual's experience of illness. "There are two important parts of me," he says. "There is the physician and there is the musician. Music connects me with the importance of being replenished spiritually. And that is something that as a physician I must never forget. The patient before me is a human being with the same joys, sorrows, and complexities as myself. Doctors have to listen to what makes one person different from the other and constantly evaluate that distinction in order to figure out what makes one treatment work better for one person and not the other."

He introduces our team to Audrey and Ed Taylor. Audrey, who is fifty-eight, works in computer graphics. She is about to experience one of the most traumatic events in medicine—open heart surgery. Dr. Delbanco will follow her through the experience and interpret it for her and her family: her husband, Ed, a retired firefighter; their son, Ed, Jr., an MIT graduate with a degree in engineering, who now runs his own small construction company; and their daughter, Ruthie, an elementary-school teacher. Audrey's ordeal will test the family. How they manage their collective trauma, Delbanco explains, can affect Audrey's recovery from the surgery. "The hospitalization of a loved one is a crisis for the whole family. Families can interfere with medicine or they can be the medicine. I would say that respecting and facilitating family bonds may be more crucial to a patient's survival than the latest diagnostic procedure or therapeutic innovation. All too often they are left out of the picture. As doctors, we don't get into the house anymore. And we don't get that larger context in the examining room.

"If we physicians also thought of ourselves as medicine," he says, "we would treat people differently. The more informed you are as a patient and the more your family understands what is happening, the more you and they will be able to make wiser decisions. Information is hope. The terrible doctor robs the patient of hope. As physicians, we have to treat the body and appeal to the mind—the patient's and the family's."

This rings true to me. When I was growing up, our family doctor in Marshall, Texas, instinctively knew a lot about healing and the mind. When he asked, "How are you feeling?" he was interested in more than our stomachaches or fevers. He lived down the street, went to the church on the corner, knew where my parents worked, knew our relatives and family history—and he knew how to listen. He treated the patient holistically before anyone there ever heard of the term.

That was years ago. Today the practice of medicine in an urban, technological society rarely provides either the time or the environment to encourage a doctor-patient relationship that promotes healing. Many modern doctors also lack the requisite training for this kind of healing. As Eric J. Cassell writes in *The Nature of Suffering and the Goals of Medicine*, "Without system and training, being responsive in the face of suffering remains the attribute of individual physicians who have come to this mastery alone or gained it from a few inspirational teachers." Healing powers, Cassell continues, "consist only in and no more than in allowing, causing, or bringing to bear those things or forces for getting better (whatever they may be) that already exist in the patient." The therapeutic instrument in this healing is "indisputably" the doctor, whose power flows not from control over the patient but from his or her own self-mastery. Modern physicians have mastered admirably the power of the latest scientific medicine. To excel at the art of healing requires the same systematic discipline.

Talking with different doctors during this journey, I realize that we do need a new medical paradigm that goes beyond "body parts" medicine, and not only for the patient's sake. At a time when the cost of health care is skyrocketing, the potential economic impact of mind/body medicine is considerable. Thinking about our medical system as a "health care" system rather than a "disease treatment" system would mean looking closely at medical education and our public funding priorities.

On this first stage of my journey, I realize that the subject of healing and the mind stretches beyond medicine into issues about what we value in society and who we are as human beings. As patients, we are more than lonely, isolated flecks of matter; we are members of families, communities, and cultures. As this awareness finds its way into hospitals, operating rooms, clinics, and doctors' offices, perhaps it will spread further, as well. Healing begins with caring. So does civilization.

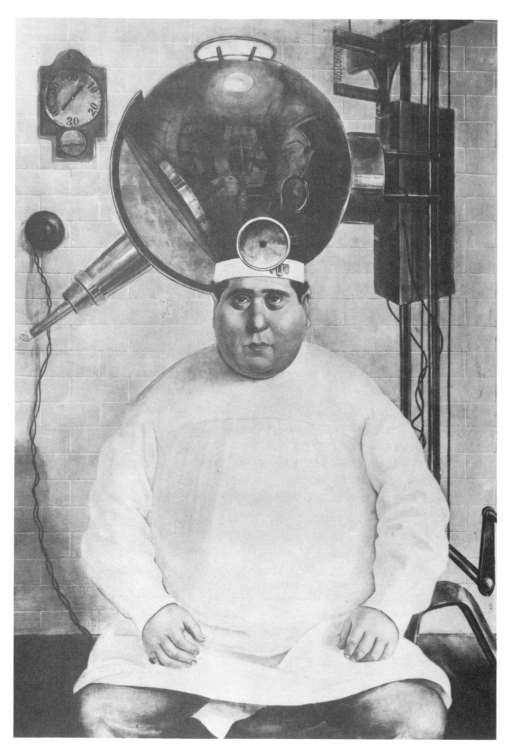

Otto Dix, *Dr. Mayer-Hermann*, 1926

THE HEALING ROLES
OF DOCTOR AND PATIENT

Thomas Delbanco

THOMAS DELBANCO, M.D., is Director of the Division of General Medicine and Primary Care at Beth Israel Hospital in Boston, Associate Professor of Medicine at Harvard Medical School, and Director of the Picker/Commonwealth Program for Patient-Centered Care. He is a founder and past President of the Society of General Internal Medicine. Dr. Delbanco has brought renewed attention to primary care in academic medicine; he is currently working on projects to strengthen and enrich the doctor-patient relationship.

MOYERS: Watching you with your patients, I get the sense that you treat the body and appeal to the mind. Is that a fair characterization?

DELBANCO: I hope I'm addressing both the body and the mind. But they're so intertwined that it's hard for me to differentiate. I know more about the body than the mind. It's probably the easier to study and that's what we learned in medical school—ninety-five percent body and five percent mind. But I'll tell you, once you're in practice, and you're taking care of real people, it becomes much closer to fifty-fifty. One's important one day, and the other's predominant the next day, and they're always mixed up. So appealing to the mind, as you put it, is an interesting notion, but I don't think I'll buy it.

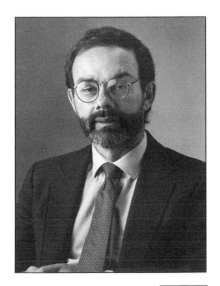

MOYERS: You don't buy it? But you're appealing to something other than just the physical, mechanical parts that make up the human body.

DELBANCO: I'm drawing on the person as a unique individual, and that's much more a function of his or her mind than her body, absolutely—

MOYERS: Wait a minute. What do you mean "a unique individual"?

DELBANCO: Well, people are bloody different one from another. That's actually what makes the fun of medicine. It's not so much that their bodies are different, it's that their minds are different. So in that sense, we focus very hard, or we ought to, on what their minds are about and how that interdigitates with the rest of them.

MOYERS: Interdigitates?

DELBANCO: Yes. When someone's belly hurts, I ask very quickly what's going on in the mind as well as in the abdomen. When someone is depressed, I think also about what might be going on in the body that's leading to the depression. Mind and body are inextricably woven together. Every primary physician knows that. Studies show that probably half the visits to us in the office are for things related to mind issues rather than body issues. We'd better be educated in both if we're going to serve those patients well.

MOYERS: What do you want to know about a person's mind when you become his or her doctor?

DELBANCO: I want to know what they bring to the table. I want to know what they want from me. I want to know what kind of person they are, so I'll know how they filter what I say. I think doctors are actually chameleonlike. I find myself a very different person with different patients.

MOYERS: Like journalists.

DELBANCO: Well, no, I see you people as generally pretty aggressive. But I'm sometimes very passive and laid back, and say "Tell me more." With other people I'm rather directive, and say "Do this, do that." With some patients I'm rather gruff and distant, and with others I'm warm and cuddly. I do this unconsciously. At one level maybe I'm play-acting and not being myself, and maybe that's not the right thing to do. But at another level it's my sense of what that patient wants from me, what kind of doctor he or she wants me to be.

I think there may be two kinds of doctors—those who are very different with different patients, and have a sense of what the patient wants, and then vary themselves to meet that; and others who are very much the same with everyone. My own sense is that those who adapt to different people attract a more varied group of patients.

MOYERS: Why do you need to know so much about the patient beyond the physical?

DELBANCO: I can't manage patients, or consult with patients, or even help patients if I don't know what makes them tick. What their serum potassium shows me is very little in the context of the whole person. They may be terrified to hear that it's low. They may be relieved to hear that it's low. They may have no interest at all in hearing that it's low. I have to have a sense of how they want me to convey information to them. Do they want me to tell them what to do? Do they want to tell me what they want to do and have me comment on whether I think it's wise or not? Do they want me to be directive or consultative? There are an awful lot of different roles I can have, and I can't possibly guess which one you'll choose. So I've got to know what you bring to the table, what your culture and beliefs are, what values you hold, and who you are, particularly if a big thing is going on. I don't think that's so true if you have a sore throat.

MOYERS: Do you think what you know about a patient's life-style and mind makes a physical difference to the patient?

DELBANCO: We don't really know, but my guess is that it does. I certainly know that if I'm ill, I want my doctor to know what I'm about. And certainly it makes a big difference to patients in a life-or-death situation to know that I know what they're about and what they believe in and what they care about. That probably makes a difference not only in the process of their care, but very likely in the outcome of their care and how they feel afterwards.

We did a study of patients who had suffered cardiac arrest and discovered that when we sent people home, half of them sat there paralyzed by fear that it could happen again. It had never entered our minds to talk to patients about the probabilities of having another cardiac arrest or what they could do to prevent it. So it made an enormous difference in their outcome that we didn't really know what made them tick. If we'd understood that, we could have helped them a lot.

MOYERS: Are you saying that their fear has an effect on their bodily well-being?

DELBANCO: I'm sure of that. Now, the scientific evidence is still very scant. I can't prove it. But I suspect that most doctors believe that very strongly.

MOYERS: But haven't good doctors always known that?

DELBANCO: Oh, yes, we're not talking about a new rocket science here. I learned this from my mentors. We had teachers in medical school whom we followed around to the bedside just to watch the way they talked to patients.

MOYERS: What does a good doctor do in relation to my feelings or my mind that helps in the healing process?

DELBANCO: First of all, a good doctor listens to you—and then addresses what you're feeling. I have a vivid recollection of an incident with the wife of someone I trained with. The wife had a weird set of symptoms, and we were very worried about her. She wasn't functioning well. So we sent her to our professor, whom we admired. When she came out, we were all waiting with our fingers crossed. "Well, what's the prescription?" And she said, "He tells me I've got to get a washing machine. I'm working too hard at home." That was the diagnosis.

Another time I remember presenting a patient to this mentor, spending fifteen minutes in the best medical-school style, going through this symptom and that symptom and this finding and that finding. At the end of it he said, "Well, Delbanco, do you think she's sick?" I sat there thinking, "My God, what is this man asking me? I've spent fifteen minutes telling him everything I've found out that was wrong, and he's saying do you think she's sick?" Well, he was reminding me that we were treating the whole person, just as he was doing with our friend's wife. You don't find the washing-machine prescription in many textbooks. But it helped her a lot. She was cured, she was brought back to health, she was made whole, if you will, by that prescription.

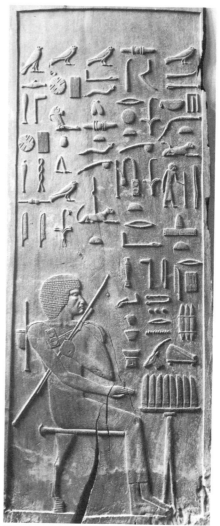

Hesire, Egyptian physician, 2700 B.C.

MOYERS: There's an old notion that the body hurts, and the person suffers.

DELBANCO: Right. Disease and illness. We can look at disease, but illness is what you feel.

MOYERS: What's the difference between disease and illness?

DELBANCO: Disease is looking at your liver and saying "It isn't quite right, Bill. And that heart doesn't sound quite right to me." Illness is how you are feeling. If you feel fine, and I think your liver and heart aren't quite right, what kind of negotiation should we make? If you're smoking, and you're happy with it, and I can list 400 things that can happen to you as a result of smoking, do I write it down on my chart and say "Problem—smoking" if you don't think it's a problem?

MOYERS: What would you do?

DELBANCO: I would write down "Smoking. Moyers doesn't think it's a problem." And we'll come back to it.

MOYERS: On the assumption I come back to you.

DELBANCO: Yes—and you may not. I may say, "Bill, you're a journalist, and you've got an occupational disease—you're drinking a little too much. I'd like you to cut down on it." And you may say, "The hell I'm drinking too much! I don't like you, and I'm going to get another doctor." I'll take that risk because I think that drinking is a big problem and that if we intervene early, we can make a difference.

MOYERS: I would come back to you, though, because I think you're good medicine.

DELBANCO: Yes, the doctor can be good medicine. Alcoholism is an interesting example here because there is little science in how to treat it. We know AA helps a lot of people, but we can't study it because it's anonymous. We have medicines, we have psychotherapy—and then we have the doctor. If I'm your doctor, I might say, "Bill, I think you're drinking too much, and I want you to stop. Come back once a week and tell me how you're doing." I have plenty of patients who've stopped drinking this way. So I think you can argue, in that sense, that the doctor in himself or herself can be good medicine.

MOYERS: When we say that the doctor is the medicine, are we saying that the doctor is a substitute for aspirin?

DELBANCO: I think often we're not only a substitute for aspirin, but maybe a safer substitute. Part of the illness you may be feeling is fear. We often have the privileged role of dispelling uncertainty and sometimes even fear.

MOYERS: How does fear cause a physical reaction?

DELBANCO: We have some insight into that. For example, if I'm driving along on a highway on the edge of the speed limit, and I hear a siren behind me, my knees might begin to shake, and my pulse could get faster. My adrenal glands are pumping out epinephrine—the flight-or-fight response. There is a real physiological response to fear. If the policeman passes by and goes after someone else, the fear passes, and I feel better. But there are also other, more general fears, a gestalt of the mind, if you will, that we know very little about.

MOYERS: What do you mean by "gestalt of the mind"?

DELBANCO: The mind is so complex. I know what the brain looks like—I've seen it on a table, I've seen it laid open. But the mind is well beyond any medicine

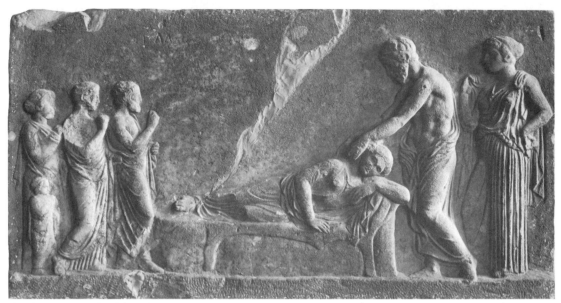

Asclepius, god of healing, 200–400 B.C.

I've learned. And yet I know it's an integral part of medicine and a part of the person I have to address. That's both a frightening and fascinating aspect of what I do—to try to take into account that vast thing about which I understand little and yet that so much affects the people with whom I'm working.

MOYERS: Are we talking here about something more than a placebo effect?

DELBANCO: I don't know. The placebo effect is wonderful medicine. Placebo means "I shall please"—I'm going to help. It's cheap, although if you make a sugar-pill placebo and charge a lot for it, it works better than a placebo for which you charge very little. And if you have certain colors on that pill, it may work even better. The placebo is one of the most powerful medicines we have. It's very hard to tell sometimes whether what we're doing is more than the placebo effect.

For example, suppose I tell you, "Bill, you've had a rough year, you've been doing a lot of reporting, and I want you to relax more. I'm going to give you some techniques that will help you to relax." Then I give you a couple of techniques, one which we know produces physiological relaxation, and another one that is a sham relaxation technique that doesn't really work. I don't know if the sham technique is going to work any less well than the one that's been studied physiologically, because you're going to expect to get better, and so the sham technique is very real medicine for you.

MOYERS: So if I think I'm going to get better, something is happening there between the mind and the body. We don't know what it is, but it's happening. Is there a short way, in your experience, to describe the mind/body relationship?

DELBANCO: When people talk about the mind/body relationship, I think primarily about what makes one person different from another, what makes a person an individual, what makes that person recognizable to me—not just the physical state, but who they are as people. The mind/body relationship is a fascinating marriage between what people say, think, and feel, and their physiological processes. The mind modulates what goes on in the body. We know more about the body than the mind, or we think we do. Actually, we know incredibly little about the body, either—but it's staggering how much we have to learn about the mind. In a sense, I don't even want to learn about the mind because the mind is part of the mystery of you, and I like that sense of mystery.

MOYERS: Do you probe as if your patient presented a mystery to be solved?

DELBANCO: No, it's a mystery to register. I don't think I'll solve it, but I think I'll register it, and I'll understand it to the greatest degree I can. And my understanding of it will affect the way I work with you as a patient.

MOYERS: If hospitals were to act on the basis of what you say, how would they change what they do?

DELBANCO: We would take a much more organized inventory of each individual as he or she comes to us—what you want, what you expect, what your fears are, what you're worried about when you leave us.

MOYERS: That's interesting, because usually the inventory I fill out asks "Have you ever had this illness before? Have you ever taken a drug like this or a drug like that?"

DELBANCO: That's the doctor's review. That's what I can do in my sleep, standing on my head, having been up all night, and having drunk too much wine. I can do the review of systems, going from your heart to your gastrointestinal tract to your kidneys to your this and that—it's a patter song. I learned it the first thing in medical school, and I'll always be able to do it. What we don't ask and what I'd like to see us ask is how is Bill Moyers different from other people?

MOYERS: But why do you want to know that? What difference does it make to my healing while I'm in that hospital?

DELBANCO: It makes an enormous difference. It helps me talk to you in ways that are helpful to you. For example, you may want to be told everything about what's wrong with you. Or you may not want to know anything about what's wrong with you. You may want me just to say, do this, do that. You may want your family very involved in your care. Or you may want me to keep your family at a distance. You may want to endure pain because you're tough, and you think it's good for you to hurt a little bit. Or you may want to feel no pain because you're afraid of pain, and it makes you sick, which might affect your response to medicines and other things. I've got to know what makes you tick. I may know a lot about your disease, but I don't know how you experience your illness. The attitude with which you confront your illness will make a real difference in how you do over time.

MOYERS: What have you learned, from both your clinical experience and your research, about the stress we feel when we go to the hospital?

DELBANCO: I've learned that we usually underestimate it. For instance, if I talk to you when you get to the hospital and tell you ten facts, if you remember one, you'll be

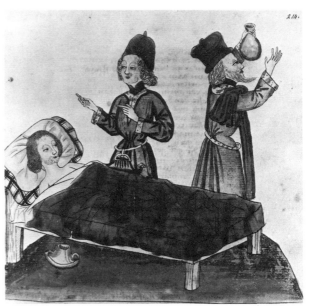

Merchant at the Bed of his Lovesick Friend, 1467

lucky. We've been so struck by what we've discovered that we've sent medical students to be hospitalized incognito, to experience what it's really like to be ill. They sign in as patients and make up illnesses—which is an interesting ethical issue in itself—and then they go through the first couple of days of hospitalization. They come out thunderstruck by the stress they experienced, even though they were not ill.

MOYERS: What did they feel?

DELBANCO: They felt terrified, and passive, lying back in bed and letting people do things to them in ways they normally would never have thought of doing. And they felt depersonalized, that people didn't treat them like human beings. The stress that patients go through is quite extraordinary. We tend to underestimate it or forget about it.

MOYERS: How do you explain that? Hospitals are supposed to be nurturing environments.

DELBANCO: Hospitals are nurturing environments, but they're also very big shops with tons of people working in them. A sociologist called Goffman talks about "total institutions"—for example, mental hospitals, concentration camps, prisons. Goffman points out that there are two kinds of people in those places: those who are there involuntarily and those who choose to work there. The way they both keep sane is by separating from each other. They develop their own kind of language, and their own styles of communicating. For example, patients may talk to each other in ways they'll never talk to those caring for them.

Meanwhile, the people who work in hospitals, even with the best intentions, and even though they are nurturing people, will tend to separate from those they care for. You can see how this happens when you look at what our students go through about the second year of medical school. At about that time they begin to read about awful illnesses, and then if they feel a lump here or a bump there, they'll say, "Well, here I go, I've got the symptoms of this or that terrible illness." Over time, we begin to get over this—but there's always the lingering thought: "My gosh, there but for the grace of something go I." So we keep our distance from the person that we're lucky to be different from.

MOYERS: The last time I went to the hospital for an extended stay, I felt as if I left myself outside.

DELBANCO: I've had patients say similar things. Some, by the way, are very happy about it. They come into the hospital and say, "You know, it's the first time in my life I can lie back and relax and have other people take care of me. I've been running this house for thirty years. I've been doing this or that, and now I'm going to be passive, and I like that." Others go crazy and say, "My gosh, I've been controlling myself all my life, and I've been controlling my environment. Now I get into this strange place, and I lie here, and I can't control anything." Some of them literally go crazy and begin to imagine things or see things on the wall. They have what we call a temporary psychotic episode, which we know will go away when they return home.

MOYERS: Why don't more doctors perceive what it's like to be a patient in the hospital?

DELBANCO: I think doctors have more understanding about that than the public gives them credit for. When I was a resident, a psychiatrist at Columbia wrote the first paper discussing how people go crazy in the intensive care unit. And now we expect it, so we can give appropriate care and reassure the families.

MOYERS: What causes someone to go crazy in the intensive care unit?

DELBANCO: That's a good question. I have a theory about it, which has never been tested, but which has to do with dreams. You know, everyone dreams. Some people remember their dreams, some people don't, but we all dream. We can see that by looking at the eye movements during sleep. If you wake up someone while their eyes are moving, they'll say, "Yes, I'm dreaming." Now if you sleep eight hours a night, that's plenty of sleep. But if I awaken you every time you dream, even though you still get a normal total amount of sleep, you'll become crazy. In two or three days you'll begin to imagine things, to see things on the wall. I have a sense that you're not allowed to dream in a hospital.

MOYERS: They keep poking you and giving you something.

DELBANCO: Yes, they keep moving you around and doing things to you, and you don't get to dream. That may be one of the reasons people go crazy in intensive care units—but, as I say, I haven't studied it.

MOYERS: Do you think that modern medicine, as it is practiced in the hospital, is adequate in the face of suffering?

DELBANCO: I don't think we're ever adequate. We're better, and we have more insight into what we do than we used to, but we've got a long way to go. I've been involved in some studies in which we ask patients what they experience in the hospital. We've done it now in a sample of sixty hospitals around the country, picking patients at random. And we're not adequate. Almost a third of our patients told us they didn't know what they could or couldn't do when they went home. A lot of them pointed out that their pain wasn't managed in a way that they thought was adequate. We have a lot of deficiencies. I think we're getting better at looking at what we're doing and trying to work on it and listening to our patients in ways we haven't before. But no, we're not adequate.

MOYERS: What I am taking away from this is that the patient-doctor relationship is the core of mind/body medicine in the hospital.

DELBANCO: Well, not just in the hospital. People have been talking about the mind in medicine for a long time. In fact, they used to do it a lot more before we had so many technological things we could do to patients. Sometimes the technology gets in the way of the patient-doctor relationship. If I'm so busy trying to figure out what test to schedule next or what consultant to get, I may be in danger of forgetting who you are and what you're experiencing. Technology has distanced us from our patients, and we don't like that. We want to get closer to you, and one of the ways to do that is to talk with you about who you are and what you want from me and what I want from you.

MOYERS: What about your patient, Ms. Taylor, for example? What do you want to know about her?

DELBANCO: How is she going to recover? Is she going to feel whole again after she leaves the hospital? Is she going to feel the things she used to love to do are still possible for her to do? Can she take those long walks with her husband again that she missed, or is she going to be scared that the first time she gets a twinge, she'll have to stop? How she responds to that first walk or the third walk will determine how she lives after that. And I have a lot to do with how that works, because how that

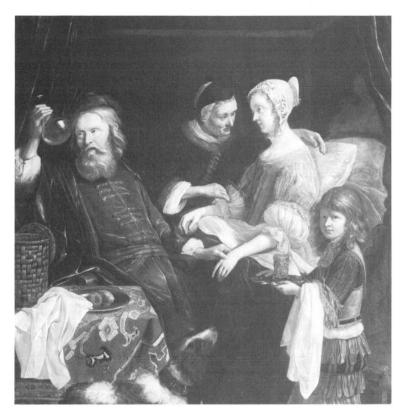

Jacob Toorenvliet,
The Sick Woman,
1647

heart will feel is not going to be merely a function of how well the surgeon cleans out her vessels or replaces them. It's going to be a function of what she brings to her rehabilitation, what I teach her in the hospital before and after about her illness.

MOYERS: At your first meeting with Ms. Taylor, you asked Mr. Taylor to be there. Why?

DELBANCO: I have trouble seeing patients in isolation. We learn more from people when we see them in context. We don't make home visits much anymore, although the best place to learn about people is in their homes. We learned that as students. I used to ride around in an ambulance when I was an intern at Bellevue, and I've never forgotten some of those experiences of seeing the patient in the home. Seeing Ms. Taylor in the context of her family is very helpful. I have a much better sense of what she's like and the environment in which she works and who brings what to the table. For example, she likes her husband to help translate. Her son, who's a scientist, is a very accurate translator. Her daughter feels things very strongly and can translate her mother's feelings to me. So all of these family members are very expert witnesses to what Ms. Taylor is experiencing.

MOYERS: Are you suggesting that illness is not only a crisis for the patient but possibly for the family, too?

DELBANCO: No "possibly" about it. Often we're blind to what the family has experienced because we don't draw them in as quickly as we should. But it's a tremendous crisis.

MOYERS: What were the Taylor family's greatest concerns?

DELBANCO: Well, some of the family members were afraid that she'd never get off the table, which is a rational fear. No surgeon can say to Ms. Taylor, "I promise you're going to be fine." That isn't the way the world works. She has real heart disease, which is why she has to have an operation. And that heart disease is life-threatening. So the concern ranges from "she's never going to get up again" to "she's not going to be the mother I knew" or "she's not going to be the wife I knew." The work she used to do and the money she used to bring in—maybe that's gone in the future. Those are very lively fears in the family that we're often blind to because we never hear about them.

MOYERS: That seems so commonsensical, and yet including the family like this places a great burden on the doctor.

DELBANCO: Well, doctors have never been paid for time very well in this country. A surgeon may get paid by each stitch he puts in, but society hasn't figured out a very good way in our current system to pay me for my time. To the degree that doctors are driven by money, which, thank God, they usually aren't, they'll avoid taking time to talk to a family. Time is expensive.

MOYERS: Do you assume that people do better if they're given more information?

DELBANCO: My general assumption is that people should be more informed. I'm a better doctor if I'm more informed, and I think patients are better patients if they're more informed. Of course, that's a general assumption. Some patients are terrified by information. There are others for whom a little knowledge is a very dangerous thing. It's hard to generalize about people, but when in doubt, it's better to know more than less. For example, we have studies showing that if patients get a lot of education before the operation about what to expect in the operation, how to manage pain afterwards, and what kind of stresses they will feel, then they will have a better postoperative course. And while there's not that much science yet that tells us the answers to all these questions, virtually every doctor knows that when patients understand what's going on, what they can or cannot do after leaving the hospital, what the natural history of the evolution of the recovery will be, what they can do to aid in that recovery, what warning signals to watch for so that they get help earlier rather than later—all of that will have a real impact on the recovery.

MOYERS: What do you think you did for Ms. Taylor and her family?

DELBANCO: In a way, it's amazing, but I found myself just a few hours before the operation still explaining to them why the operation was necessary. I explained what was going on in her heart, what the vessels do, how the pump works, what we're trying to fix, what could happen if it isn't fixed. I'm educating them in a way, but I'm also dispelling uncertainty. Uncertainty is the worst illness. The fear of the unknown can really be disabling. Even if the news is bad, people feel better if the uncertainty is dispelled.

MOYERS: And did Ms. Taylor benefit from this kind of straightforward communication?

DELBANCO: I hope she did, although you can never be sure, because people like to please doctors. She might say "Yes, it was helpful" whether it was or not.

MOYERS: But if she thinks it's helpful, the placebo effect might make it really so.

DELBANCO: You know, it's a strange business. I was in Germany recently, visiting a hospital where they were treating people homeopathically. In the U.S. medical world, we don't believe in homeopathy—you know, giving people minute doses of substances that we feel have no effect whatsoever. Eighty-five percent of the pneumonias in that German hospital are treated with homeopathic medicines, and only fifteen percent were treated with the antibiotics that I've been trained to use. And the doctors at this hospital think their patients do well. Now they haven't studied it in the way that I like to study medicine. And maybe homeopathy has nothing to do with this, maybe it's all placebo. But whatever it is, it's powerful medicine because their patients with pneumonia get better. The natural course of illness is also to get better. So how do we learn and really understand this? Do the patients get better on their own, do they get better because of the placebo effect, do they get better because of a homeopathic medicine, or do they get better because of penicillin? It's hard to sort it out sometimes. But we can't just dismiss it.

You know, what changed us a lot was acupuncture. We used to curl our upper lip in academic medicine and say, what's that stuff? And then Reston of the *Times* went over to China and was operated on using acupuncture anesthesia. And we sat up and said, "Hey, this is weird, we'd better be more open-minded." Then we began studying it, and we found little chemicals running around in the body, and we said, "Aha! So that's what's going on here." We have a scientific explanation for acupuncture now, or we think we're on the edge of it, so we feel better about it.

Well, we should be more open about an awful lot of different kinds of healing. What we do is still much more art than science, although we glory in the science of what we do. And we should glory in it. Our science is progressing at a fantastic clip, and you and I are going to be the beneficiaries of that. But our art also has to progress.

MOYERS: When you say it's art, what do you mean by that? You're a violinist. Is there a relationship between the art of music and the art of medicine?

DELBANCO: Because of my fascination with music, I often think in the metaphor of the relationship between art and medicine. I don't know exactly what makes Bach tower over all those people in Germany at the time who were writing very similar music. I know I come back to him time and time again, and I don't want to listen to the others. In the same way, I know who the great doctor is and the also-ran. And the difference between the great doctor and the also-ran is not how much he or she knows, but what he or she brings to the patient as a human being. Knowing this makes the analogies between the art of music and the art of medicine more explicable. I see the people who rise above the others, who serve as mentors—they have something extra.

MOYERS: In the same way that I don't know why the right note from that violin can bring tears to my eyes, I don't know why the right word from a doctor can bring hope to my heart. But it does.

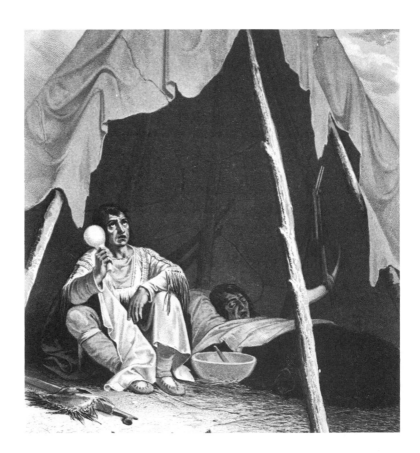

Christian Schuessele, *A Medicine Man Curing a Patient,* 1851

DELBANCO: Well, that's part of the mystery of medicine, isn't it? And it's part of the art of medicine too, and what makes it so exciting to be a doctor. I think the magic of a doctor-patient relationship, if it works well, is to make that connection. I'm working hard now at trying to find an organized way to understand what doctors and patients want from each other.

MOYERS: You want to change the doctor-patient relationship?

DELBANCO: Yes—in a sense I want to bring it back to what I think it once was, but in another sense I want to move it forward. I want patients much more actively involved in what goes on, and to report on what we do well and what we do badly or indifferently. My goal is to listen to them and eventually to have them work with me in improving myself. For example, I think it makes sense to have a few of my patients sit down and say, "Tom, you're a very nice guy, but between you and me and the lamppost, I think you could do this a little differently, and you could do that a little better." Doctors listen to patients very hard, and that gives us all collective hope. We're much more apt to listen to our patients than to the administrators or the federal regulators or the state because we do care about our patients a lot. But we've never really taken advantage of that fact and asked patients to honestly critique what we do. We do that now with our students—we expect our students to critique us, just as they expect us to critique them. I think we can change the doctor-patient relationship so that patients can help us get better, just as we're supposed to help them get better.

I'm very encouraged that in our medical schools now we're spending a lot of time talking about the doctor-patient relationship. We're videotaping our students and asking patients to come back and tell students what they think of what the students did. We're bringing in people in recovery from different illnesses to be interviewed by students and then to critique the way the students talk to them. I think we're changing the way we're imprinting our young people. My hope is that the doctors of the next generation will not just check off your heart and your lungs and your liver, but will also be just as eager to see what you're about as an individual and how you're different from someone else and then to interact with you in that way.

MOYERS: But what about the doctor who doesn't have your personality or your passion, or who doesn't play the violin? Is this a possibility for those doctors?

DELBANCO: We can all change. When I grew up, we were told that teachers were born, not made. Now we're running courses in which we teach people to be better teachers. People who are pretty bad teachers are becoming good ones, and people who are pretty good teachers are becoming better ones. So I'm not going to sit here and say that doctors can't change. Doctors want to be close to their patients. Doctors are very angry about the walls that have come up between their patients and them. They need ways of coming closer. And I think one of the ways that we can

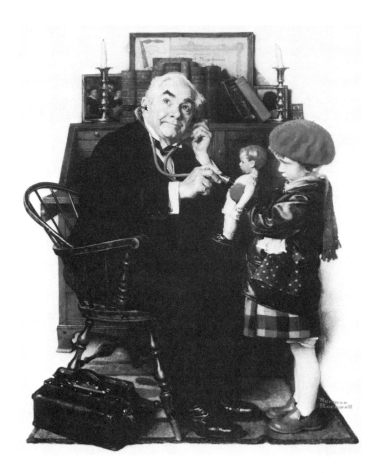

Norman Rockwell,
Doctor and Doll,
1929

come closer to our patients is to treat them as individuals and to talk about ourselves as individuals.

MOYERS: But look, we're in the modern world. Doctors are overburdened, over-busy, overworked, overrun.

DELBANCO: When I was an intern, I was up every other night, and I had very little help. I did everything myself. Today interns are on call only every fourth or fifth night, and they have other people drawing blood and doing tests. And they're depressed. They're unhappy, frustrated, and spend a lot of time wondering whether they should go on in medicine. I loved what I was doing. What was the difference? I think one of the big differences is that I was much closer to my patients. I didn't have a hundred tests in the way, a hundred things to schedule and order, a hundred rules to follow. I had very little more than my stethoscope and a few tests and quite a lot of time with people.

It's easy to look back at the good old days and say, "Well, let's bring them back, and everything will be fine." I can't do that, I know. But I can remind myself of the positive attributes of the good old days. And I can work hard to bring some elements of them back and rescue medicine in that sense. One of the ways to do that is to work very consciously and very hard to become partners with those for whom we care. We can do that better than people in the old days did because we understand more not only about the body, but also about the mind.

MOYERS: I think it was Sir William Osler who said that faith in gods cures some; hypnotic suggestion, others; and faith in the common doctor, still others.

DELBANCO: Yes, and doctors had better learn about all three of these elements to move us forward. You know, it's fascinating that if you look in the dictionary, healers are defined as people not trained in the medical arts. But if you look up "doctor," do you know what it says? "Someone who's a practitioner of the healing arts." Look at the paradoxes in that strange opposition the dictionary gives us. The fun of being a doctor is being trained in the science of medicine and in the art of medicine, and then bringing those elements together with the mystery of being a healer. That's a hell of a privilege.

MOYERS: But how do you bring mystery and art together with science?

DELBANCO: Let me give you a musical analogy. If I'm going to play the violin, I have to know some very concrete things. I have to know where to put my fingers, how to draw the bow, how hard to push, how quickly to draw, and so forth. To a certain degree there's a science of violin playing. But if I want to make the music really speak to you, then I have to do something that goes beyond just these mechanics. Medicine is no different from that. I've got to go beyond the technical aspects of this test and that part of your body. I've got to somehow try to understand your spirit and maybe even touch it at times.

What fascinates me about violins is how different each of them may be from each other. You look at three violins, and at one level they look very similar, but, my gosh, are they different! One works for this kind of music, another satisfies how you feel at this point in time as opposed to that point in time, a third speaks to a different type of impulse. And that's so like patients. The bodies at one level seem very similar to us, and we understand their physiology similarly. We know what can go wrong in them, and what can go right. And yet when you go beyond that to the unique person that makes up that individual patient or that individual instrument, they are so different.

The way music can touch my spirit is intoxicating. And if I can do that with a patient, if I can relate to a patient in an artistic way, a way that takes into account what they're about, I'm pretty sure I'll be a better doctor to them. That mixture of technical expertise and the art of medicine is what gives me the best chance of helping a patient deal with an illness and be healed.

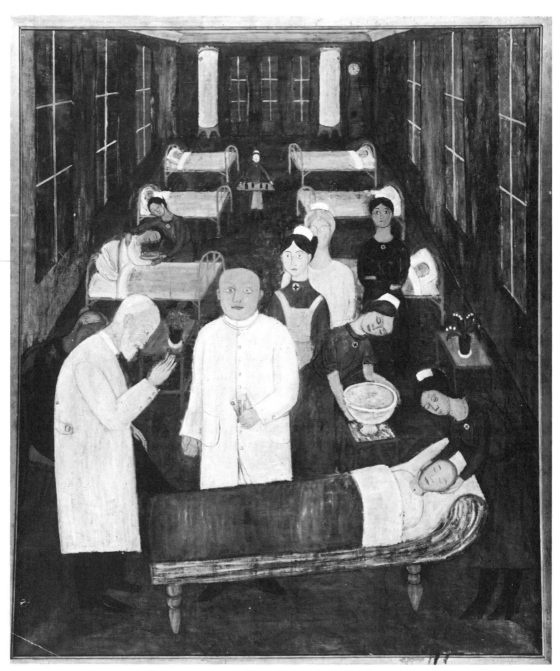

Hilding Linnqvist, *Hospital II*, 1920

THE HEALING ENVIRONMENT

Ron Anderson

RON ANDERSON, M.D., is Chairman of the Board of the Texas Department of Health and Chief Executive Officer of Parkland Hospital in Dallas, Texas. Parkland, a public institution that serves both paying and nonpaying patients, is often rated among the twenty-five best hospitals in the United States and is trying to implement principles of mind/body medicine. Dr. Anderson is the coauthor of "Medical Apartheid—An American Perspective."

MOYERS: How do you relate mind/body medicine to what you and your colleagues here at Parkland do every day?

ANDERSON: I talk about the autonomy of individuals—what they're trying to do with their skills, or their coping behaviors, or their financial resources, and all the things that they bring to bear on an illness. I try to have people understand wholeness if I can, because if you don't understand the mind/body connection, you start off on the wrong premise. You also have to understand the person within their family and community because this is where people live. They have a disease, but they live with their illness, and if you miss that mind/body connection, then all the other things are hard to tie together.

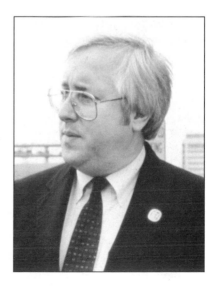

MOYERS: When you talk about wholeness, I'm not quite sure I understand what you mean.

ANDERSON: I mean by "wholeness" as whole as you can be, given the assault on your person by a disease. Your body image may have been changed, or you may have experienced grief or loss. How can I get you back to the highest state of function that I can? If I can't cure, I can care. And if I can't care, then something is very desperately wrong.

You try to bring healing to a person and help them heal themselves. Many times, if they have information, and if they're empowered through a caring milieu, they will be better able to function. The doctors and nurses won't be going home with them, so it's very important that we get them to the highest plane of function that we can. We have a saying in our geriatric ward that we've never met a patient we couldn't care for. We've met many we couldn't cure.

MOYERS: Caring is good medicine.

ANDERSON: Yes, I think caring is a good medicine. It was good medicine when my mother gave it to me. It was good medicine back before we had antibiotics, when doctors cared, and were empathetic, and talked to people. I'm afraid the technology, the wonderful drugs, and the power we have now sometimes substitute for the attitude of caring.

MOYERS: Is there a scientific basis for the proposition that caring is good medicine?

ANDERSON: Yes, but it's hard to measure. People in medicine want to get a statistical P-value or student T-test, or they want to at least see it all stacked up on the wheelbarrow so they can count it. But I know in my own practice that I see people get better because of the caring relationship. They'll tell me things they haven't told other people, things that are critical to their care plan. Caring for someone, having them understand that you really want the best for them, opens up whole vistas when you take the history in a physical examination.

I love to go on rounds and spend time alone with the patients myself and then have them tell me things that they haven't told the three or four people who've gotten a history before. You know, a lot of studies show that black and brown men, and women, in general, don't get as many sophisticated tests or go as often to cardiac surgery for the same degree of disease. The reason for that, I think, is not that people are racist but that they simply don't know how to talk with people from other cultures. They don't listen. They talk, and they don't listen. In a caring environment you're going to listen, and you're going to find out what people want, and what their value system has to say about their illness. And, therefore, you can be a better doctor because you can deliver what the patient wants, not just what your peers want.

MOYERS: Why is it important to know the values of a patient who comes in here for treatment?

ANDERSON: Well, for example, many people value functionality more than living longer. Sometimes young doctors are very fearful of death. Death itself is a failure. But to an elderly person death may not be a failure. It might be a victory if it happens correctly. It releases them. They don't want to be in a long-term-care facility. They want to have their dignity preserved. They want to be in some control. So their goals may be very different from the doctor who is going to prevent death at all costs. We have to talk to patients to see what their values are and what they would like as an outcome, because otherwise we're simply imposing our value systems on the patients.

MOYERS: Can you think of an example where knowing the value system of a patient actually helped you deal with that patient?

ANDERSON: I could give you many case studies. It happens in every patient. For example, an elderly person in the hospital who has a loved one at home whom they are caring for may actually be the more vigorous of the two. Their concern may be to get back home to care for their spouse. So when you tell them they have to stay a few more days because this is important for their care, their anxiety about the spouse they've left at home is so great that they can't really get any therapeutic benefit from those extra few days of bed rest. But you have to talk to them to know about the home situation. I'm really disappointed in house staff when I come in, and no one's talked about the home situation.

We once had a fellow who was a blue-collar worker, a truck driver, who had a heart attack. Now he might have the same heart disease as the banker in the next room—but the approach is different. The truck driver is probably going to lose his job because he won't be allowed to drive an eighteen-wheeler. His employers may not retrain him for other work. He has an enormous work ethic, and enormous financial pressures, with two kids in college. He's never gone to college, and he's trying to put his kids through college. For the banker, on the other hand, bypass surgery may be rather fashionable. People come to visit him and ask, you know, who's going to do your surgery?—that kind of thing. When he comes home, he'll have four or five months of recuperation. He hasn't lost any income. His family is pretty well set, and his kids are out of college. Now both could be totally destroyed by the disease, or both could die from the disease, but each has an enormously different illness.

MOYERS: And how does that affect your treatment of those two people?

ANDERSON: I would want to know what their desired outcome is. In both cases it may be that surgery is the best way to repair blood vessels—but what about reha-

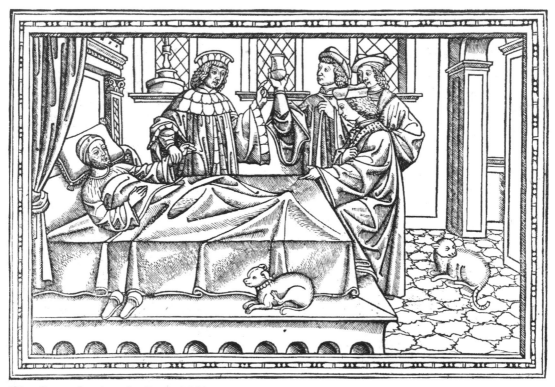

The Consultation, Italian, 16th c.

bilitation? I've got to think not only about the truck driver's heart, but also about his employability. I've got to think about how he will do when he's well. If he's unemployed, he's going to have higher blood pressure, and it's not unlikely that he'll drink more or that he'll have peptic ulcer disease. He'll lose his whole image of self because he's always worked and been self-sufficient. The other person in this example doesn't have the same threat to his self-image. Yes, he's scared because he's had a heart attack, and he knows he might die. He has special needs, and he may have grief, and he may be very concerned about the future, but a lot of things are taken care of because of his station in life.

MOYERS: How does this kind of concern help you define mind/body medicine?

ANDERSON: In my view, mind/body medicine is really the art of medicine. We've done very well with science in medicine, and I'm very proud of what we've been able to accomplish with that. But we've set aside the art of medicine. You know, years ago, physicians were almost mystical, priest-like people. I'm glad we've given that up, but even so, people want that healing presence. They want that concern. People intuitively know there's a mind/body connection.

Also, there's a lot of evidence that we're programmed to see what we believe. It's very important to know what belief system is operating and to understand differences. I look at patients as a mosaic. I hate to see hospitals blend them into little ingots and make them all be the good patient. They're not all the same. I want my physicians to understand that and understand the patients' connection to themselves, their families, and their communities. It's my world view, and I think it's a correct world view, not just for medicine, but for education and so many other things in society. It seems to satisfy patients a lot more when you deal with them as mind/body. They don't seem to complain as much that the system isn't caring for them. It's more dignified, and they have more power, more control. And it's more fun.

MOYERS: So mind/body is the art of caring.

ANDERSON: I think it's the art of understanding the whole person and not just the physiological system. In medical schools we deal with diseases and tissues and organs and body systems. But when you put the art in medicine, you deal with persons and with their families and communities. You have to have that connectedness. You deal with the spirit.

MOYERS: Do you think, medically, there is a spirit in a human being?

ANDERSON: Oh, sure. I think the spirit is extremely important. You see people with cancer who give up and those who don't. I've seen AIDS patients live much longer than anybody could have ever anticipated. There's a thread here that I see, but that's hard to quantify. My own grandfather had lung cancer from smoking tobacco for years. When he was diagnosed, my little brother had just been born. The cancer was terminal—he couldn't have radiotherapy or anything else, and everyone told us he had only six months to live. But he said, "I've educated all of my children and all my grandchildren until they got into school. I've given them my value system, and I'm going to give this boy my value system, too. I'm going to swing him, and I'm going to take him hunting, and I'm going to tell him all the stories I've told my other grandchildren, and I'm going to see him into elementary school." And he did. He lived for six more years. You see, he had a very positive attitude, and a goal.

I see that kind of story over and over. And, on the other hand, I also see Native Americans, eighty-year-olds, who decide to die when it is the right time. They've talked with their families, and they're resolved about this. I remember that as a young intern, when I first saw this, I said, "This can't happen. There's no reason for this person to die." But the attending physician, who had worked with Native Americans for forty years, said, "But she will die if she wants to." I couldn't understand that, but since then I've seen it happen time and again. People can't quantify this, so it isn't sexy. You can't study it in the test tube. But you know that it's real.

MOYERS: How can you be sure it's not a placebo effect—you know, the power of suggestion, the response of belief?

ANDERSON: I'm not sure that the placebo effect is bad. When somebody has a placebo effect, that doesn't mean that a chemical isn't working. The person's own endorphins, enkephalin, dopamine, serotonin, and norepinephrine are doing something for them as a consequence of a caring and healing act. On the other hand, I hate to see people use placebos instead of taking care of someone's pain. Sometimes it's a disservice to the patient to use a placebo because it's misleading them, it's lying to them. I think it's better to create a partnership and understanding and to try to deal with what their real pain might be. Pain may be a way of asking for something else—your time, or your attention.

MOYERS: The placebo effect demonstrates the impact of belief on the physical body. If I believe I'm getting better because of what I think they're doing to me, my body may say amen to that.

ANDERSON: There's no question that your body and your mind tied together can help you fight infection. People who are depressed, or who have just lost a loved one, are more likely to have congestive heart failure, and to have to come into the hospital. They're more likely to have other illnesses that we think of as preventable illnesses. Part of it is caused by a lack of self-care, but I think part of it is also a kind of turnoff of the immune system.

MOYERS: But how can you teach the art of medicine, as you call it, to young medical students, who are hurrying to get it all done, facing a twenty-hour day, knowing that they are judged on the number of patients they deal with, how many charts they check, and how much they study? Can you really expect them to stop and dwell on these issues?

ANDERSON: In my own practice I've found that it takes more time if I don't do this. It's like preventive medicine—if I deal with the patient's problems and anxieties and concerns ahead of time, I actually make the therapy plan and the outcome better for both of us. But I think we beat out of our medical students and our house staff officers a lot of compassion and empathy and a lot of their willingness to understand the person. They are told to understand the disease, and that's what they're tested on. We have wonderful disease models, and we're getting more of them all the time. Everyone talks about curriculum overload for medical students. The didactic portion of their training is going to beat them up here. Then, when they get to the wards and see a harried faculty member and harried senior house staff, they may develop the attitude that the patient is the enemy.

One of the reasons that many physicians don't want to do primary care in this country is that they're trained in hospitals where they don't understand the patient as that patient lives in a family and a community. They don't have any continuity with the patient over time. Any physician who takes care of patients for ten or fifteen years cherishes that relationship. Medical students don't see that. They just see an intensive care unit with the technology, and they're beaten down by that. It's easier to write a prescription instead of stopping to talk with a patient. One of the things I tell medical students is that writing a prescription is not the end of the social contact with the patients. Many patients don't need a prescription, they need you to talk to them. They need you to visit with them, particularly the elderly person who comes in. Somehow that offends the house staff officer, who says, "She just wants social contact." What's wrong with that if it's healing?

MOYERS: And is it sometimes healing?

ANDERSON: Sometimes it's much more healing than prescribing a medication to handle anxiety. The drug they get for anxiety may build up in their system so that they get sluggish, for example, and then they may fall and break a hip. Sometimes it's better not to give medicines, but to depend on a patient's relationship with a church or community or doctor.

MOYERS: But if patients are seen as the enemy, for whom are hospitals organized?

ANDERSON: Traditionally, hospitals have been organized for doctors, for auxiliaries, for insurance companies—everybody but the patient. They've taken on "the total-institution format." The total institution is like a concentration camp or a jail or even a place that was created to service a need, but that is overwhelmed with volume and stress and strain and people not dealing with their own feelings. Public school systems may be the same way. Hospitals should be places created for the service of patients. We should be patient-centered. We ought to deliver care as best we can within a very clear value system. Sometimes we forget that. Doctors should be customers of a hospital, but not the only customer.

MOYERS: Isn't it too much to expect young doctors to master this mind-boggling array of technological knowledge and to practice the social and personal skills as well? Isn't it enough for them just to be competent and efficient?

ANDERSON: Being competent and understanding your field is the basic premise for ethical practice. If you're not competent, you may really care, but you can be really dangerous at the same time. So you have to stay competent in your field. But if you're going to be in a care-giver role, you've got to pay attention to the underlying relationship with your patient. Maybe it's okay for a radiologist, or an anesthesiologist, who puts you to sleep and doesn't talk to you, to simply be competent in their field. But for an internist or a geriatrician or a pediatrician, or a family physician, it's imperative to have that understanding, that skill. It's really not that hard to do. It doesn't take more time.

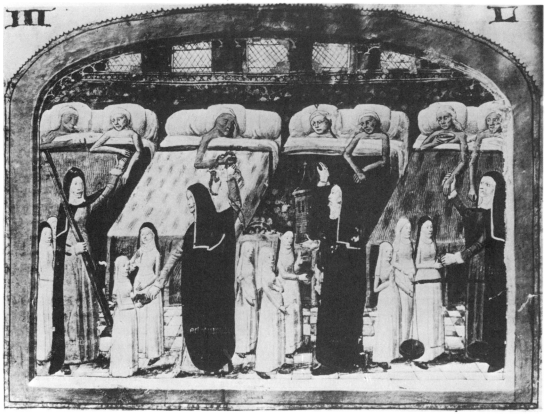

Hospital, French, 14th c.

MOYERS: Why have we lost that skill? I remember my family doctor, Dr. Tenney, down in Marshall, Texas, who brought that caring to his treatment of our family.

ANDERSON: Some would say that caring is all they had in those days. They didn't have penicillin, and they didn't have the technology that we have today. They were empathetic at the bedside, and they patted your hand while you died. But I don't think that's really the case. I think they did very well with the tools they had in those days, and we do much better with the tools we have now. But sometimes we almost have to protect patients from the technology that we have. To do that, we have to know what they want and what they expect.

To answer your question, I don't know what's happened to that caring other than that the system sometimes takes it out of the young men and women who come into medicine. They don't come spoiled. But they become too busy and get concerned about other needs in society—cost, access, reimbursement, and all the other things that you're always fighting.

Although we have advanced technology and spend a lot, this nation is not satisfying its patients. We're the only country where the more we spend, the less people are satisfied with health care. There's a reason for that—patients tell us that they want a more personal relationship with their doctors. They may like their individual doctors, but they don't like organized medicine. You hear that all the time. Many of them don't even like their individual doctors, although they say, "Well, you know, he's good at what he does"—but they wouldn't invite him over to dinner.

Patients are so intimidated that they don't feel like they're a part of the team. But as we shift to more chronic disease models, we've got to have people who are able to help take care of themselves when they go home. Chronic diseases have to be dealt with as illnesses in the community and in the family.

MOYERS: What kind of illnesses do people bring to Parkland?

ANDERSON: We get an array of everything at Parkland, from the very serious trauma injuries to diabetes and hypertension and asthma. We also get the premature, high-risk pregnancy cases, and we have the tiniest little neonates that you can imagine. We take care of all flavors of society and all socioeconomic levels. That's one reason I love being here. It really is a mosaic of society. But that makes it tough when we talk about giving patient-centered care, because every patient is a little bit of a new twist.

MOYERS: I can see how a private hospital could afford to streamline its services according to the individual, but how can you put these practices into a huge public hospital?

ANDERSON: Many of the hospitals that think of themselves as patient-centered or customer-centered are really dealing with amenities, not with empowerment. What we're talking about here is creating a system of choice in a public hospital setting so that the day after universal health insurance, if it comes, we would be attractive, we would be a system of first resort, a system that had cared even when people didn't have choices. I really think that's how we will survive. I think it's going to help us with our taxpayers if they can understand what we're about, and I think it will help encourage business to make an investment in the infrastructure. I think there are spinoffs that make patient-centered medicine a very sound business plan as well as a right way to practice medicine. Private hospitals may be doing it for more market share, but we have more market share than we can stand. So we're doing this because we think that the value of the individual person demands it. The integrity of this institution has to be based on how we dignify the care and provide services we think are socially just and empower the people we care for.

MOYERS: When you use the word "empowerment," what do you mean?

ANDERSON: Well, in most hospitals we take your clothes away and give you a little gown with the back out of it. You may lose your dentures. Jewelry and other things that make you feel like a person are taken away. And you're supposed to be a good patient, therefore, you're obedient. Patients don't need to be obedient, they need to be able to complain, and to ask questions and to assert their point of view. You need to have a partnership, even though it can't be an equal partnership. *We* need to be the advocates for our patients in this partnership. That means they have to be empowered to complain without the fear that if they complained, they might lose their care.

MOYERS: But you want to empower them for more than complaint, don't you?

ANDERSON: We want to empower them to learn how to take care of themselves when they go home, because they're going to be part of the health care team. Now not every patient can do this, but where you can, you develop a partnership with patients so that they can go home and understand the medication, for example. Or, if they have side effects, and you need to change the medication, then they become the ultimate decision-maker at home, and the doctor is the diagnostician, the person who initiated the therapy that was negotiated.

A case in point here might be a young man with hypertension. One drug is twenty dollars a month, and another, which is a little bit better in terms of side effects, is eighty-five dollars a month. If I prescribe the eighty-five-dollar medication, he can't afford it, and he feels guilty. I may have his blood pressure controlled, but he doesn't necessarily feel better. If the man has to feed a family, provide transportation, and worry about his children's education as well as everything else, this sixty-five-dollar difference a month is a lot of money to him. If you talk to him about what the side effects are, he may still choose that twenty-dollar-a-month medication because his health is dependent upon nutrition and how he feels about his family and how he's providing for his family.

MOYERS: Do many patients have stress?

ANDERSON: Our patients have enormous stress. We take care of many people who are uninsured, and many people who are charity patients, funded by our county, and they're very stressed by the financial implications of their care. They may have been very proud people who've always worked, maybe at two or three jobs, and this is terribly stressful for them. They don't know what's going to happen to them, and that's very stressful.

Of course, that kind of stress is true across socioeconomic lines. When you're in the hospital, you're vulnerable. Something's happening to you. You're changing. You become aware of your own mortality. You know you're not in control of everything. And so that's a stress, a big stress. And if you add on unemployment, or homelessness, or an alternate life-style with people discriminating against you, or old age,

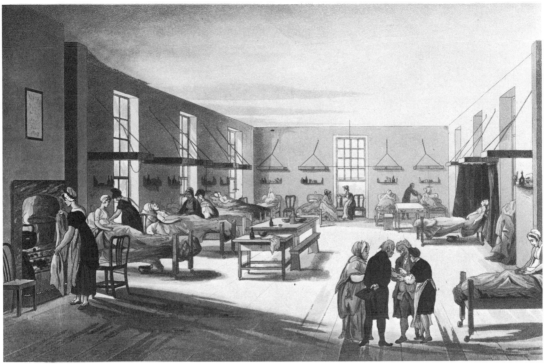

Augustus Pugin and Thomas Rowlandson, *Middlesex Hospital,* 1808

where you may be wondering whether you are supposed to die and get out of the way, there's even more stress. This kind of stress is best handled by talking with the patient, not by prescribing medication for anxiety.

MOYERS: Is stress the primary condition that mind/body medicine addresses?

ANDERSON: Stress is only one of the conditions, but it's an important one. Obviously, it's been one that many people have dealt with for centuries. But even with stress, the situation of the person has to be taken into account. It's not just that this person is different from the next person but that the person's attitude varies during different stages of coming to terms with their illness. If you have a young man with Hodgkin's disease, for example, he'll change as he goes through the various steps in his process—he'll go through anger and then denial and then bargaining and then on to resolution and understanding and acceptance. Every step along the way, you have to modify your approach to some degree because although the patient is the same person, the circumstances are changing.

MOYERS: How about your ward for premature babies? It's highly regarded. Does it come under your mind/body umbrella?

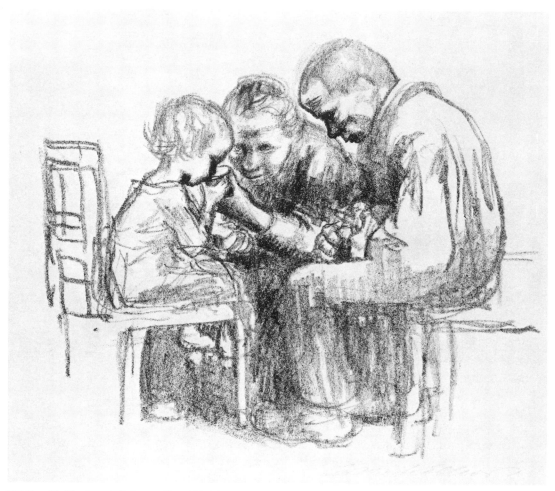

Käthe Kollwitz, *Visit to the Children's Hospital,* 1926

ANDERSON: Yes, although it may be hard for people to understand how you can deal with this little baby of one or two pounds in terms of mind/body. You know, is this really a person? It is a person. You'll see people trying to stroke and touch and provide stimulation for these babies so that they develop normally, or as normally as possible.

But you're dealing not only with the baby but also with a mother and a father and maybe a grandmother. Many times, when the baby has been there months and months, tied to all the technology, the family has a difficult time. They're scared to take the baby home. They think, how can I take the place of all this equipment? How can I take the place of all these nurses? Will I be sufficient to the task? Sometimes they're very scared to bond with that child. You can see that in the reticence on the part of the mother to take the baby. But that's something we can work through and help them with. We even have a room there so that they can come and spend an hour or two and take care of the baby, with a nurse right outside the door. That's important so that they know they can do it. One of our jobs is not just to focus on the baby but also to encourage that family to keep focused on each other and to support each other.

MOYERS: You're not content just to save the baby.

ANDERSON: Well, we have to send that baby home, and we may have spent a fortune on it. We're not worried just about the first twenty-eight days of life but about the first year, the first five years. You don't want to drop the ball just because the high-tech intensive care is over. You also have to arrange for the ongoing and comprehensive care of that child. And the best care-givers are the family.

MOYERS: But we don't normally think of hospitals that way. We think of them as dealing with crises of medicine, but not with a long-range strategy of social and personal and family care.

ANDERSON: When you think of a disease, you can think of the hospital. But when you think of an illness, you've got to think of home and family and community. Hospitals need to tie these together. For example, when the baby isn't going to go home, and you know it, the mind/body experience for the family is extremely important. Families need to be able to hold and bond with a child who's not going to make it. Commonly, we'll have a family come in when a child is being taken off a ventilator so that they can share that experience, even though it's a very negative outcome. It's their child, and they need to deal with that loss. The artificiality of the tubes and machines can be taken away for a short time so that they can have their child, even so briefly. The way they deal with this experience is important to their grieving later on. When this happens, we try to have some sort of support group for the family. Even with trauma, where you have an adolescent son killed in a car wreck, or someone who's going to be changed forever because of a spinal cord injury, you have to work with the family. After the patient leaves the hospital, everyone has to be able to deal with the illness. We can be very competent in dealing with the trauma, or the disease, but until we deal with the illness and the wholeness of that individual, we are not good doctors.

MOYERS: This is a very ambitious agenda for a public hospital using the resources of burdened taxpayers.

ANDERSON: Everyone talks about cost—but the cost of this approach is less, especially as you go out in the community to care for people. Community care costs a fraction of what care costs in hospitals, where there is sometimes a mindless application of technology, particularly at the end of a life. Mindless technology costs us a fortune in this country. My own view is that you can deliver care of higher quality for the patient within their value system at a lower cost. Patients may not want some of the things that we do. We do what's competent, but we need to be conscientious, and we need to let patients be fully informed. I'm not talking about pulling the plug, or anything like that, simply because it's more cost effective. I think it was Woody Allen who said that death is the greatest cost container of all. That's not what I'm talking about. I'm talking about quality within the patient's value system, not my own. Many times we spend a lot of the money because we focus on the disease and don't want to get involved with the human or emotional side. But that doesn't create better health care. So I think it's our job as a public hospital to be good stewards of taxpayers' money, and this approach is better stewardship.

MOYERS: You've set up community clinics around the city. Why?

ANDERSON: The community clinics focus on prevention. If we can prevent something completely, or find it so early that we can secondarily prevent death and disability, we can save money as well as deliver a higher quality of care. Many of the problems Parkland has to deal with are not going to be solved in a test tube. We have wonderful scientists next door, who are also clinicians, and they win Nobel Prizes — but the problems we're talking about stem from behavior. Teenage pregnancy, for example. Transmission of the HIV virus. Penetrating injury from gang violence. Drug-related activities. There are ways we can intervene to decrease the numbers of behavior-related illnesses that cost us a fortune. Community Oriented Primary Care is out where people live, and it talks to them about what they want. It deals with issues of hopelessness and helplessness, which create an environment from which violence and teenage pregnancy and lots of other things are derived.

MOYERS: It's right there where people live every day.

ANDERSON: And it's their community. I had an interesting experience once when I was talking to a group of people about empowering the community. One of the members of the community came up to me afterwards and said, "You know, I'm an old man, so I hope I'd not have lived long enough to have one more white man come and empower me." He's absolutely correct. I don't empower anybody in that community. That community can empower itself if we provide the right milieu, the right type of health care system that isn't so irrational, but which is all tied together and takes care of a whole family. In most cases you have to go over to this part of town to get women, infants, and children care, and then over to another part of town to get your well baby cared for, and then back to Parkland for sick-baby care. At the community clinic we take care of the whole thing in one place.

MOYERS: What do you mean when you say the community is empowered?

ANDERSON: It's empowered to talk about what it wants from the health care delivery system. It is able to complain. It is able to advise. There are advisory boards there to talk to us about what they expect of us as deliverers. If you look at our mix of physicians, you'll see many more women there than you'll see here at the hospital, and many more physicians of color. Children out there will see an African American internist, and they'll say, "You know, I want to be a doctor. You think I could be a doctor?" There's a mentor there they can talk to. Instead of being passive recipients of health care, they're active participants in their health care.

MOYERS: You keep coming back to the impact of environment on health.

ANDERSON: You know how the environment of Eastern Europe has been devastating to the health of the people. And in parts of this country there's a sense of hopelessness and helplessness that leads people not to take care of themselves. When people have very little self-esteem, they place themselves in harm's way. I think Dallas just topped 440 murders this year.

MOYERS: A record.

ANDERSON: And it's been a record every year for four years. We're seeing the wounded who survive, and ours is a record every year, also. What can we do about this? Part of what we can do is to deal with the hopelessness and helplessness, to let people feel that they can contribute and control and set their own course and their own future. They haven't felt that. And so a lot of this violence is a kind of lashing out at themselves. In some inner-city communities, from which we get so many of the illnesses, the environment is boiling. We just wrote an article for the *Journal of the American Medical Association* called "Medical Apartheid: An American Perspective."

MOYERS: It's clear you think that your medical students ought to understand the importance of their patients' experience in their communities.

ANDERSON: I think that's the definition of the good doctor now. I want them to be good doctors. I want them to understand because they'll be more effective. They'll do a better job.

MOYERS: What do you want them to know?

ANDERSON: I want them to know about the patient and about where a patient lives. I want them to know why compliance might be a problem. Compliance means the patient is doing something you've asked them to do. If compliance is a problem, I want my medical students to understand why the patient is having difficulty participating as a partner.

MOYERS: You want your medical students to know the values of that patient.

ANDERSON: What I want them to know is the person. The patient's a person, not the cholecystectomy in Room 245, you know. For example, I got a call about an eighty-six-year-old man whom I knew fairly well and who was being cared for by a young physician in another hospital. He had terrible diabetes and peripheral vascular disease, and they needed to amputate his legs. He asked, "What are my chances if you took my legs off?" And they said, "Well it's a fifty-fifty deal even if we take your legs." And he responded, "That's not good enough. I don't want to be bed fast. I came in walking, and I don't want to be dismembered. I know I may die, but I'm not afraid to die. That's all settled. I have that taken care of." And the doctor says, "But you're going to die." He says, "I know I'm going to die. I'm eighty-six years old."

The physician was very uncomfortable with that, and so he transferred the patient to our hospital, where we helped care for him during what I think was a very dignified period of time for him. And he did die. To him, it was a victory—so much so that he and his wife both thanked me. They appreciated that we handled his pain, we took care of those kinds of things he felt needed to be taken care of. He was very

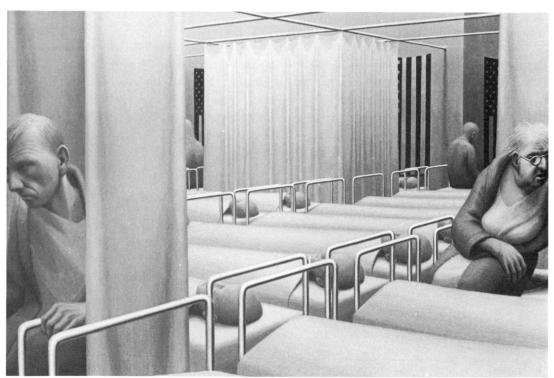

George Tooker, *Ward*, 1970

concerned about being a burden to his family and others, but the main thing was that he didn't want to be dismembered. It wasn't the kind of life he wanted to live. Now to the young physician, it was life or death. But to this eighty-six-year-old gentleman, it was life on his conditions. He wasn't afraid of death; he was afraid of being disabled.

MOYERS: You didn't cure him, and you didn't give him extra years, so what did you do for him?

ANDERSON: It's important to give life to years, not just years to life. We cared for him. And death in that case might have been a healing, although we hate to say that. We're fearful of death. We fight it in our society all the time. But to this man, with his religious background, this was a healing experience. It was what he wanted, and what he expected the doctor to do.

MOYERS: He wasn't just a body to you.

ANDERSON: No. And it was really important where he felt his soul was in relationship to God. That made death okay for him. I tell house staff officers, "Regardless of your religion, never, never take away that strength, that ability to handle a crisis, that ability to handle a loss. That's a very powerful thing that some patients have." Sometimes house staff will walk out into the hall and say, "How in the world can they believe that?" Or "How in the world can they behave that way?" And then, later on, they'll sometimes come back and ask me, "Could we talk about it?"

There's an old samurai axiom that the greatest samurai is the one who first conquers himself. Our fear of death sometimes really gets in the way of understanding that eighty-six-year-old man, who was very rational and well put together. What he asked us to do was very ethical. His death was not our failure. While we were in consultation, he said to the physician, "You can't really save my life. You can prolong my death, but you can't save my life. In my religious system I've already been saved. It's all handled. I will not be disfigured."

We once had a doctor on staff who told a Cambodian woman that she had a kidney infection. In her belief system the kidney is very important, so having a kidney infection is like having an infection of the soul. Now you can't have a little infection of your soul, that's a life-threatening thing. So she was very, very concerned. She went home and gave away her possessions, the family came in and wailed, but three days later she was still, miraculously, alive. So they called the doctor back and said, "Why is she still alive?" And he said, "Well, she's just got a little kidney infection, why shouldn't she be alive?"

Meanwhile, of course, we had put enormous stress on this woman and her family because we didn't communicate or try to understand her value system. Now, I can't make scholars of culture out of my house staff, but I can try to have them get an interpreter there to be sure they don't communicate poorly to someone.

We need to acknowledge personhood and belief systems. Sometimes people will say, "I put my care in the hands of the Lord," and the house staff officer will say, "I'd rather have a competent neurosurgeon." Generally, you can get someone to come around to the right medical decision without attacking their religion. And if you attack their value system or their belief system, usually they'll dismiss you. They may not be able to get rid of you in a public hospital, but they've clicked you off. You don't really understand, so they'll decide not to talk about that anymore.

MOYERS: And then you can't help them heal.

ANDERSON: You can't help them heal nearly as well as you can if you understand their value system.

MOYERS: I saw Native American artifacts on your office wall—how much have you been affected by your interest in Native American medicine?

ANDERSON: I've studied Eastern philosophies, and the martial arts, and I have a Christian background as a Baptist. But I also find a lot of spirituality within the American Native culture that is very compatible for me and for healing.

MOYERS: You're in charge of one of the largest public hospitals in the country, and you're saying that Native American culture has something to do with the way you practice medicine and heal?

ANDERSON: Yes. I've seen physicians who are very competent in the Anglo world fail in an American Native world, particularly when it comes to psychiatry, or things that require understanding culture. I remember one time when I was helping the Indian Health Service recruit physicians, that all the doctors on the recruiting trip took to the road while the medicine men did the healing paintings. That was a little demeaning to some of these fellows. They didn't understand. We had lots of trouble getting people placed until we recognized the value of the healer. We recognized the medicine man's role in public health, and we taught them public health and emergency medicine so they could handle prehospital care and help the physician. And they handled the psychiatry.

MOYERS: What do medicine men know that we don't know?

ANDERSON: They know about the spirit of man. They don't know the technologies and even the disease theories that we know. But they know about wholeness and try to deal with that. When they talk about the medicine wheel, they're talking about circles. We think in straight lines and in squares and boxes. But there are hardly any squares and boxes in nature. If you look through a microscope, you don't really see microorganisms that are square, you see round things and spheres and spirals.

For some reason, American Natives think of things in a continuum, generation to generation. They have an attitude of kinship that's unbelievable. And when they adopt you into their society, the feeling of fellowship is a very sacred bond. They also have a sacred bond with their environment. They see things whole, and they try to travel that circle. They see the spirit as part of life, not separate from it. In every aspect of life they deal with the combined mind/body.

We have an astronaut cardiologist at the medical school who says that what impressed him most in his NASA flight was the thinness of the atmosphere around the earth. He said it looked like it was a few millimeters thick. And he realized how

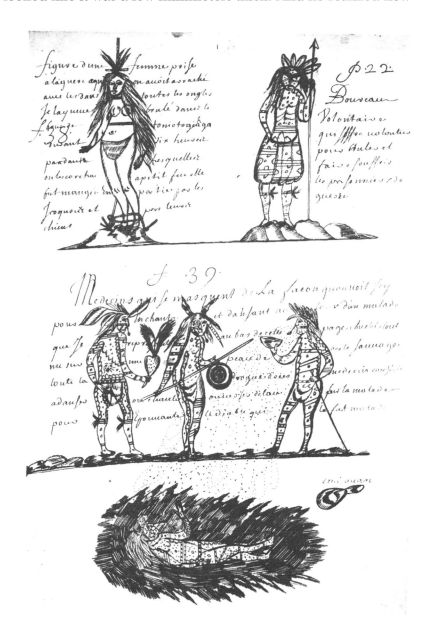

Louis Nicolas,
*Indian Curing
Scene,* ca. 1700

fragile things were. The Indians knew that too. They didn't kill all the buffalo for their tongues and their hides. They had reverence for those things that they had to take for food. They saw that their spirit extended into other animals, and they had a bond with those animals.

MOYERS: But that seems like a world so foreign to Parkland Hospital in Dallas, Texas, in the mid-1990s.

ANDERSON: It's a world foreign to many people because it's not "science," it's how we interact with other people. If I had a sense of kinship with African Americans, Southeast Asians, and Hispanics in this community, I would see that they had the opportunity to do well because it would benefit me.

MOYERS: And it would make our society more whole.

ANDERSON: Absolutely.

MOYERS: Would it be correct to say that for a good doctor, nothing that heals is really foreign?

ANDERSON: Well, I'm not sure. Something might be healing in some folks' definition of healing that I wouldn't find acceptable. I think that's why we talk about being value-driven. It's not just the patients who bring values to the table—we have values too, and we have to be sure that we don't compromise those.

Sometimes it's difficult to understand the other person's world view, and that's where you have to try harder. If you can't see that other world view, then many times you will fail, because you will try to give them the answer that you want, or that your family wants, the answer that you grew up with as a Protestant, a Catholic, a Jew, a Muslim. Whatever your world view, you'll want to try to solve problems within that view.

MOYERS: You used a term with a colleague of mine—"resurrection medicine."

ANDERSON: When patients come in, literally at death's doorstep, and you're trying to pull them out of the jaws of death, you're practicing resurrection medicine. It's exciting. We spend a lot of money on resurrection medicine, and we write a lot of articles about it. We get tenured as professors, and we feel good about that when we go home. But the question is, why do we have to practice resurrection medicine when we can practice preventive medicine? Why is this person in a diabetic coma? Could we have interceded somewhere so that we didn't have to literally save the man's life, but so that the man would have been saving his life daily?

We used to think we were very good because people were so sick, and we resurrected them. But now we are stepping back and asking, "Why are they so sick? Maybe that's our fault. Maybe this is a medical system, not a health care system." That's why we made the step out into the community. We're tired of having to practice resurrection medicine. We're good at it, and it's still exciting, and we still write our papers—but it's not the only way. We have to go out and build those clinics and decrease the amount of deferred maintenance on humankind before we start trying to pull away from any tertiary support. We've got to care for the person who's been shot, and for the tiny, tiny baby, but we also need to do something else on a parallel track to prevent the pipeline from funneling all those patients down on to our campus.

MOYERS: You know, you're dealing with what in some quarters would be called "life's unmentionables"—the very people the majority of society detests for their burden on taxes, and for their social and personal and sexual behavior. You're dealing with the outcasts, in a sense. How long can you get away with that?

ANDERSON: I've made it a life decision. There are those who want to lend a helping hand and make people whole, and there are others who say, "Well, if we help people too much, we'll make them more dependent," and they'll stand off and not do very much. It's pretty easy to stand off because we have the attitude that you should pull yourself up by your own bootstraps. But in Texas, forty percent of those people who need to pull themselves up by their own bootstraps are children. Many others are frail, elderly people who don't have insurance because the employer won't purchase insurance or can't afford to. So we're the insurance policy for those persons. And while we take care of folks that no one else wants to talk about, my attitude is that this isn't Parkland's problem, it is our community's problem. It's also our community's opportunity. If the children who drop out of school would stay in, they would make a tremendous contribution to society. And if they aren't salvaged, they'll make another kind of contribution, and it will be very expensive.

I don't want to be the conscience to this community. I'm not the honest man with a lamp at all. It's just so obvious that this is the thing that needs to be said because these patients are all equally valuable. They are the building blocks of society. You know, modern medicine, with all its technology, can be a wonderful thing. It can make people more functional, and it can extend life, but it can't stop us from dying. We may have enormous breakthroughs in technology, but we also know a lot already that we aren't applying. These are public health things. These are primary care things. These are things we're having difficulty persuading our young medical students to do.

I think we need to humble ourselves a little bit and realize that we don't need many more transplant surgeons, we need people who deal with fundamental things. If we really value human life, how can we not invest in prenatal care? How can we not invest in the children's programs or preschool education? Programs that work when done competently enrich people and make them better able to contribute something back to society. It's foolish to talk about the cost of medicine and doctor reimbursement all the time and not be addressing those things that can make individuals and communities whole.

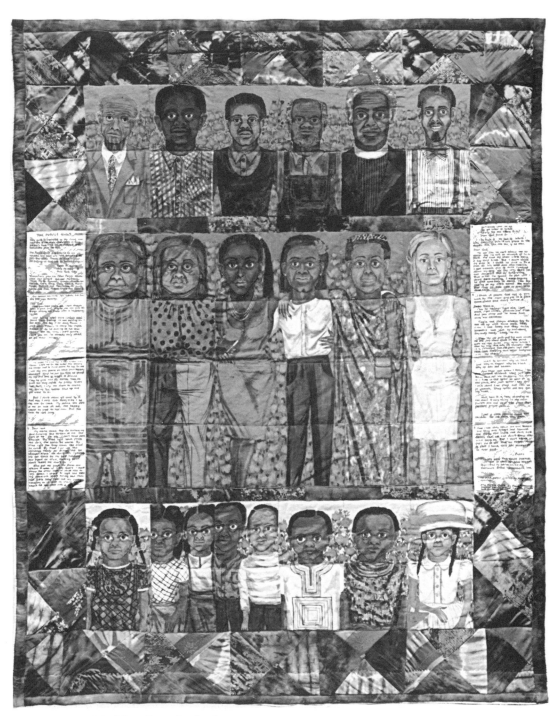

Faith Ringgold, *The Purple Quilt*, 1986

HEALING AND
THE COMMUNITY

David Smith

DAVID SMITH, M.D., is Commissioner of the Texas Department of Health. Formerly he was Senior Vice President of Parkland Memorial Hospital in Dallas, Texas, and the Chief Executive Officer and Medical Director of the Community Oriented Primary Care (COPC) Program of Parkland Memorial Hospital. In addition, Dr. Smith is a pediatrician and on the teaching faculty of the University of Texas Southwest Medical Center at Dallas.

MOYERS: You call your clinic a "Community Oriented Primary Care Clinic"—what kind of community is this?

SMITH: Well, it's a diverse community, primarily African American, but with pockets of Hispanics as well. But the people no longer own this community—they lease it. For the most part, it's a working community, with many people just trying to make it so they can go somewhere else.

MOYERS: What common illnesses do these people experience?

SMITH: Of course, the common illnesses vary by age and by ethnicity. But we see a lot of diabetes, and we see

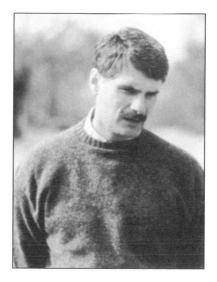

a lot of strokes that could have been prevented through dealing earlier with high blood pressure. We see a lot of children who haven't been immunized because the system has failed them, so they get diseases like measles. And we see individuals with large ulcers and sores that should have been taken care of much earlier. Also, we're seeing more and more asthma.

MOYERS: These illnesses seem so physical in nature that I wonder if mind/body medicine has anything to do with a community like this?

SMITH: Every aspect of those illnesses has a component that relates to mind. The healing process, the motivation to seek help, the understanding of how they got into that state in the first place—all these involve the mind. We know that in the healing process of anything from an ulcer in diabetes to asthma, the mind is very intricately involved with whether the patient gets better or worse. You can actually make yourself more ill. We know there are many different chemical aspects of the body that are controlled by the mind. In fact, you can put patients in a position where they'll actually get worse, even despite the best "medicine."

MOYERS: The popular cliché of mind/body medicine is that it's a luxury for affluent people who can afford it. How can you bring it into the lives of these people, who don't have the resources of the middle or upper middle class? Can you teach it to them?

SMITH: I don't think you teach it. You allow them to learn it. To teach it to them is not going to work. We have to allow them to develop the skills by using more culturally relevant models. We've got to bring in African Americans and Hispanics to work with these families. We've got to be part of the community. For chronic diseases particularly, we've got to find ways to encourage the patients to follow through. Follow-up loses priority for these people because they have so many other things to deal with. We've got to use outreach people who are knowledgeable about the community, and we've got to allow the families to be more involved as part of the treatment team, and we've got to encourage individuals to take more responsibility for their own care.

MOYERS: What does culture have to do with one's attitude toward mind/body medicine, using the mind for dealing with or preventing illness?

SMITH: Well, take religion, for example. It's a very powerful force in this community. So the church is a very appropriate place to begin mind/body medicine. And in fact, we frequently use church leadership and church congregations. For example, when we have terminal patients, and the quality of life becomes an issue, or in the rehabilitation of people with an injury or a chronic disease, we often turn to the church, which becomes part of the therapeutic process.

MOYERS: Some skeptics think of mind/body medicine as a set of fringe practices, like acupuncture, herbal prescriptions, massage—all of those relatively esoteric things. But that's not what you seem to mean by it here.

SMITH: No, it's really very basic. It's bringing a whole body together to prevent disease or to help the healing process.

MOYERS: But do you come to this community and say, "You're responsible for your healing, so you've got to use your mind to influence your body"? How do you do it?

SMITH: First you inform. Patients generally aren't even aware of what is going wrong. They aren't told why they're sick, and so they can't be as effective a part of the healing relationship with the doctor. Perhaps as doctors we aren't comfortable developing the kind of relationship with people that would help them heal themselves. Mind/body in many ways is a relationship between the person who's providing care—not necessarily a doctor—and the patient, and then between the patient and the part that needs to be healed.

MOYERS: Are you just talking about the old-fashioned bedside manner of a doctor who comes around and visits you when you need him?

SMITH: That's part of it. But you also need to feel that you have some control in relation to your own body and your illness.

MOYERS: So if you're not talking about acupuncture, or herbs, or massage, or meditation when you talk to these people about their minds and healing, what are you talking about?

SMITH: They have a right to be able to deal with their own disease, to be able to take care of themselves, and to understand what's going on.

MOYERS: What do you mean?

SMITH: We've traditionally not informed people well enough for them to be aware of what's going on. We've not empowered them so that they can help us take care of them. For example, we bring people who are wheezing with asthma into the emergency room, and we give them some wonderful medicines. We say, "Take these pills, and go home, and I'll see you back in two weeks." We don't talk to them about the fact that emotions can affect asthma, or that mold, and the pollens coming off trees, and other environmental factors can affect it. We don't talk to them about the screens that aren't on their houses and that should be. We don't take into account the fact that landlords don't put filters in the furnaces or change them frequently, or that the electrical outlets aren't working, and so they can't use their breathing machine. We simply give them the pills and tell them to come back in two weeks.

MOYERS: And if they can't afford the pills, they don't get them.

SMITH: That's correct. We're talking about a prevention partnership in which the patient is empowered to be a partner with you in the healing process. And if that doesn't happen, you're going to fail, particularly in a community like this, because there are so many variables that can make that person ill.

MOYERS: Stress, financial worries . . .

SMITH: Yes, or even the failure of the transport system to get them where they need to go. There's a lot of stress in the community.

MOYERS: So you and your colleagues don't tell them, "Well, let's talk about mind/body medicine. You need a little course in meditation, or some herbs."

SMITH: No, they'd probably throw us out of the exam room if we did that. We talk to them about the healing process—and it's not just the physician who talks to them. We have other health people who work with us: social workers, for example, and nurses who come out to their homes to work with them. When I see a patient in the emergency room, I initiate a mind/body process in which the patient is the most critical player. In fact, most disease processes that we see get worse if we don't allow the mind to be part of the healing process. For example, if we don't try to decrease the stresses in a patient's life, we'll have a tough time controlling that patient's blood pressure.

MOYERS: People who can afford it use biofeedback to learn how to control stress.

SMITH: In this community, people use their religious faith to get outside of their stressful world. These folks don't have time to suffer burnout, and they can't afford burnout. That's a middle-class term. To find relief from stress, these people turn to family, friends, and religion. We need to foster these because the people in this community have tremendous stress. People get blown away in front of their own houses. Crack deals are going down out in front of their houses. Cats and rats and dogs are running through their houses. The water flows through their homes because they have poor drainage. They're chronically worried about where the next dollar's coming from, or where the next meal's coming from, not to mention how to pay for health care, which is way down on their list. Their stress is incredible, and they don't have the opportunity to get away from it. We need to be aware of that stress, because a pill will not make the difference in the disease processes we're seeing.

MOYERS: So you start where people are. You don't try to take them to some spa or retreat.

SMITH: No, it's done in the home. We return to the home and the community. Community is the key word, because a lot of the resources for these families are within this community.

Mary Cassatt,
Mother and Child,
1889

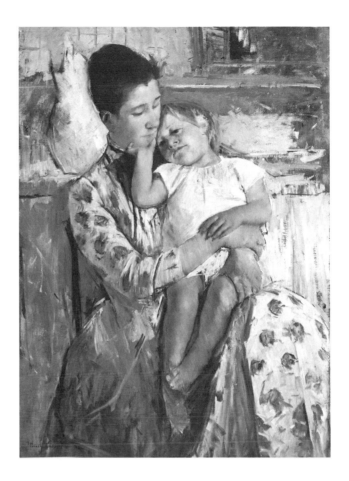

MOYERS: Where do these people go for primary health care, or do they even get primary health care?

SMITH: They really have not been getting good primary health care. For one thing, since most of them work, it's difficult for them to use the services available in the traditional nine-to-five setting. We force them to choose between ignoring health care, or losing a day's wages to go get it. Children have to leave school to get health care, which sends a message that school is not that important. But, of course, those are the traditional messages we've put in our medical system.

MOYERS: Do most of these people see a doctor on a regular basis?

SMITH: No. Because it's so difficult for them to get health care, they often put things off. Then, when they really feel sick, they go to the emergency room at Parkland Hospital. Up until recently, that was really the only thing they could do.

MOYERS: But isn't it difficult for a public hospital to provide the care these people need?

SMITH: In fact, we don't. We end up putting band-aids on things. We take care of the acute problem, but we can never deal with the more complicated things, like prevention. A lot of the people who come to us with medical ailments are suffering from much deeper psychosocial problems.

MOYERS: By psychosocial you mean . . .

SMITH: By that I mean that they've got problems in their environment, either physically or emotionally. They can't put food on the table. They can't keep a roof over their heads. They're suffering from abuse or neglect.

MOYERS: How do you explain the phenomenon that medical care is not available in communities like these?

SMITH: I think part of the reason is that the incentives are all wrong. The incentives right now are for keeping health care in a centralized area. We offer health care in a wonderful medical center in the middle of the city and force everyone to come to us. We make it convenient for the providers of care, for the doctors and nurses, but not for the patients. We think that's great. Perhaps there's even a feeling of omnipotence because of it. But we should be reversing that trend and taking health care back out to the community.

MOYERS: So in centralizing medical care in a big place like Parkland, we're in effect denying people like these regular access to medical care.

SMITH: Yes, and we create other barriers as well. We talk about the financial barriers all the time in medicine, but what about the other barriers? In fact, we make these people crawl over each other to get health care. It gets so crowded in the clinics and emergency rooms that patients usually have to wait for hours.

The other day a child complaining of an earache was brought to the emergency room at Parkland. About eight hours into the wait, he felt better, and the mother said, "I might as well go home." What had happened is that the eardrum had burst, and the fluid had started to drain out of it, releasing the pressure. The problem hadn't been solved. The child now has a hole in his eardrum and is certainly at risk for not being able to hear as well, and to do as well in school, and could have chronic hearing problems for the rest of his life.

MOYERS: What finally brings people to a place like Parkland?

SMITH: Well, the condition just gets unbearable—often to the family more than to the individual with the condition. People continue to put off seeking help, and stoically bear the pain and suffering, until eventually the family or neighbors will bring them into the emergency room.

MOYERS: So they wait until there's a crisis before they reach out for the kind of medical care they truly need.

SMITH: Absolutely. And this is one of the reasons we began setting up these community health clinics. Parkland was overwhelmed by people coming in who needed help. There would be something acutely wrong, and all we were doing was just patching them up and giving them band-aids and pills. We were seeing more and more people who were sicker and sicker. We couldn't get to the front end of the problem and try to decrease the number of people coming in by offering preventive services.

So the real philosophy here is to take health care—not just medicine, but comprehensive health care—back to the community, and to try to eliminate some of the barriers that we see. When patients try to get access to health care in a centralized health campus or medical complex, they face barriers such as transportation, child care, school, loss of wages, or the fact that they have to wait eight to twelve hours for care.

MOYERS: So one of your goals was to bring health care back to the neighborhood.

SMITH: Yes, but not just by setting up our main campus in the neighborhood. We also need to deliver health care in nontraditional settings. We should be providing services in laundromats, in schools, in churches—and we are, even in places that are within walking distance of this facility. At first that might seem rather absurd. Why would you build a nice facility and then take your staff two blocks down the street to the high school? Because that's where the kids are. Why should I pull them out of school? Why can't I be there for them? Why can't I deal with the PTA that meets there every third Tuesday and take care of the parents and the other children?

So, yes, one of our goals was to bring health care back to the neighborhood. But another goal was for us to bring a different array of talent to health care—for example, outreach people, the old-fashioned public health nurse, translators.

MOYERS: Translating from English to Spanish, and Spanish to English.

SMITH: And in some of our sites, translating Vietnamese, Laotian, and Cambodian. If patients call at night, there's a bilingual answering service. If around forty percent of your patients are monolingual Spanish, it's no good having an English answering service. You see, we had to bring a different team to this community if we were going to make any difference. If we just put another hospital out here, where we were waiting for people to come to us, but we couldn't provide outreach and some culturally relevant skills, like translation, we were going to be in trouble, and no better off than we were before.

MOYERS: There's something rather old-fashioned about this. You're talking about the kind of care I got as a kid over in East Texas, when Dr. Tenney and others would pay house calls—their presence was . . . healing.

SMITH: That's right. It is very old-fashioned. We've become technocrats and turned away from this kind of health care, but we really need to come back to it.

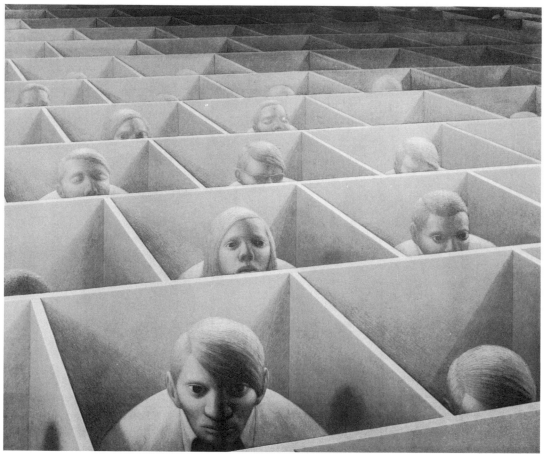

George Tooker, *Landscape with Figures,* 1966

MOYERS: Why did we turn away from it?

SMITH: Because the incentives are all wrong right now. We pay for the high tech, catastrophic side of health care.

MOYERS: All the gadgets.

SMITH: All the gadgets. You create a gadget, we'll pay for it tomorrow.

MOYERS: Yes, but I have to tell you, I like some of those gadgets. I've been helped by them.

SMITH: Oh, no question that we need those gadgets, too, because they do wonderful things. But there's not a good balance. We're investing in new technology, but at the same time, we're not investing in prevention or in understanding what makes people tick or why they got sick in the home that's across the street here. We don't know that. And then we don't go back out to see if we can change some of the things that may have precipitated the sickness. These things are very fundamental and basic. But the incentives aren't there.

First of all, we're not even taught how to function in that environment. We're taught in a centralized, mechanized, medical model, not a health model. We don't look at the entire spectrum of health care approaches, including prevention and rehabilitation. We say, "We can cure you," and we give you something to make you better—but then we throw you back out in the environment, which we don't understand very well, and you get sick all over again. The incentives for a health model rather than a medical model just aren't there.

MOYERS: And is reimbursement one of the incentives? Medicare and Medicaid and insurance companies will reimburse you if you put one of these people in the hospital with the big gadgets, but they won't reimburse you for coming out here and talking about prevention, the environment, stress, and taking responsibility.

SMITH: No, they won't. We are perverse in the way we look at incentives. The incentives are back-loaded. Pay me now, or pay more later. In this society we take care of our cars at the front end by changing the oil filter and doing other preventive maintenance. But our health care system offers no incentives for the preventive things, or for getting you to understand how you can avoid coming to our emergency room. We don't reimburse for prevention, and we also don't train people to do it. We don't use the right setting. We don't train out here, for instance, we train in the large, centralized medical center, away from the patients, and we make them come to us. It's artificial.

MOYERS: So by the time people come to you, it's almost too late to help them.

SMITH: The statistics show that's what's happening. There are rising rates of asthma deaths in communities like this. When we can't even deliver a simple vaccine that can prevent measles, then we've got a problem in the system.

MOYERS: These people don't have family doctors?

SMITH: No, they don't. What we're really trying to set up here, as much as anything else, is not a clinic, but an expanded practice. People can see the same person every time they come in. They also become attached to some of those different talents that we have here. They may be attached very closely to an outreach person, or to a VISTA volunteer, or to a social worker. It's even a little better than the family doc, because we bring a broad array of skills and services to bear on their problems.

MOYERS: And do they find it helpful to have the same doctor every time they come in?

SMITH: Oh, absolutely. They're amazed: "You mean I get to see the same doctor? You mean you aren't going to have somebody else every time I'm here?" Because that's what they get in a training setting—residents in training, rotating every month.

MOYERS: Will Medicare, Medicaid, and third-party providers reimburse you for these "marginal" folks like nutritionists and social workers and translators?

SMITH: Marginal?

MOYERS: I was using that facetiously.

SMITH: My profession wouldn't like to hear this, but these people are probably as important or more important than the physicians in this scheme of things. If they weren't here, we wouldn't be as effective. So we absolutely need them. The problem, traditionally, has been the one you've just cited. No, they're not covered by Blue Cross–Blue Shield, Medicare, or Medicaid. We're seeing some improvement, but not enough to pay for what I call "nonreimbursable staff." But we can't afford not to have them. And we do need health

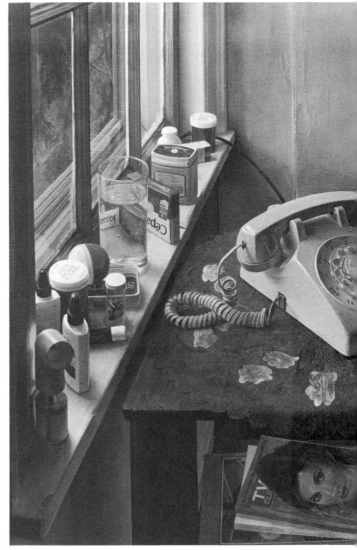

Catherine Murphy, *Bedside Still Life,* 1982

care reform that will allow us to keep them. Who pays for this now? The taxpayers of Dallas. The fact that we have support through that process and the fact that we write over thirty grants a year is how we keep these people.

MOYERS: But an overburdened taxpayer might ask, "Why should we pay for other people to do what they ought to do anyway—take care of themselves?"

SMITH: You can look at it two ways. One involves doing what's right. But if you want to take another, self-serving approach, you could say, "If I don't get those kids measles shots, measles will cross over into the middle class section of town"—which it did. So we want kids in this community to be protected against measles so that everyone is. Another example: if we can prevent a stroke that's going to come to $100,000 in intensive care costs, doesn't it make sense to invest $200 a year in health maintenance? One way or the other, you're going to pay.

MOYERS: How do you compare the cost of treating people here as opposed to the cost in a traditional hospital?

SMITH: We've actually looked at that and found that at Parkland, if you go in for an acute problem, say a sore throat, it will cost you $120 to $125 to be seen by a doctor. If you go to one of Parkland's seven community-center sites, it will cost somewhere around forty-seven dollars by the time you walk out with your prescription. In the meantime you may also have seen a social worker, a health educator, and maybe even stuck your head into the dental department. But forty-seven dollars. It could even be less if we didn't have the overhead associated with keeping our funding sources intact. I've got to keep grant writers, for example. And each of the funding sources insists on using its own forms. But still, the cost savings for coming here rather than to Parkland is immense. And that's not even measuring the potential impact of preventing a really bad outcome, like a stroke in a patient with high blood pressure.

So the approach here is not only cheaper, it's more comprehensive. If you want to use the car analogy, what we do here is not only take care of the noise or vibration in the car, we'll go ahead and change your oil and deal with the fact that the radiator needs to be flushed. We don't wait until we have to deal with you in a catastrophic or resurrection mode.

MOYERS: Resurrection mode?

SMITH: We want to save you. We want to feel like we're in *M*A*S*H*, and we've just done something that's going to bring you off the table, and you'll look at us and say, "Oh, Doctor, you've saved me." We don't feel as wonderful about doing prevention, even though it's cheaper. What happens in the resurrection mode is that we end up paying more later, and the patient is worse off because the condition has gotten more serious in the meantime.

MOYERS: But then why doesn't the health care system recognize the need for the kind of preventive care offered by people like nutritionists, psychologists, social workers, and translators?

SMITH: I wish I had an answer to that question. I don't know, because prevention

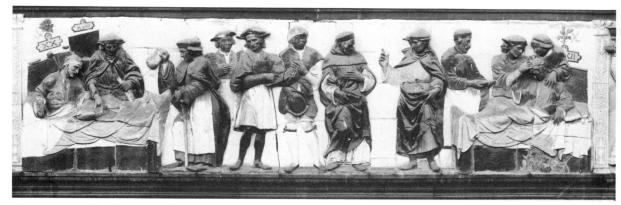

Giovanni della Robbia, *Visiting the Sick,* 1525

is just common sense. It's just common sense to embrace strategies that save money and save lives and help people be more functional and enjoy life. One of the things we know is that seventy-five percent of these people work. Who is going to be our labor force in the year 2015? It's going to be predominantly brown and black. And if we don't start investing in these folks, we're going to have to do one of two things—export jobs or import labor. So it's in our best interest to have some solutions to the health care crisis in communities like this.

MOYERS: When did you know that you were doing something right here?

SMITH: I think we first knew we were doing something right when patients began to come to us who had a choice, but who had heard through word of mouth, which is the most wonderful way to get things across in these communities, that something different was happening here, and that they could get the kind of care they needed.

MOYERS: They chose you.

SMITH: Yes. Another incident happened just recently at Parkland Hospital that made us think we might be doing something right. We had a patient in from one of our health centers, and the residents were all clustered around her, and the attending doctor was about to pontificate over the case. He leaned over her bed and said, "Mrs. Jones, who's your doctor?"—expecting her to say that one of the residents was her doctor. But she said, "My doctor's Dr. Irvine."

"Who's that?" asked the attending physician.

"Well, that's my doctor out in east Dallas at the community clinic. He takes care of me. In fact, he was just in here to visit me."

The doctor chuckled and gestured to the residents and said, "Well, who are these folks, then?"

She said, "Well, I just don't know who these folks are. I think they're in training, and they're trying to learn to be like Dr. Irvine."

MOYERS: Or any one of your "family" doctors.

SMITH: Because that's what the people really value. They've got somebody that's consistently there for them, not a doctor who is simply walking in and out of their lives.

MOYERS: But why is it important to these people to have a family doctor?

SMITH: Most of them want consistency and somebody who will listen. They don't want someone moving in and out all the time, who isn't available for them. They also want someone who's in their community. If I establish my practice in their community, I'm not making a value judgment against the place. If I make people go to a different side of town to see me, I'm communicating that I really don't want to have my office over where they live. They appreciate our being in their community.

The other thing I think they appreciate is that the rest of the staff is also there to listen. It seems as if they're getting special attention. People like that.

MOYERS: Is that just a personal preference? Or is it really a factor in health and healing?

SMITH: It's really both. For many patients it is a personal preference, but then you can use that relationship to help in healing the individual.

MOYERS: But what difference does it make if I know the doctor, or the doctor knows me, as long as he or she actually helps me?

SMITH: It gets back to the trust issue, and it also gets back to the issue of mind and body. There's a comfort level when someone is willing to listen and when you have a relationship with that person. One of the stresses we don't talk about much is the stress of seeing a doctor. When a doctor doesn't care, is cold, doesn't have time to talk, and runs in and out of the office, and if the staff is too busy filling out forms to pay any attention to you, there's stress. You've come in already stressed, and the situation is more stressful. And what happens then? You aren't comfortable, and the treatment will not be as effective.

MOYERS: But given the choice between cure or comfort, I'd choose cure. I would take today's longevity over the lifespan of a hundred years ago. I'd take childbirth today over what my grandmother had to go through. In other words, no matter how expensive these gadgets are, I don't want to give them up just to feel more comfortable about health care.

SMITH: No, but we have to look at whether we're continuing to see progress in these areas. I would venture to say that we're not. We're losing ground in longevity in African American males, for example. And we've lost ground on improving longevity in Hispanic women and African American women. They're not living as long as we would expect when we compare them to the Anglo population. So longevity isn't moving forward the way it once did.

MOYERS: And if we believe the surveys that tell us how unhappy people are, longevity itself is not the only goal.

SMITH: Yes—are we adding life to years, or simply years to life? Are we feeling good and enjoying life, or are we living to be ninety-five, but miserable? Again, mind/body.

You know, you can cure people, but if they're still dealing with the environment that contributed to the problem, the stress will continue, and the problem will return. We see that often with asthmatics. We improve them to the point that they can go back home, but if we don't deal with what's going on at home, they're going to be back. So we haven't made any real difference, we've just created a dangerous cycle of sickness and temporary relief.

MOYERS: You have a son who's an asthmatic, but he's also a champion swimmer. Have mind/body interactions helped him?

SMITH: Very much so. People with a disability like asthma will often worry about whether they will be normal human beings. When you have a chronic disease, you can wonder why you have it. My son, for example, wondered if this disease was a kind of punishment. We had to deal with that because emotional stress would actually precipitate wheezing. So we had to do more than just give him the pills and the breathing machine that he needed to make his asthma better. We had to talk it through so he could be comfortable and more forward. And he did. He decided he was going to do something about this disease, and so he got involved in swimming. And while swimming may have expanded his lung volume and all those wonderful physiologic things, perhaps the most important thing it did was to give him confidence.

MOYERS: You're absolutely convinced the mind plays a role in healing.

SMITH: Oh, no doubt. There is no doubt whatsoever.

MOYERS: What do you need to know about a person who comes to you for help if you're trying to deal with that individual in a mind/body sense?

SMITH: It may sound silly, but you need to know everything about them. What are the strengths, both of the individual and the community? Who's out there who can help them? What are their religious beliefs? Religion is very important to healing here. A lot of our Hispanic patients go to *curanderos*, or lay doctors, who do things that some people would describe as witchcraft. We have to understand that a

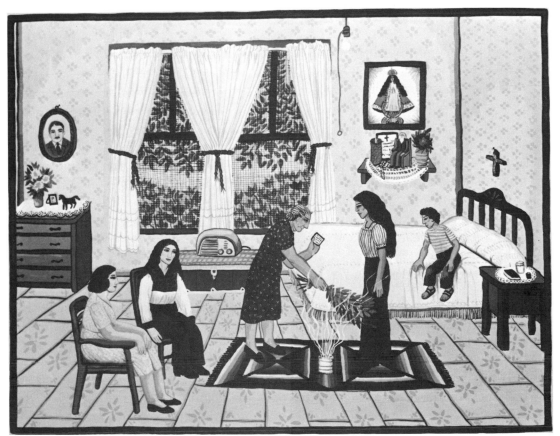

Carmen Lomas Garza, *Curandera* (Faith Healer), 1977

patient may have a relationship with one of these people, because if we say, "You guys need to get rid of those teas, and quit lighting those candles, because we can take care of you," we've lost it. They're not going to get better.

MOYERS: Why not?

SMITH: For one thing, they won't take our medications. For another, sometimes the *curanderos* will prescribe teas that actually have medicinals in them. One of them is foxglove tea, which contains digitalis, a substance that makes the heart beat better. If we know a patient is on foxglove tea, we need to make sure that we don't overdose that patient with Digoxin.

MOYERS: So to practice mind/body medicine, you need to know about a patient's faith, family, and culture.

SMITH: Absolutely. You have to understand where the patient is coming from and build on that.

MOYERS: In reporting this story, I keep running into doctors like you, who say that we have to begin to see the whole patient. What do you mean by that?

SMITH: Our traditional focus is on individual body parts. We look at your lung, we look at your kidney, we look at your stomach, we look at your brain. You've got a different doctor for every organ. We never put it all back together for you, let alone for ourselves. Then what we do is treat the particular organ system. We send you off on what I call "the organ express." We're not thinking of you as a whole, so you think maybe you shouldn't either. Maybe you should just focus on your kidneys — but it's very confusing. Because another doctor has given you a pill for your heart, and you don't know how the medicine for the kidneys might affect the heart. You might ask your kidney doctor, but you'll get the reply, "Gee, I don't know, I'm only the kidney doctor."

MOYERS: Why doesn't the medical profession see the whole patient now?

SMITH: Well, we used to see the patient as a whole. We used to do home visits. We used to spend a lot more time understanding and really living in the communities that we served. And I guess "served" is a good word. But we've seen the pendulum swing all the way over to a compartmentalized medical focus. We've become experts in particular areas, but we're not experts on the entire human being. We really don't like the unknown, and mind/body medicine is full of unknowns, so you have to have an open mind as a health care provider to practice it.

MOYERS: But your definition of mind/body medicine strikes me as just plain, old-fashioned common sense.

SMITH: It is, and that's the way the patient needs to understand it, too. We need to listen to the patient and work with the whole human being. Patients will sometimes tell you things that seem totally out of context, which you might be tempted to dismiss. For example, they'll talk about the fact that they had to change a flat tire on the way over here. But if you listen, you find out that the tires are all bald, and they haven't been able to do anything about it, and that before coming here, they had to take their epileptic child somewhere else to take care of his seizure problems, and it's been very difficult for them.

MOYERS: So by the time they get to you, they are tense and distraught.

SMITH: And if you make them wait, or if you don't really understand or listen, they aren't going to be as cooperative as you would like.

MOYERS: So how medicine is delivered can often affect the very process of healing that medicine should be all about.

SMITH: Yes, you can really make the condition worse if you don't pay attention to the interrelation of mind and body.

MOYERS: Listening to you, I'm wondering, why aren't more hospitals setting up clinics like this? Why aren't more hospitals incorporating mind/body techniques, or at least mind/body philosophy, into what they're doing?

SMITH: I'm not sure. Many of them have been in such a reactive mode, worried about reimbursement, and keeping the physical plant up, and so many other things, that maybe they're not thinking. Also, most hospitals are worried about keeping their beds full. But we're in exactly the reverse situation. We'd like to have a few of them empty, and we'd like to get a lot of the people out of the emergency room because we have too many, and because as good health care providers, we know we're not doing the best for them in that crowded setting.

MOYERS: Do you think people out there are ready for mind/body medicine?

SMITH: Well, it depends what you mean by the people out there. I think the patients are ready for it.

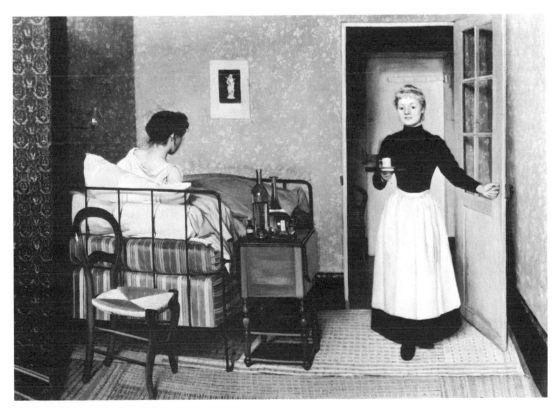

Félix Vallotton, *The Sick Girl,* 1892

MOYERS: It seems to me, as a reporter, that people are ahead of the medical profession in many respects.

SMITH: Not only are patients ahead of us, but I think business is beginning to get ahead of us. It doesn't make good business sense to keep paying for making sick people well when we could have prevented the illness in the first place.

MOYERS: Change the oil now for ten bucks and save a thousand-dollar ring job.

SMITH: Absolutely. We're paying for the thousand-dollar ring jobs every day in our large hospitals. What we aren't doing is changing the oil filters.

MOYERS: But in many cases, the oil filter, metaphorically, is in the mind or in the patient's relationship to the environment and the community.

SMITH: We take patients out of context too often in medicine. We bring them into nice buildings like this one—but hospitals are artificial environments.

MOYERS: Are you saying that the community is the best place to practice mind/body medicine?

SMITH: Absolutely. The best place to do it is out here in the community, because here we can use the strengths of the community. You know, we talk about the failure of our communities, but one thing is very clear: there are incredible strengths in these communities, mainly in the individuals. You see it in the people here who are trying to force the drug dealers out, or the ones who are working together to force landlords to make improvements on their homes, or the ones who are trying to get the city to do something about the flooding, or the ones who make sure that their neighbor gets to the doctor. You've got to understand the strengths of the community, because they're really there.

MOYERS: You're talking about a whole new way of seeing health.

SMITH: Well, I don't know if it is or not. Maybe our ancestors were a little smarter than we are about some of these things. If you were the family doc, you lived down the street, and you knew what was going on. You knew the fact that the plant around the corner had laid off workers, and you knew whether certain problems in a patient were related to substance abuse. Even Native American medicine, which was a very effective form of health care, created a healing environment. And what we have to do now is reestablish a healing environment in our communities.

II

HEALING
FROM WITHIN

"The physician is only nature's assistant."
— G A L E N

They are your everyday, garden-variety Americans, twenty-five of them, and they are sitting in a circle on the floor, their legs tucked beneath them, or on folding chairs. Their eyes are closed. They are eating raisins. Three raisins each, one at a time.

"S-l-o-w-l-y," says the man in the center. "Lift one raisin slowly to your mouth. Chew it v-e-r-y s-l-o-w-l-y." He pauses and surveys the circle. "Observe your arm lifting the raisin." Pause. "Think about how your hand is holding it." Pause. "Now put it in your mouth and think about how it feels there." Pause. "Savor it." Pause. "Notice any thoughts, either negative or positive, that you have about raisins." Pause. "Pay attention to your salivary glands." Pause. "Your jaws." Pause. "Your teeth." Pause. "Now notice your tongue as you slowly, s-l-o-w-l-y, swallow the raisin."

I have been eating my own raisin, s-l-o-w-l-y. At first I felt silly, sitting here on the floor, my legs crossed under me, my eyes closed, deliberately masticating a dark purplish red shrunken piece of fruit. But something odd happened as I chewed. I tasted the raisin—truly tasted it. I have eaten raisins all my life, gulping them down, straight from the box, gobs at a time. But the actual taste of a single raisin, savored in its own right, as if it were the first, last, or only bite, is a new experience, one that concentrates the mind.

I open my eyes. The others are still chewing. I remember what brought them here. Madeline, the housewife, said she has a panic attack every time she gets stuck in traffic. Ed, the truck driver, has started to experience heart flutters on his rounds. The doctors can't find anything physically wrong with his heart, but he is scared, and the stress of the fear is getting to him. Mary, the accountant, said she suffers terribly from migraine headaches. Dan, the carpenter, told how his days are barely livable since his accident. He is in constant pain, can no longer jog or play ball with his kids. And he is struggling to find a new way to make a living. The first time I saw him, the pain in his eyes made me wince.

I glance at him now, see his brow plowed like a field, and look away. Then I look back. He is concentrating on his raisin. So are the others, drawn into the circle as if they were wagons in an old western, huddled against the night.

In the center is Jon Kabat-Zinn. Trained as a molecular biologist, he is an assistant professor of medicine at the Massachusetts Medical Center and founder of its stress reduction clinic, one that several hospitals now use as a model. His patients have been referred to him by other doctors, who have been unable to treat their pain.

The pain is crippling—the pain of multiple sclerosis, heart disease, rheumatoid arthritis, migraine, hypertension. This circle is these patients' court of last resort. Now, instead of swallowing pills, they are eating raisins.

What's the point? I ask.

"They're really meditating," Kabat-Zinn answers. "Only we don't call it that. The word *meditation* tends to evoke raised eyebrows and thoughts about mysticism and hocus-pocus. Even though the words *medicine* and *meditation* sound alike, we don't want to scare people away. So we call it 'stress reduction.'"

It is, he will explain, an exercise in mindfulness. *Mindfulness* is Kabat-Zinn's favorite word. He says most of us live with our minds on auto-pilot. Without really realizing it, every one of the people in this circle is actually practicing an "eating" meditation, mindful of the raisin, living in the moment, becoming aware of something other than their pain.

Once a week for eight weeks Kabat-Zinn teaches patients a variety of techniques and experiences. They will learn to "scan" their bodies, moving consciously through the painful areas until they can "relax into their discomfort." They will learn yoga, arching into a ball, raising their pelvises, stretching their arms over their heads, lifting their heads and feet while lying on their stomachs. At first, groans and grunts fill the room. But by changing their body language, their physical posture, says Kabat-Zinn, they can change their attitudes and feelings, including their attitude to their suffering.

Over six thousand people have completed the clinic's program. Each patient is expected to attend the two-and-a-half-hour session each week and to practice at home, forty-five minutes a day, six days a week. In a follow-up study, 72 percent of Kabat-Zinn's patients report moderate to significant improvement in their condition after one year. As I learn from one of Kabat-Zinn's colleagues, Dr. John Zawacki, many of these were people who had been "so overwhelmed by anxiety that they couldn't even sit still" when first referred to the clinic.

I look at Dan again. He is swallowing his last raisin. Because his head is lowered, I cannot see his Adam's apple at work, but I can tell that he is guiding the raisin down, purposefully. The deep furrows in his forehead have almost disappeared. He opens his eyes and slowly turns this way. Our eyes meet. For the first time since I joined the circle, he smiles. Later, he will tell me that on the third raisin, his pain seemed to lessen. At least he wasn't as conscious of it, or as afraid of it. "The fear of pain," Kabat-Zinn tells me, "is often worse than pain itself."

Cut to California. Palo Alto. Stanford University. Another circle of people. All women. And David Spiegel, a psychiatrist. These are his patients. All have metastatic breast cancer, which kills most women within two years. They have agreed to participate in a research project, the second of its kind that Spiegel has conducted. The first produced an unexpected result that Spiegel now hopes to repeat.

In the original study, Spiegel, intending to assess the "often overstated claim . . . that the right mental attitude will help to conquer cancer," randomly divided eighty-six women into two groups. Half were given standard medical care. The other half received that same care—radiation, chemotherapy, drugs—but were also asked to meet once a week in a group therapy session. Spiegel had hypothesized that they would show an improved quality of life. He was right; the women reported less depression, anxiety, and pain than those in the other group. What startled him some years later, when he was reviewing the study after all but three of the women had died, was the discovery that those who took part in the group psychotherapy had lived twice as long after they entered the study as the group that received only standard medical care.

Spiegel had been extremely rigorous about the design of the study. He consulted with other scientists and with skeptics and showed them his findings, asking them to poke holes in his methods and conclusions. They couldn't.

What could account for the results? Spiegel is cautious and warns that the results may not be the same in this repetition of the experiment. "Something in the group appears to have helped these women live longer. But what that is, I don't know." He cites numerous studies which show that people with many social ties live longer than people who are not connected to other human beings (married cancer patients, for example, survive longer than unmarried patients). The sense of social alienation that many cancer patients still suffer, Spiegel says, "is a terrible thing, and a danger to their mental and physical health." By coming together regularly, patients help one another overcome loneliness and isolation. The women grow to care for each other. They form a support network that extends beyond the session; they visit each other in the hospital, go out to eat together, call each other during the week. Even those women who have a strong supportive network outside the group find that they can say things about their cancer within the group that they cannot say elsewhere. "When a topic is too painful for one woman to deal with directly, she can benefit from hearing another woman pursue it. The act of merely being with and interacting with others who face a similar experience," Spiegel says, "serves to buffer the traumatic effects of facing an illness on one's own."

I watch our film of the sessions as the women talk about death, and I wonder how such a head-on confrontation of mortality can have a therapeutic effect. Having read the self-help literature of positive thinking, I know that many people look upon contemplating the worst as a self-fulfilling prophecy. Spiegel disagrees. Death can be handled better when it is broken down into a series of problems, he says. What the women are doing is "detoxifying dying," which is important because "most patients told us they were not so much afraid of death as they were of the process of dying—the pain, diminishment, and loss of control."

He asks the women to write down, in order, the ten most important aspects of their lives—ones that define who they are. They do so, listing personal qualities, people they love, special pursuits they enjoy, and experiences they cherish. Then he asks them to erase each item, slowly, one by one, and to consider what remains when first one thing drops away, then another. The women close their eyes. They can see themselves changing as the disease progresses.

One woman weeps. She has a six-year-old son whom she will never see graduate from high school. She has told her son, "Mommy will be going away." Spiegel suggests that this could imply she is leaving by choice and that the boy might feel responsible for her departure. She decides to tell him that "there may come a time when Mommy can't be with you, but I would always be with you if I could." Later she will write him a series of birthday cards up to his eighteenth birthday, as a way of trying to support him after she is gone. Writing those cards charges her remaining months with significance. This, says Spiegel, is crucial. "They assess what is important in the time that is left, and discard what is trivial."

We will never know which aspects of Spiegel's work may have extended the lives of the women in the first experimental group, and it will be years before we know whether the current group is so fortunate. But the implications of the study are provocative. They suggest that some techniques, although no cure for cancer, may help cancer victims, and that others summon from within the individual valuable resources in fighting illness.

During this journey I met others whose research, like Spiegel's and Kabat-Zinn's, opens us to the possibilities of mind/body medicine. Even children can be taught to use the power of their imaginations to affect their bodies, as Karen Olness has demonstrated in teaching children biofeedback techniques to cope with migraine headaches. Talking with Dr. Olness, I also learned about the intriguing case of a girl who was conditioned to react to the smell of a rose and the taste of cod-liver oil as if they were a powerful drug. Olness herself underwent surgery using only self-regulation techniques—basically, her imagination—as an anesthetic.

The power of the mind is astonishing, and yet we know so little about how it works. When I asked Dean Ornish about how he had managed to reverse heart disease in patients, he told me that a low-fat diet and moderate exercise were important, but at least as important was stress reduction through yoga, meditation, and group support. Ornish refers to his work as "emotional open-heart surgery."

Common themes run through these discussions: the importance of social support; the value of expressing feelings; the doctor-patient relationship; the power of metaphor; the importance of grieving; the facing of death. In gaining a sense of control over our medical treatments, in making conscious choices about how we spend our lives, and in allowing others into our sufferings, we are releasing innate healing capacities that make us nature's allies in our own recovery.

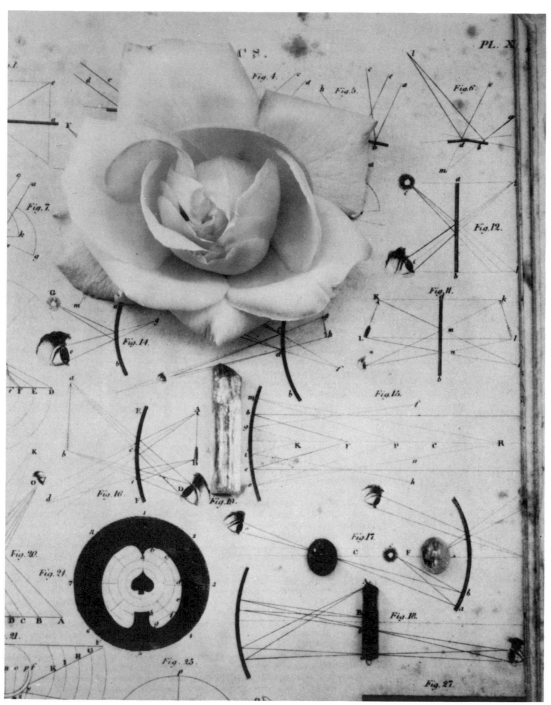

Olivia Parker, *Contact*, 1978

SELF-REGULATION AND CONDITIONING

Karen Olness

KAREN OLNESS, M.D. is Professor of Pediatrics, Family Medicine, and International Health at Case Western Reserve University. Olness has demonstrated that children with migraine headaches can learn biofeedback techniques that can reduce the number of migraines.

In Dr. Olness's clinic, I met a lively ten-year-old, Mika Crass. Several months before, Mika had begun to suffer from severe migraine headaches, and no drug was able to stop the unpredictable round of intense, debilitating pain. As I watched, Mika's hands were attached to a computer that measured the electrical resistance of her skin. As the resistance diminished, a design on a computer screen grew smaller. Using this feedback, Mika has learned to recognize when her mind is relaxed. By regularly practicing this same self-regulating technique, she has been able to ease the pain of her migraines.

MOYERS: What are you trying to teach children here?

OLNESS: Many of the children come here to learn self-regulating strategies to deal with chronic pain. Mika, for example, was able to learn how to reduce the frequency of her migraines and also how to reduce the discomfort when she did have migraines.

MOYERS: What's the scientific basis for that?

OLNESS: Well, the tendency to have migraines is a genetic or a biologic condition. Like many such conditions, migraines can be triggered by certain external events—a certain food, perhaps, or fatigue, or a hormonal change. Although we don't know the specific cause of migraine, we do know from controlled studies

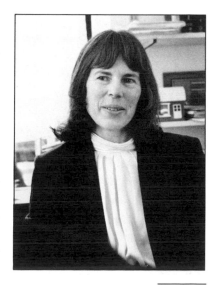

that regularly practicing a relaxation imagery exercise results in far fewer migraines than taking conventional medicine for the same purpose. We know this because we compared a standard treatment for migraine in children with the use of relaxation imagery and other self-regulating strategies. Children trained in self-regulating techniques did far better than the children with the medication, and certainly better than the children who were on placebo, and received no treatment at all.

MOYERS: What did you teach Mika to do?

OLNESS: We asked Mika to think about what she likes most, which is tennis. She imagined playing tennis, connecting her brain to her arms and legs and moving appropriately on the court.

MOYERS: It seems to me you're trying to tap into the children's imaginations.

OLNESS: Yes, but we're very careful not to prescribe what they should imagine. We talk with them to find out what they're interested in, just as we found out that Mika was interested in tennis. And we will then ask them to think about something with a context that they like, enjoy, or understand. An example would be a child who likes to play outside. You find out that the child enjoys playing outside in the snow, so you ask the child to imagine putting on very nice warm mittens. "Think about those nice warm mittens, and then see if the image on the screen gets smaller. Or, if you don't like my suggestion, think of your own way. How would you imagine warming your fingers?" And they will say, "Well, I thought of putting a candle under my fingers. I put my hand just above the flame, and then the temperature went up." It's fun to watch their creativity.

MOYERS: Do you teach self-hypnosis to these children?

OLNESS: Yes, I teach self-hypnosis to the children, but I think that needs some definition. In the course of their normal day-to-day play, children probably go in and out of a hypnotic state. But the term "hypnosis" is somewhat scary to people. Many athletic teams use a format identical to ours, but call it a biofeedback exercise, or a relaxation exercise. A relaxation exercise may induce a temporary altered state of awareness. In fact, in most biofeedback exercises there is a self-hypnosis component, although it's not always called that.

In our work with children and self-hypnosis, we always emphasize their control and mastery. We say, "I can coach you, I can teach you, but this is something that belongs to you. You can use it when you wish, but you don't have to use it if you don't want to."

We're very careful to be sure parents do not remind children to practice. Parents remind children to do a lot of things. It's a lot easier, however, for a child to fake doing a relaxation exercise than practicing the piano. And if a child decides that this is just another thing which is the parents' agenda, we haven't much confidence that the child will practice effectively. So we're very careful to say to parents, "This is something that is in the control of your child, so please don't remind him to practice. We can discuss how he will remind himself to practice. But he must be in control of this, or it's not going to work."

MOYERS: When biofeedback first emerged, we had great expectations for it. We thought it might even deal with major illnesses. But the use of it has been rather limited so far. Some people can do biofeedback effectively, and some cannot. What does that say about the mind?

OLNESS: It says that to become successful takes a lot of practice. It took me two months of daily practice to develop what I would call excellent skills in pain control. Children learn much more quickly.

MOYERS: Did you develop these skills for your own personal use, or just professionally?

OLNESS: Well, both. Initially, I developed them just to see if I could. Then I had a few experiences in which I needed them, and they were very useful. For example, I had surgery and used my self-regulation of pain as my anesthesia.

MOYERS: Literally? Under the knife?

OLNESS: Under the knife, right. This was all videotaped by my colleagues. I had a skiing accident and tore the ligament in my thumb, and it had to be resutured. It was about a forty-five-minute procedure.

MOYERS: With no anesthesia?

OLNESS: I had no anesthesia.

MOYERS: What was going on in your mind?

OLNESS: I was focused and concentrated. That's the essence of self-hypnosis— concentrating one's attention in a different way.

MOYERS: When you were lying on that operating table, and they were suturing up your hand, what images were you seeing?

OLNESS: I was thinking about a favorite memory, which is being on the farm where I grew up. I remembered the feeling of lying in the grass, looking up at the heavens, and seeing a bit of the barn. Images can be wonderful. They can obviously also be frightening if we have negative images. But during the operation I simply focused on my image of the farm during the entire procedure, and I was extremely comfortable. I was perfectly conscious of what was going on outside, but I wasn't very interested in it.

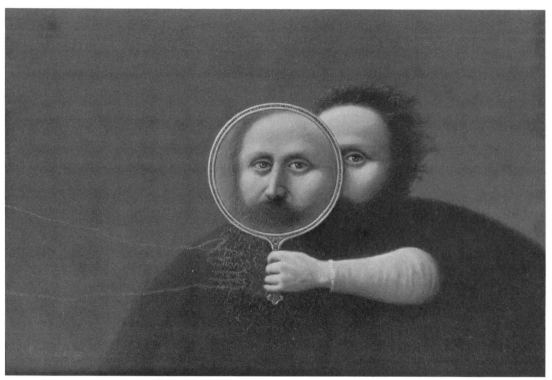

Alfredo Castañeda, *When the Mirror Dreams with Another Image,* 1988

MOYERS: What did you learn about your mind from that experience?

OLNESS: I must tell you that it was a very reassuring experience, because I had taught this for years, and I wondered whether I could use this technique if I really needed it—and I could. I felt the way I suppose a person does when he or she has finished a marathon. Although it was a mental achievement, my feeling was akin to that of winning a race.

MOYERS: So the essence of self-hypnosis is not magic, it's the mind communicating with the body.

OLNESS: Very much. All hypnosis is self-hypnosis. It is a strategy to focus and concentrate for the purpose of achieving something that is in one's best interest.

MOYERS: We don't really know how meditation and self-hypnosis work, do we?

OLNESS: We don't, but we also don't know how some medications work, and yet we use them.

MOYERS: Like aspirin. Aspirin was around twenty years, and people were using it, successfully, before anybody could explain how it worked.

OLNESS: That's right. We still don't know all the details about how it works. We're finding more and more about aspirin every year. I'm not troubled by the fact that we don't understand exactly how self-hypnosis works. And I'm intrigued with the possibility that we will be able to understand it. I hope that we will. It challenges us in our research.

MOYERS: I see, but what about us poor mortals who do not have your discipline or understanding? I wouldn't go into surgery with the power of imagery as my only accomplice.

OLNESS: That's all right. But some people, those who have adverse reactions to anesthesia, do not have an alternative. I know many examples of people who have had major surgery with self-hypnosis as the sole anesthesia. They are highly motivated. If you were motivated, you would probably be able to do this, too. Of course, some people have certain learning disabilities or other handicaps that might make it difficult for them to learn these techniques, just as they might have problems learning other things. But I think the average person, properly motivated, could certainly learn self-regulation.

MOYERS: Self-regulation—that implies the mind is in control.

OLNESS: Yes, and we emphasize that, especially with the children and adolescents who have chronic illnesses and who aren't in control of very much. They can't control when they're going to get sick or come into the hospital—but if they learn these strategies, then they can have something they control, and they can contribute to their own healing.

MOYERS: Biofeedback, self-hypnosis, meditation, imagery—what is the difference between one of these and another?

OLNESS: I don't think there's any difference in the state, but there is some difference in the purpose. Meditation is for the purpose of going within or quieting. Self-hypnosis or relaxation imagery is often for achieving a specific goal, such as getting rid of a habit or controlling pain. Having practiced all these different techniques, I think I can say that the feeling state is the same. And Herbert Benson, a professor of medicine at Harvard, found that he could not differentiate among these techniques in terms of temperature or heart rate or pulse or brainwave pattern.

MOYERS: Is there scientific evidence to support the thesis that these techniques work?

OLNESS: There are encouraging studies, but most aren't conclusive. Like all studies, they need to be replicated. There are probably a dozen studies involving adults that show some change in the immune system in association with what I call intention. But it would be much too soon to rush out and expect to cure a certain disease on the basis of our immunology findings thus far. I would hope for many replications, I would hope for detailing the process by which people achieve changes in their immune function, and then I would very much hope that these findings would be applied in the clinical setting. When we understand exactly the process between the thought and the physiologic change, that is, the warming or the cooling of the fingers, ultimately we will be understanding how images are constructed and how they impact a neurotransmitter.

Once I had a four-year-old patient who did very well on one of these biofeedback exercises. After it was over, he said, "But I want to know, how does the thinking get down to make my fingers warm?"

I answered, "We don't know, but when you grow up, maybe you'll figure it out."

And he said, "I'm a smart boy, probably I will."

That was about fifteen years ago, so maybe he's ready to figure it all out.

MOYERS: Do you think we will find the scientific basis for the claim that how we think affects our health?

OLNESS: I think we're very close to having the tools to do that. My intuition is that whatever energy is associated with the construction of images and the process of thinking transmits a message to a cascade of body processes. That's not a very precise answer to your question. But I have felt that for a long time, because I have for so long observed the impact on physiological responses when children use their excellent imaginations. Jacob Bronowski once said that all civilizations have failed in one area—they have limited the capacity of imagination of their young. I think we are at some risk of doing that in this society, too.

MOYERS: Being a journalist, skeptical by craft if not by nature, I find it, well, preposterous to think that what I imagine can affect my immune system or the heat of my body.

OLNESS: I, too, came to this research with a great deal of skepticism. And I remember when I first shared my work demonstrating that children could increase and decrease their skin temperature, a professor of pediatrics said to me, "I wouldn't believe that even if I saw it." And that's exactly the point of view I had when I went into this research years ago. But I find it exciting now to see that, in fact, changing images does affect physiology. I have no doubt about that any longer.

MOYERS: We're just on the shore of this untraveled country.

OLNESS: I would say we're on the surface waves, and we have yet to plumb the depths.

MOYERS: But where do you think those depths will take us?

OLNESS: I think that with new technology and new tools for measuring intricate happenings within the brain, we will come to understand how changes in thinking or changes in images translate to changes in body function. And when we have that understanding, then we will be in a position to give specific instructions to people with illness on what they might do to help themselves.

MOYERS: Do you have any sense where that place is that the mind and the body meet?

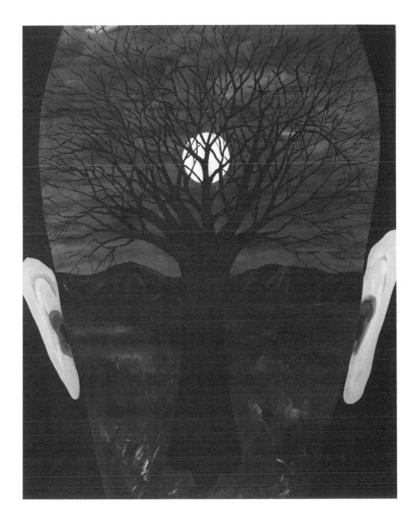

Jonathan Borofsky,
*The Moon in My
Mind at 2,998,773,*
1986

OLNESS: I don't have a precise sense, but I feel strongly that images and the minute energy associated with images that connects with neurotransmitters or information-transmitting molecules is where the mind and body meet. But, of course, to answer that question, we need far more sophisticated tools than we have now.

MOYERS: It seems so hard, though, to test these experiences clinically, to repeat them, and to get enough evidence.

OLNESS: Yes, the studies that we've done so far have been very difficult, with many tedious aspects and many complications. But I think we must continue with the research. I think it's as important as any other area of health science research.

MOYERS: In part, because technology can only take us so far.

OLNESS: That's right. Another important aspect of this area is that many of us have been in the habit of inadvertently conditioning ourselves negatively. It would help if we simply knew how to reverse that, if we knew what habitual images were not in our best health interests. That in itself would be a great advance in our understanding of this area.

MOYERS: Do you imagine ways in which more people can benefit from these self-regulation strategies?

OLNESS: Well, I think it would be wonderful if every child, beginning at age six or seven, could have an opportunity to be hooked up to a biofeedback system, maybe some sort of computer game that was cued to a physiologic response. Then, early on, children would have the experience, "Aha! I change my thinking, and my body changes." I think that's a generic concept that we should give our children as early as possible in life.

MOYERS: The sense that I can take control.

OLNESS: That I can take control. And that by changing my thinking, I can be in control of a body response.

MOYERS: You've heard the claims in some quarters that if you can imagine your good cells attacking your cancer cells, you can cure the cancer. Is there scientific basis for that?

OLNESS: I don't think so. In fact, I have a concern that people may feel guilty for having cancer and not being able to make it go away.

MOYERS: The victim is blamed.

OLNESS: That's right. It is certainly important that people with chronic illness do whatever they can to involve themselves in being in control of something—by diet-

Mary Frank,
Night-Head,
1971

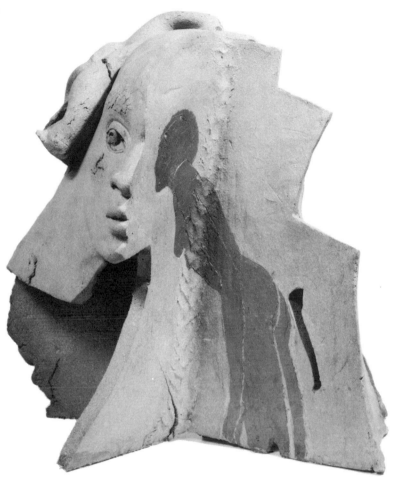

ing, for example, or by doing relaxation exercises. But there's so much that we don't know about most chronic illnesses and so much we don't know about how medications work that I think we are quite justified in assuming that there are likely to be some significant clinical outcomes from the forefront research in cyberphysiology.

MOYERS: What do you mean by "cyberphysiology"?

OLNESS: The word "cyber" derives from the Greek. It means "the helmsman" or "the steersman." It means being in control of some aspect of one's physiology or body processes. I think it's a good generic term for all the various training strategies. For example, athletic coaches who use some of these mental training strategies are in fact using a cyberphysiologic training strategy.

MOYERS: So you're on the deck with your hand on the wheel, and your mind is the rudder?

OLNESS: Yes, that's right. The mind is the rudder.

MOYERS: Is that also true in the case of Marette, the girl who came to you for help with lupus?

OLNESS: Yes, Marette had severe lupus, which is a chronic condition that affects many parts of the body, including the kidneys. She wanted to learn some self-regulation strategies to control her pain and anxiety and to help her feel more comfortable.

MOYERS: Was she in a lot of pain?

OLNESS: Yes, not only from the disease itself, but also from the numerous procedures she had to undergo. By the time I saw Marette, her disease had progressed to the point that her life was in danger. Because it was an emergency situation, we contemplated putting her on an experimental drug that had the effect of suppressing her immune responses.

MOYERS: You thought the drug would help fight the lupus?

OLNESS: Yes, we did, although we knew the drug would create severe side effects. Now it happened that I had just read a recent article by Bob Ader, who had used the same medication in an experiment with laboratory animals with lupus. Ader had given the animals saccharine-flavored water at the same time that they were given the drug. After a few pairings, the animals were simply given the saccharine-flavored water without the drug—and physiologically, the animals responded in the same way.

MOYERS: As if they were getting the drug?

OLNESS: Yes.

MOYERS: What did you think was happening in Ader's experiment?

OLNESS: I think Ader was making a very clear case that the pairing of various taste and smell stimuli with drugs eventually results in those stimuli triggering certain responses.

MOYERS: So the rats were conditioned to act as if the substitute they had been taking was the real thing.

OLNESS: That's right.

MOYERS: And you thought that perhaps you could do that with Marette?

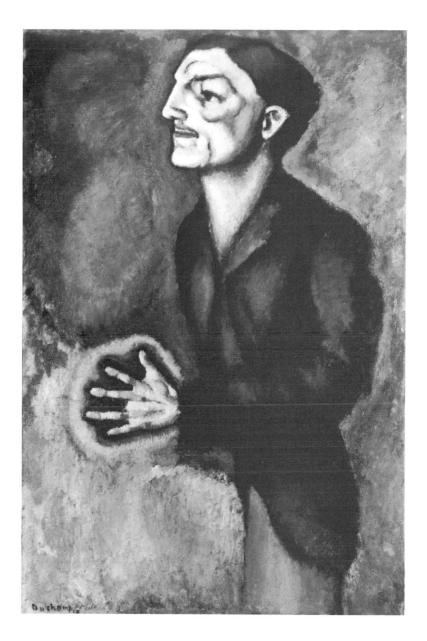

Marcel Duchamp,
Dr. Dumouchel,
1910

OLNESS: We thought it was possible. I shared Ader's article with Marette's mother, who saw the parallel immediately. She wanted everything possible done for her daughter, so she called Bob Ader and asked if it would be unreasonable to use the same strategy with Marette as he had used with the laboratory animals. He was encouraging, so we spoke with Marette's primary physician, who agreed. Then we had an emergency meeting of our Human Subjects Committee to get permission to try this approach, and we began the very next day.

MOYERS: Exactly what was your concern for Marette?

OLNESS: We were about to give Marette a toxic drug, and we hoped that by pairing the toxic drug with what we called a "conditioned stimulus," we could reduce the amount of the drug that she would require.

MOYERS: What do you mean "conditioned"?

OLNESS: Let me give you an example. Suppose a child with cancer is receiving a drug that causes nausea. And let's say that on the way home from the treatment, his mother buys him a certain flavor of ice cream. Because of his nausea at that time, he will associate the ice cream with nausea and become negatively conditioned to that particular ice cream flavor. We see that happening with children again and again. They may not even be consciously aware that was how their aversion started.

For example, I have an aversion to a particular Norwegian pudding that my mother would give me when I was ill. I cannot tolerate that pudding although it is supposed to be a delicacy. I have been conditioned to associate that pudding with illness. I think initially I wasn't aware of the linkage. It was only when I was older and thought about it that I realized how I came to dislike that pudding. As humans, we are often conditioned in ways that we don't understand. I don't think Marette, for example, was conscious of the way she was being conditioned.

MOYERS: Exactly what did you do with Marette?

OLNESS: We gave Marette a taste stimulus. Dr. Ader's advice was that the stimulus should be relatively unpleasant so that it would be unforgettable and that it should be something to which Marette had not previously been exposed. So I asked my colleagues and my husband and various friends, and I went around tasting various vinegars—and we finally came up with cod liver oil.

MOYERS: I know why you chose cod liver oil—it tastes terrible. I haven't had it for forty years, but I can still remember the taste. I didn't eat fish for a long time after using cod liver oil.

OLNESS: I remember it, also, all through my childhood. But we also gave Marette a pungent rose perfume.

MOYERS: You mixed those?

OLNESS: No, we gave them simultaneously. Marette sipped the cod liver oil as she was receiving her intravenous injection of the drug. And we uncapped the perfume. Subsequently, whenever Marette received the drug, we did the same sort of conditioning. That is, at exactly the same time she was receiving the drug we had her sip the cod liver oil and smell the pungent rose perfume.

MOYERS: Why did you choose a taste and a smell?

OLNESS: We knew from research that taste and smell are most easily conditioned. We felt that by using both a taste and a smell, we might double our chances of success. Also, we weren't certain whether Marette as an individual was more likely to be conditioned to the taste or the smell, so we used both.

MOYERS: How long did this go on? Did you give it to her every day?

OLNESS: Initially, we gave the perfume and the cod liver oil at the same time Marette received the drug. After three pairings of the drug and the stimuli, we gave Marette the scent and the cod liver oil without the drug. Over time, we gave Marette less of the drug than we would have given to a child who was not undergoing such conditioning, and Marette did equally well.

MOYERS: Her body would "think" that it was getting the drug and react as if it were, even though what she was getting was your concoction.

OLNESS: That's right. Marette did very well, but after a year she could no longer bear to sip any more cod liver oil. She was nauseated at the sight of cod liver oil, and she was unable to swallow it. She said she began to feel nausea as the spoon of cod liver oil came toward her lips.

MOYERS: But didn't you want her to associate the substitute with a positive response?

OLNESS: What we wanted was for her to associate it with the correct physiologic response. We were not as concerned with how she subjectively felt about the taste or the smell as whether or not the sensors from her taste and her olfactory apparatus would convey signals to her brain to respond as if her body were receiving the drug.

MOYERS: So her body would then fight the lupus, but without the side effects from the drug.

OLNESS: Yes, that's what we hoped for.

MOYERS: But weren't you sending the body mixed signals, with a foul-tasting liquid and a sweet-smelling fragrance?

OLNESS: I think we were sending mixed signals to Marette's consciousness, but I'm not sure we were sending mixed signals to whatever system triggers the conditioned response. In retrospect, however, if I were to give Marette another taste, I think I'd choose something more pleasant.

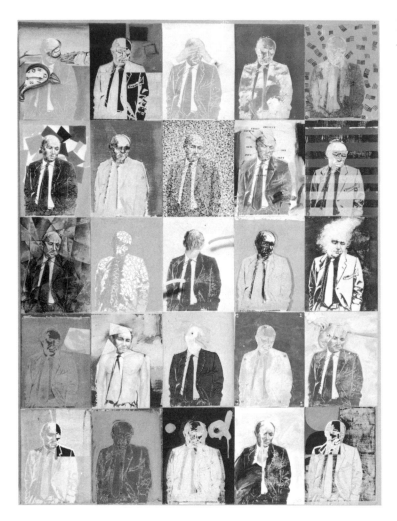

Paul Giovanopoulos,
Man 2, 1987

MOYERS: But even though the cod liver oil was unpleasant, her body got the message and responded as if she had received the powerful drug.

OLNESS: Her clinical response suggests that is what happened—but remember, this is one child, and we certainly can't draw valid conclusions on the basis of one case.

MOYERS: So you're not urging me to give up the medication I'm taking.

OLNESS: No, I'm not, but I am saying that if you sipped something with a particular and unusual flavor whenever you took the medication, it is possible that whenever you tasted that flavor again, your body would respond as if you were taking the medication. That could be positive, but it could also pose a risk if it's happening willy-nilly, without your knowledge.

MOYERS: Do you have any way of measuring the mind's role in this?

OLNESS: Not yet, but I hope that we will in the next century. It's very important that we understand what happened in a case like Marette's. I think it's also very important that we look into the conditioning that probably is occurring without our knowledge, and that we understand what might be the positive and negative effects of that conditioning. For example, a lot of people in this country are taking medications, and it is possible that some of the effects of those medications are being conditioned by environmental stimuli. We need a lot of research in that area.

MOYERS: If Marette's case is supported by further research, what are the implications for mind/body medicine?

OLNESS: We might use fewer drugs, and that means less cost for people as well as fewer side effects.

MOYERS: When you were working with Marette, do you think you were trying to teach her body or her mind?

OLNESS: I really don't see them as separate. I think we were teaching her unconscious mind to a greater extent than her conscious mind—and the unconscious mind is inextricably connected with the body. We have demonstrated that a simple change in a thought process is reflected in a physiologic change. In Marette's case, we were not impacting a conscious thought process, we were influencing those nerves connecting her tongue and her nose to her brain. As a result of that conditioning, we hoped that her brain would send signals to various parts of her body to respond as if she were receiving the drug.

MOYERS: And by "conditioning" you mean the body is taught to respond to certain stimuli?

OLNESS: Right. It happens without our conscious awareness.

MOYERS: Without our mind?

OLNESS: With the unconscious mind. We are conditioned without our conscious awareness all the time.

MOYERS: And so the trick is to find out how to employ our conscious mind, our aware mind.

OLNESS: Yes—to take charge and to say, okay, if I'm going to be conditioned, then I'm going to be in control of that.

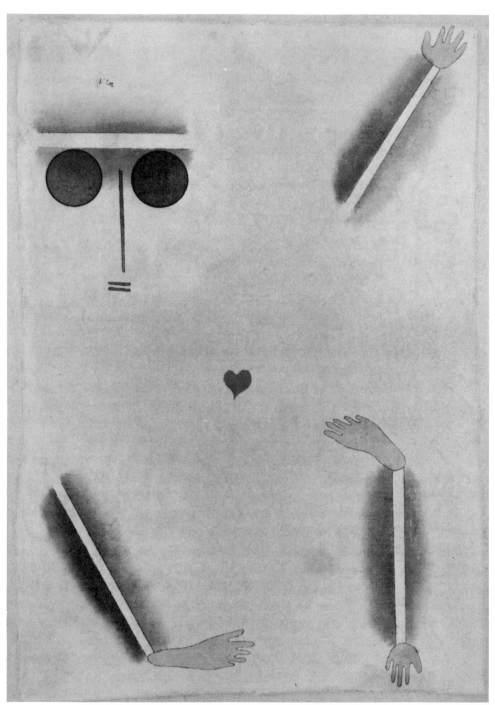

Paul Klee, *Has Head, Hand, Foot and Heart*, 1930

CHANGING
LIFE HABITS

Dean Ornish

DEAN ORNISH, M.D., is Assistant Clinical Professor of Medicine and President and Director of the Preventive Medicine Research Institute at the School of Medicine, University of California, San Francisco, and an attending physician at the California Pacific Medical Center in San Francisco. His research has demonstrated for the first time that coronary heart disease can be reversed without the use of drugs or surgery. He is the author of *Dr. Dean Ornish's Program for Reversing Heart Disease.*

I had read about Dr. Ornish's scientific studies showing reversal of serious heart disease using a combination of meditation, stress-reduction exercises, group therapy, walking, and a vegetarian diet. Our conversation took place at a retreat for heart patients where Ornish had just given a lecture in which he showed slides of computer-analyzed coronary angiograms and PET scans and talked about the results of his research.

MOYERS: You have studied the effects of these life-style changes on heart patients. Exactly what did your study show?

ORNISH: Our primary objective was to discover whether arterial blockages can begin to reverse over a one-year period.

MOYERS: What do you mean "reverse"?

ORNISH: Over time, the coronary arteries, which feed the heart with blood, can get clogged up with cholesterol and other deposits. The process is a little like rust building up in a pipe. Until recently, it was thought that the clogging was only going to get worse over time, so that the best you could do was to slow the process down, or, if

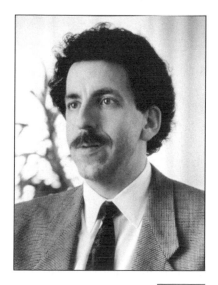

the arteries were very badly clogged, to do bypass surgery without really affecting the process itself. But our research showed that in 82 percent of the patients who went through our program, the arteries actually became less blocked. The blood flow to the heart improved, and as a result, the chest pain diminished markedly—by 91 percent, in fact.

MOYERS: But didn't about half of the people in the control group—those who didn't follow your program—get better too?

ORNISH: The majority—53 percent—got worse. Only a few patients in that group actually got better, and they were the ones who, on their own, changed their life-styles the most. In both groups, we found a direct relation between how much people changed their life-style and what happened in their arteries. We also found that the women tended to do better than the men. We had only a few women in the study, but all four of the women in the comparison group showed reversal, even though they were making only moderate changes.

MOYERS: How many people are there in your current study?

ORNISH: There were 41 patients who finished the first phase of the study, which looked at results after one year. Now we're following these patients for a three-year period, which is almost completed. So far, in many cases, we're finding that the longer people stay on this program, the more improvement they show, while the people in the comparison group tend to get worse and worse. The two groups are beginning to diverge even more over time.

MOYERS: But your group includes the most highly motivated people, the most ambitious, those who really want to make a change, and whose will to do this is intense. Isn't that going to bias the outcome?

ORNISH: To an extent, that's true, but remember how people were recruited to this study. We designed the study to take only people who had just had an angiogram for reasons unrelated to our study. We asked these people if they were willing to follow the program and take another angiogram a year later. It's the worst time to recruit someone for a study, because they've just been through the angiogram, which is a kind of X ray movie of the heart—an uncomfortable, invasive, and risky proce-dure. But about half the people we asked said yes even before we knew whether the program was going to help them or not. And only one patient dropped out during the first year. So more people may be willing to change their life-styles than many doctors may believe.

Now you could say, "Well, 50 percent of the people you asked said no," and that's right. When people don't want to change, I don't hesitate to use drugs and surgery, because my goal is not to get people to change, it's to do the best scientific research that I can, and to show what is possible and what works, and to what degree and for whom; and then, as an educator, to tell the public, "Here is what we did, and here is what we found, and here is how you can do it if you want to." You see, I think it's very paternalistic for doctors to say, "Oh, my patients would never do that." Even the American Heart Association has said that since people won't follow a diet that's as strict as the one in our program that we shouldn't even tell them about it— even though we now know from a number of studies that when people with heart disease followed a 30-percent-fat 200-milligram-cholesterol diet, as the Heart Association recommends, the majority got worse rather than better. To me that's analogous to saying, "Well, we know you won't quit smoking, so we're not even going to tell you to try. Just smoke two packs a day instead of three." We don't tell people that, even though it is hard to quit smoking. What is true and what is easy are different issues. My role as your doctor is simply to say, "Here are the facts. It is your decision, it is your life, and whatever you choose, I will support."

MOYERS: I appreciate that. Nonetheless, it is a very small sample to draw such large implications for the rest of us. Aren't there more studies to be done? Don't you need to enlarge the sample, and repeat it over and over?

ORNISH: In science, all studies need to be replicated. I hope to continue to do more research, and, also, other people are starting to replicate our studies. Of course, if you want to be a real purist, nothing is ever really proven, because you can always find weaknesses to criticize in any study, including ours.

But the size of the sample really isn't the issue. If you randomly divide people into two groups, and give one group an intervention, then you have to distinguish whether the difference between the groups at the end of the study is a real finding or simply the result of chance. What determines that is the degree and consistency of change and the accuracy with which you're able to measure the change. The more significant the degree of change, the more likely it is that the change is not due to chance. We are using new tests that are very accurate, and very reproducible, and we are giving people a very intensive program, so the changes are fairly large compared to, say, those found in drug studies. So many of our patients changed in such a consistent and significant way, as measured by the standard statistical methods, that the likelihood of the differences between groups being due to a random chance was very small. Also, our findings are not in a vacuum. There's a whole body of animal studies, of epidemiological studies, and of other clinical trials using cholesterol-lowering drugs that is consistent with what we've found.

MOYERS: But do you really have to put people through this boot camp to get these results? For example, studies show that Japanese who move here and change their diet develop heart disease. Other studies show that Europeans who could eat only vegetables during the Second World War because there was no meat lowered their rate of heart disease. Couldn't you have the same effect on heart disease simply by changing the diet and spare these poor souls this ordeal you're putting them through?

ORNISH: I'm not sure I would call it an ordeal, or that they would either. We have gotten to a point in medicine where it is somehow considered radical or an ordeal to ask people to stop smoking and manage stress better and walk and eat a healthful diet. And it is considered conservative to saw people open and bypass their arteries or to slip balloons inside their arteries and squish them, or to put them on powerful drugs for the rest of their lives. So I think our priorities are a little topsy-turvy.

Now I want to make clear that I'm not against drugs or surgery. In a crisis they can be life-saving. And in my own practice I never tell people, "You have to follow this diet, you have to come through this program, you have to meditate." Because even more than feeling healthy, I think we want to feel free. And you can't feel free if someone is telling you to do something, even if it is supposedly for your own good. That goes back to Adam and Eve, when God said, "Don't eat the apple." We saw how effective that was—and that was God talking.

MOYERS: Right. But you do tell them that these techniques can possibly reverse their heart disease. You believe that, don't you?

ORNISH: Well, I was skeptical when I began. I did not do this research to prove that heart disease could be reversed, but simply to see what would happen. As a scientist, I am curious. But I did not assume, as some people did, that it would be impossible. I reasoned that since no one had ever really looked at it scientifically, whatever we showed would be of interest. As it turned out, we showed that there often was reversal. Our statistical analyses indicated that each component of the program played an important role. We found a direct correlation between the amount of overall adherence to the life-style program and what happened in the arteries, and in secondary analyses we found that adherence to each part of the program was also directly correlated with what happened in the arteries.

Now, unlike most things we do as doctors, the worst that can happen if someone practices stress management, for example, is that they can manage stress better. This is not like putting someone on medications that can have serious side effects, both known and unknown.

MOYERS: In this study, did even small changes in artery function actually make a difference in the health of these people?

ORNISH: If you talk with them, they'll give you a clear yes. There are several reasons for that. On a technical level, in a critically blocked artery the blood flow through that artery is a fourth-power function of the diameter of that artery. In other

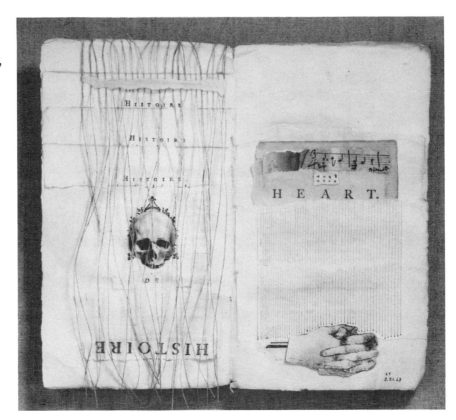

Lenore Tawney,
Heart, 1968

words, even a small change in a critically blocked artery has a relatively big effect on blood flow to the heart.

MOYERS: Sort of like a Roto-Rooter.

ORNISH: In a sense, yes. And life-style changes can improve blood flow to the heart through other mechanisms, too: the arteries can dilate; blood clots are less likely to form; and new arteries can begin to grow around the blockages. In many cases, in our earlier studies we measured significant improvements in blood flow to the heart in only a month. Subjectively, most patients will tell you that their chest pain began to diminish in a few days to a few weeks. Now we know from looking at studies of bypass surgery and angioplasty that the major benefit that you get from those approaches is a reduction in the amount of chest pain people have. No one has shown that angioplasty, where you blow up a balloon in the artery and squish the blockages, can prolong life or prevent heart attacks. Also, the three major randomized control trials of bypass surgery have shown that with the exception of a very small subset of patients who have critically severe disease, bypass surgery does not prolong life either. The major benefit is improvement in how people feel and the reduction of chest pain. Now, if we can show—as we have in three separate studies—

that through life-style changes alone, not only do people feel better, but that they *are* better, then to me, life-style change is a valid alternative to cholesterol-lowering drugs and surgery. And people need to know that they have alternatives.

MOYERS: When you look back at all your data, can you identify the major determinant in the reversal of the heart disease?

ORNISH: No. Each part seems to play an important role. For one patient, who may have been on a high fat diet but who manages stress well, the diet change may be more important. For another, who's under a lot of stress but who eats a decent diet, the stress management may be more important. But if I had to choose one factor that I thought was most important, I would say it is dealing with the deeper issues of what really motivates us, and what brings us a sense of contentment and peace and well-being. Even when you try to get people to take medications to treat high blood pressure or to lower cholesterol, you find that after a year, a fairly small percentage of patients are even taking a pill, much less changing diet or life-style. In other words, providing people with health information or giving them a prescription is not usually enough to motivate them to make life-style changes or even to take their pills.

MOYERS: I understand that. But if we can't identify the major determinant, then science can't say how it works. And if we can't say how something works, it becomes very difficult to take it out of the small group you have here to the larger community.

ORNISH: That problem is inherent in any behavioral study because you're never simply changing one factor. You can do that with drug studies because you can give the comparison group an inactive pill. The person who gives the pills and the person receiving them don't know who is getting the real drug and who is simply getting a placebo. But it's not that simple if you are putting someone on a diet or if you are teaching them stress management or exercise. Clearly, they know who is getting it, and so do we.

The other problem is that ideally, in science, you try to have just one independent variable—the drug, for example. Then you have a dependent variable—the blocked artery—and you say, "After a period of time, if there's an improvement in the artery, the drug must have been the cause." But even in drug studies we find that is not often the case, because when you are dealing with people, you are never really changing just one variable. We might like to fool ourselves and think that we are, but more often than not we are changing a variety of factors. Let me give you an example. People sometimes say, "Well, why don't you just put one group on a diet, and another on stress management, and a third on exercise, and compare them?" But that assumes that you are able to separate these factors. If you put a group of people on a diet, you are not just putting them on a diet, you are making them part of a group, and being part of a group is supportive in itself. You're giving them a

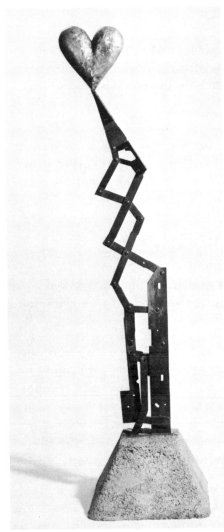

Jim Dine, *The Six Foot Heart Machine,* 1991

sense of meaning, a sense of empowerment, a sense of control over their lives—and that is very effective stress management.

From another perspective, sorting out all the variables doesn't really matter that much. As the old Amish proverb says, "When you're making vegetable soup, you don't ask whether the peas or the carrots are more important." We can say that, taken as a whole, our program causes certain measurable benefits. But if we try to separate what factors cause which benefits, we are on shakier ground.

MOYERS: Have your findings taught you anything new about the human mind?

ORNISH: What I have learned may not be new, but it is new to me. I began this work with a certain degree of skepticism. But what I am coming away with is an appreciation for how powerful the mind is in affecting our health, for better and for worse. As physicians, we can, deliberately or inadvertently, increase the negative effects of the mind on the body—but we can also use the mind to have a healing effect on the heart.

MOYERS: You told the people at this retreat to maintain a healthy skepticism.

ORNISH: I think a certain skepticism is by far the healthiest approach. You can have enough faith to say yes, this is worth trying—but don't believe it until you experience it for yourself. You know, seeing is believing, but in many ways our beliefs affect what is possible. Believing is seeing. If science can open the door by showing that these approaches have worked in other cases, then people might try what they otherwise would dismiss as too strange or too much of a bother. Then, when they begin to feel better, as most people do during the course of a week, the experience is taken out of the realm in which someone has to cajole them or convince them to do something. They find they have more energy, or less chest pain, or perhaps they begin to glimpse what it means to feel a sense of inner peace, or well-being, or perhaps their communication with their spouse or people in the group begins to improve. Those are the kinds of things they can carry home with them, which ultimately can be more meaningful to them than what we can show them with PET scans and angiograms.

MOYERS: Why did you begin this retreat with a talk on science?

ORNISH: Science opens the door to talking about other dimensions—such as the emotional, the psychosocial, or even the spiritual—that are more difficult to prove, but that, in some ways, are even more important. There's too much skepticism and too many biases against these nonscientific dimensions. In science we tend to believe what we measure, so if we can show cholesterol and blood pressure measurements, and pictures of arteries getting opened, and PET scans showing blood flow improving, then it makes it easier to talk about other issues we can't measure.

MOYERS: I can understand the effects of diet and exercise on the heart. But your program also includes meditation and group therapy. Do you think there is a scientific basis for the psychological aspects of what you do?

ORNISH: Up to a point. The technology for assessing heart disease is so advanced that we can measure the effects of the mind on the heart with greater precision than we can measure the effects in other areas. For example, if you put people under emotional stress, even just having them do mental arithmetic, you can use PET scans to measure decreased blood flow to the heart. Because heart disease is still so prevalent—it kills more Americans than all other diseases combined—it's a good model for looking at the effects of mind/body interventions not only on the heart, but, by extension, on many other illnesses as well.

MOYERS: The people I've talked to here are so desperate that they don't care how you help them, they just want you to do it, and they don't need to understand the scientific basis. How do you deal with that?

ORNISH: Well, I think that any time a person is in pain, there's an opportunity for transformation. As a doctor, I'm not really trained to take advantage of that but rather just to kill pain as quickly as I can, with drugs, with painkillers, or with surgery, if necessary. But within that pain is the opportunity to do something more than just killing the pain. In most cases, the pain is there for a reason, so simply dealing with the pain without addressing the underlying causes is a little like clipping the wires to a fire alarm while your house burns down, and then going back to sleep. In many ways, the physical chest pain, or angina, of heart disease is just the tip of the iceberg. There is emotional pain as well. So what we try to do here is to use that pain as a catalyst for transforming not only behaviors like diet and exercise and smoking, but the more fundamental issues that underlie those behaviors.

Telling people who feel depressed, disempowered, and isolated, and who don't like their lives, that they're going to live longer if they just stop smoking, or eat less meat, isn't always terribly motivating. Many people are more concerned with just getting through the day than with whether they'll live to be 85 instead of 84—unless they're 84. They often use alcohol, cigarettes, overeating, and overwork to cope with or split off these painful feelings. So unless we address the underlying emotional pain, isolation, and unhappiness that so many people carry around, it's very hard to motivate them to quit smoking or modify other behaviors, which are adaptive in the short run even though self-destructive in the long run.

When I was a medical student, the chief of pulmonary medicine smoked, and one of the chief cancer specialists smoked. It wasn't because they didn't know any better. Providing people with health information is important, but it's not usually enough to motivate lasting changes in behavior unless we also deal with the more fundamental issues that motivate us. Working at that level brings us to the psycho-social and even spiritual dimensions, and that's why I think it's so important to address those, as well as the behaviors. When people learn to experience inner peace—when we work on that level—then they are more likely to make and maintain life-style choices that are life-enhancing rather than self-destructive.

MOYERS: Do you find, nonetheless, that people respond better if they know more of the facts?

ORNISH: Oh, absolutely. It takes what we're doing out of the realm of California, mystical, warm, fuzzy, flaky, touchy-feely, and puts it into the realm of science. Showing people there's a rational basis for what we're advising them to do begins to motivate people to change. So that's where we begin.

MOYERS: But how can you be sure that it isn't the will to believe that is causing them to change their life-styles, and not the scientific facts?

ORNISH: As doctors, everything we do has a component of belief. We believe in the effectiveness of what we prescribe, whether it's drugs or surgery or life-style changes, or we wouldn't prescribe it. And we've known since medicine began that the doctor's belief in the effectiveness of the treatment plays a powerful role in motivating the patient's behavior. Likewise, the patient's own belief also plays an important role in the healing process. So, in a sense, you could say that everything we're doing here involves trying to change a person's belief system, to make people aware of new possibilities. You know, until Roger Bannister broke the four-minute mile, everybody thought it was impossible. Once one person did it, suddenly it became fairly routine for people to do that. In our culture, science determines the belief system. So we work within that high-tech system to prove how powerful these very low-tech, ancient interventions can be. People say, "Gee, so-and-so reversed his blockages, I've seen that in pictures of his PET scans and angiograms. Maybe I can do that." Then a whole new world opens up that helps make these changes in life-style possible.

MOYERS: Well, it's true that science is the motivating force for a lot of people, but religion is for others. Do you take that into account?

ORNISH: We work within a person's own religious or cultural belief system. So, for example, if we teach someone to meditate, we don't have everyone chanting in Sanskrit. If they're Catholic, they can meditate on a Hail Mary prayer, or use rosary beads. If they're Episcopalian, they can use "amen." If they're Jewish, they can use the word "shalom." If they're atheists, they can use the word "one." It doesn't really matter. Working within the belief system strengthens the order that it provides, and at the same time it expands the belief system to encompass new possibilities.

MOYERS: I know people who, for a couple of weeks after their heart attack, did everything the doctor said. Everything. They were scared to death—or scared away from death. But once they got back on their feet, and the world looked pretty normal again, they went right back to their old habits. How can you be sure these people won't do that? You're asking a lot of discipline from them.

ORNISH: Most health practitioners try to motivate people to change out of fear— you're going to be dead if you don't change; you're going to get a heart attack; you're a time bomb—all these terrible images. That doesn't work very well. My father is a dentist, and when I was in elementary school in Dallas, he used to come and show us these terrible pictures of tongue cancer. They were so horrible that after his talk, we would all make jokes and go out and have a cigarette. That taught me that trying to get people to change out of fear is not very effective. Although we know at some level that we may get sick and die, it is too terrifying to think about, and so we tend to deny it. For the first one or two weeks after someone's had a heart attack, you have their full attention. Then the denial begins, and you lose it. You know the old joke, that denial is not just a river in Egypt. I think there is some truth to that. Efforts to motivate people to change out of fear don't work very long.

So instead of motivating people through their fear of dying, we try to emphasize how these approaches can improve the joy of living. We're not talking about how to live longer, or how to avoid a heart attack, but how to improve the quality and joy within your life, right now. People who come here suffering with the chest pain of heart disease notice marked improvements in how they feel within a few days to a few weeks after making these changes. They have more energy, they need less sleep, and they can think more clearly. These changes motivate them to continue with their new life-style.

The paradox is that it is often easier to ask people to make big changes than small ones. That may not make sense at first. But if you make a moderate change in your diet, you have the inconvenience of being on a diet as well as a sense of deprivation from not being able to eat everything you want, and yet you don't really feel that much better. Whereas if you make comprehensive changes in diet and life-style, as we're doing here, you begin to feel so much better so quickly that the choices become clear, and you may say, "Yeah, I really like eating meat all the time, but I like the way I feel now so much better, that the choice not to eat meat is worth it to me." I grew up in Texas, eating chili and cheeseburgers and chalupas, just like you did, and I like the way that meat tastes, and I still do. But now that I don't eat meat all the time, I like how I feel so much better that for me it's a choice worth making. One of the patients in our study had severe chest pains whenever he tried to work, make love with his wife, or exercise. Now he can do all of these without pain. He said, "I like eating meat—but not *that* much."

Also, we work not just with the behaviors, but with the more fundamental issues that need to be addressed. Support sessions address the isolation and loneliness and loss of control that so many people feel. It's easier to make changes in life-style as a group and to support each other in those changes.

MOYERS: Is there a scientific basis for the idea that optimism makes a difference?

ORNISH: It's not so much optimism in the sense of telling jokes and making light of things. But I think there is a scientific basis to the idea that beliefs are powerful. If you believe that you have some control over your life, and that you have the ability to make choices instead of being the passive recipient of medical care, or the victim

of bad luck or bad genes, then you are more likely to make changes that are going to do you good in terms both of your behavior and of the direct effects of your mind on your body.

MOYERS: You're suggesting that medicine has a lot to learn from the social sciences.

ORNISH: I think we all have a lot to learn from each other. The problem is that so much of what we do is compartmental-

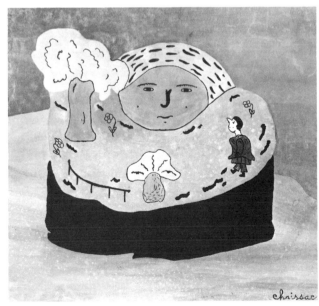

Gaston Chaissac,
Le Soleil se Lève, 1938

ized—for example, we have science on one hand and religion on the other. By definition, all of the separate, compartmentalized views are limited. But one view tends
to challenge the other view, and each sees the other as threatening. You know the
old story of the blind men and the elephant: one man has the leg, and so he thinks
the elephant is like a tree. The other is holding the trunk and insists that the elephant
is like a snake. We all have different parts of the elephant, and to the degree that we
can get together to find common ground, rather than trying to defend our point of
view and seeing all others as wrong, we can learn from each other.

MOYERS: And that's what mind/body medicine is trying to do.

ORNISH: Yes, in its best form. In its worst form, it also polarizes people by saying
that drugs and surgery are bad, and only mind/body interventions are good. They
both have their place. If somebody comes into the emergency room with crushing
chest pain, I don't teach them to meditate and feed them broccoli. I use whatever
drugs and surgery are needed to get that person through a life-threatening crisis.
But once the person is stabilized, you have their full attention. Then you can say,
"Mr. Jones," or "Ms. Smith, here is how you got into this situation. And here are
some new choices that can not only help keep your health from getting worse, but
maybe even cause it to improve." That's the kind of medicine that I find most exciting.

MOYERS: How do you think our health care system has to change in the future?

ORNISH: In many ways, the health care system is in the same crisis that patients
are in when they have a heart attack. I have heard that in Chinese, the same word
means both "crisis" and "opportunity." We are not really seeing the current health
care crisis as an opportunity.

MOYERS: By "crisis," are you referring to the expense and to all the people who
can't get access to good medical care?

ORNISH: Exactly. Our health care system involves a kind of rationing. People
don't even want to change their jobs because they're afraid they'll lose their medical
insurance, and if they don't have insurance, they know they'll lose access to health
care, or that health care costs might bankrupt them. Before health care costs were
so high, we didn't pay much attention to the health care system. But now even cor-
porations and insurance companies and the government are looking for alternatives.
We have a real window of opportunity to take a closer look at how powerful these
very low-cost and low-tech interventions can be.

MOYERS: Prevention.

ORNISH: Not only prevention, but even treatment. A bypass costs $30,000 to
$40,000. An angioplasty, $10,000—and that's without complications. Cholesterol-

lowering drugs can cost $1500 a year per person. You multiply those numbers by the 60 million Americans whose cholesterol levels are too high, and you're talking about billions of dollars every year. Last year alone, we spent 12 billion dollars on bypass surgery, even though we know that within five years, half of bypasses clog up and need to be redone. Within four to six months, 30 to 40 percent of the angioplastied arteries need to be redone—and we do four hundred thousand of those a year at a cost of four billion dollars. Now what I'm interested in studying is whether approaches like the ones we use here can be not only medically effective, but also cost effective. You don't need any special equipment. You don't need an exercise machine—we're talking about walking. You need maybe a mat to do stretching and a chair to do meditation in. This diet costs less than a conventional American diet, because meat is really the most expensive part of most people's diet.

Another opportunity in this low-cost approach is for minorities and lower socioeconomic groups and women, the only groups in our country for whom heart disease is increasing rather than declining. These are the people with the least access to drugs and surgery. Ninety-one percent of the bypass surgery last year was done on white males, generally upper-middle-class males, even though heart disease affects as many women as men. So the people who can least afford conventional medical care are the ones who can benefit most by making life-style changes.

MOYERS: So in your model of the emerging health care system, patients are much more involved in their own health.

ORNISH: Absolutely. So much of what I am trained to do as a doctor puts patients in the position of being the passive recipients of health care. They're not really doing things for themselves, we're just doing things *to* them. Instead, we could give people choices that would empower them. Knowing what we now know, if we could put into widespread practice the kinds of life-style changes that we're talking about, I think 95 percent of heart disease could be prevented. But life-style changes can happen only through the patient; they can't be done to the patient.

MOYERS: But Americans buy quickly into something that works. If your program of life-style change is as good as it sounds, wouldn't more of us be doing it?

ORNISH: More and more of us are—but it's also part of American culture that we like a quick fix. We want fast, fast, fast relief, even though it may be only temporary relief, and we want it conveniently. Now if you can really change your life-style sufficiently, you can get fast relief from the chest pain of heart disease. But that requires more fundamental change than many people are willing to do. It's stressful at first to change your life-style. So I don't have any illusions that what we're doing is going to change the world. I'm not really interested in changing the world. I'm just focusing on trying to change myself, because I struggle with these same issues, too. I've made a few steps along that path, and it's made a big difference in my life,

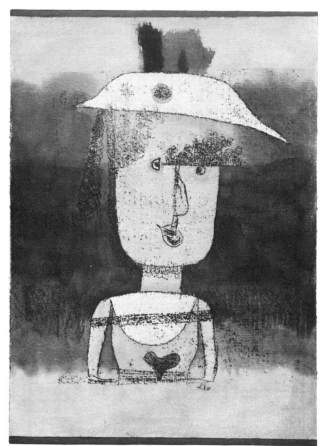

Paul Klee, *Portrait of Mme. P. in the South,* 1924

and so I'm just trying to share that with other people, and maybe it will help them, too.

MOYERS: I noticed that many of the people in the group here are middle-aged and older, and it made me think that we wait a long time, we Americans, until it's almost too late, to change our behavior.

ORNISH: If we can begin making these changes earlier in life, they can improve the quality of life that we experience, and the changes can be more moderate. On the other hand, it is never too late to begin making these changes. The oldest patient in our study, who is 77, showed the most improvement. You know, it is not about living longer, it is about living better. As I said earlier, it is not about trying to get people to change out of the fear of dying, it is showing people how they can increase the joy of living. And if you live longer, as you probably will, that's nice, too. But that's not really the reason for doing it. There's no reason to give up something I enjoy unless I get something back that's even better. But I find that when I give up certain things that I might like, like cheeseburgers, for example, I feel so much better, those choices are worth it. So it really becomes more a question of educating people, of showing them how they have new choices, new hope, and new opportunities that maybe we didn't know about before.

MOYERS: Exactly what is it you want people to do?

ORNISH: What has helped me the most, and what might help other people, is dealing with the cause of the problem. Now that is a simple idea, and some would say even a simplistic idea, but it has had a profound effect on my thinking in the area of heart disease. The farther back we go in the causal chain of events, the more powerful the healing.

And I think that's true on a social level as well. We don't always address our social problems by dealing with what causes them. For example, take the rise in street gangs. Why do we have so many street gangs now? Perhaps we do because street gangs fulfill the need for intimacy that people have. These young men don't get it from their families. In fact, they're often people from broken homes. But you can go into a gang, and suddenly, you're part of a community. So the community can be one based on heart disease, or it can be based on selling drugs—but we can find ways to channel these natural and ultimately healthy impulses we have to form communities, so that we can deal with the underlying issues instead of bypassing or ignoring them. And we can use the pain, whether it's the chest pain of heart disease, or the cultural pain of our society. We can begin to ask questions about how we got into these positions and what we can do to address the issues at a more fundamental level.

MOYERS: It's curious, isn't it, that we form our communities today around illness. Watching the people arrive here on the first weekend of your retreat, I saw these tired, frightened victims of heart disease at first reluctantly, and then rather joyously, make connections with each other and begin to talk about their illnesses. And I saw emerging there, in the relationships between these strangers, an intimacy that occurred quite rapidly. And I thought, they're being brought together by disease, and they're finding each other through pain.

ORNISH: That's beautifully said. Everybody is capable of intimacy, but many of us don't know how to go about getting it. What our culture tells us through advertising, which is a very powerful medium for communicating ideas, is that if you'll just buy this product, suddenly you'll be okay, you'll be happy, and people will like you. A beautiful woman or a beautiful man always appears in the ad to imply that what they represent comes along with the package. The fundamental problem is not that people have negative emotions but that they experience a sense of emptiness, a void.

MOYERS: People with heart attacks tell you this?

ORNISH: Oh, yes, and they will tell you that, too, if you ask them.

MOYERS: Well, I've asked them here, and they've told me, "I was eating too much red meat," or "I was working too hard, I was traveling all the time to the Far East, selling my products, buying products, going to too many dinners." One man told me he had gone to 110 business dinners last year. He didn't say, "I have a void at the center."

ORNISH: Hard work doesn't give people heart attacks. That's a myth. What we need to look at is what motivates people to work harder than they might want to. Hard work itself can be good for you. I'm not telling people they shouldn't work. But sometimes people think, "If only I can make a certain amount of money," or "If only I can get this promotion," or "If only I can get this acknowledgment, or this award"—whatever it happens to be—"then I'll be okay, then I'll feel good about myself, then people will love and respect me, then I won't feel so isolated." Those motivations are what cause the stress, which in turn can lead to illnesses like heart disease. There's an old Zen saying: "Before enlightenment, chop wood, carry water. After enlightenment, chop wood, carry water." In other words, you may do the same job, but for different reasons. It's not really what we do that leads to chronic stress and to illnesses like heart disease, it's what motivates what we do—the misbelief that somehow, something external to us is going to bring us health, and peace, and intimacy, and love.

MOYERS: You are suggesting, then, that everybody who has heart disease has a psychological problem.

ORNISH: Psychological problems are a lot more common than we think. That is not to discount the role of cholesterol, and smoking, and lack of exercise, all of which we also address here. But I don't think that's the whole story.

MOYERS: If I have a psychological problem, it's my fault, then, isn't it? Aren't you going to make me feel guilty about my illness?

ORNISH: That is one way to look at it, although I try not to do that. The flip side to that is to say that you have nothing to do with it at all, and that you're just a victim of fate, or bad genes, or bad luck. If you're just a helpless victim, there's not much you can do about your condition. But to the degree that your behaviors and attitudes are contributing to the problem, you can do something about it—and that is empowering.

We don't tell people, "Hey, you have a psychological problem, and you need to do something about it." We try to educate them by saying, "There are patterns in life that can contribute to heart disease: what we eat, how we respond to stress, whether we smoke, whether we exercise, and so on. There are things you can do in all these areas, and if you do, there's a chance you may get better." But even then, there are no guarantees. Even Mother Teresa got heart disease. So it's not that if you just are loving enough, somehow you'll never get a heart attack. There are other factors, too, but those factors alone don't account for heart disease. Taking into account cholesterol, blood pressure, smoking, genetics, and all of the other known risk factors still explains only about half of the heart disease we see. Clearly, something else is going on. My clinical experience, as well as what we're showing in our research, suggests that psychological, emotional, and even spiritual factors are important, not only in terms of how they affect our behaviors, like diet and exercise, but also in more direct ways.

MOYERS: Well, I understand that, but if more faith, hope, and love is the answer, which is sometimes what I think you're counseling, Mother Teresa would not have gotten heart disease.

ORNISH: I don't think faith, hope, and love are the whole story, nor even a major part of the story. What we're really talking about is a sense of intimacy and community. Now, there are also factors that go beyond what we know. You could change your life-style, and do everything right and perfectly, and you might still get heart disease. So we monitor patients carefully to make sure they are stable or improving.

MOYERS: Some doctors say it's just a matter of genes.

ORNISH: Genes are important, but even if your father, mother, sister, and brother all died of heart disease, that doesn't mean you need to. What it probably means is that you might need to make bigger changes in your diet and life-style than someone else might. But in our study we're clearly looking at very sick people who all have bad genes in that sense—and still, 82 percent of them showed overall reversal of heart disease. Only one patient got clearly worse, and his adherence to the program was minimal.

MOYERS: If people meditate, and participate in a group, and share their feelings, is it all right for them to have a cholesterol count of 250?

ORNISH: I don't know the answer to that. When I began doing this work I would have said no, that you would have to get everyone's cholesterol down below 200 to get reversal. But our data don't really support that idea. We are finding that if people change their life-styles sufficiently in the ways that we have talked about, they tend to show reversal even if their blood cholesterol levels don't get down below some arbitrary number. There was a direct relation between the amount they changed, and what happened in their arteries, but that was much more clearly correlated than their cholesterol levels. I am not suggesting that cholesterol is unimportant, just that these other factors may override the effect of cholesterol alone.

MOYERS: So much of what you're talking about is in the realm of religion. On the other hand, you also come back to cholesterol count and other medical considerations. Is there a new science of healing we're talking about?

ORNISH: Yes, I think there is. Thomas Kuhn's *The Structure of Scientific Revolutions* points out that humans have a hard time dealing with a universe that is infinitely complex and vast, and so we try to reduce it to more manageable proportions. We come up with theories, or structures, or views of the world, which he calls paradigms, to describe the way that the universe is. For a thousand years the Catholic Church provided the predominant paradigm in Western culture: that the earth is the center of the universe, and everything revolves around it. In the sixteenth century, an Italian philosopher named Bruno came along, and said, "Well, I don't know if that is true. I think maybe the earth revolves around the sun." People responded in the way that people often do when their worldview is challenged, and they burned him at the stake. A hundred years later Galileo came along and said the same thing, and added evidence from his telescope so that people could see for themselves that things were not the way they had thought. Eventually, the Spanish Inquisition and the Church forced Galileo to recant, but by then it was too late, because he had given people a tool to see for themselves that there were anomalies, that things didn't quite fit within the worldview that had been provided up to that point.

And so, in a way, science became the dominant worldview. If we can't measure it, it doesn't exist, and it's not real. But like the telescope, new tools are beginning to show us anomalies in our worldview. To me the anomalies are the most interesting part. But they can also be viewed as threatening. More often than not, people want to suppress that information, or they want to discredit it, or they want to kill the messenger, so to speak.

MOYERS: Is there a new model or worldview emerging?

ORNISH: You find different models emerging now. You find the holistic health model, or the religious model, or the so-called scientific model. But none of those models really gives us a complete picture. They're all powerful, and they all have their uses, but they also, by definition, all have their limitations.

What I find most interesting is to try to synthesize different models, and to find what works and what doesn't. When I speak at a major scientific meeting, I might talk about the power of yoga and meditation. But then I might find myself at a holistic health meeting, as I was recently, talking about the power of drugs and surgery. One woman said, "I have a rapidly growing breast mass, what should I do?" And they said, "Oh, you should meditate, and take herbs, and fast." I said, "No, you need a surgeon who can do a biopsy to find out what's going on." They booed me. So I never quite fit in anywhere, which is part of the problem when you're trying to synthesize different worldviews.

MOYERS: Give me a working definition, as you see it, of mind/body medicine.

ORNISH: That's a tough question, because mind/body medicine encompasses so many different things. To me, it has to do with healing that treats the body not only as though it were a machine but also takes into account that the mind has an influence on the body, for better or for worse. In a way, mind/body medicine is a kind of misnomer because this kind of healing goes beyond mind and body to some of the psychosocial and even spiritual dimensions.

MOYERS: Psychosocial?

ORNISH: Psychosocial has to do with the context for healing. An individual does not exist in isolation from everyone and everything else, but exists in the context of a community, family, workplace, religion, and so on.

MOYERS: You called mind/body medicine "an ancient intervention." What do you mean?

ORNISH: These techniques have been around for thousands of years in one form or another. You find them in every culture, every religion, and every group of people. Sometimes they are a little hidden below the surface, buried in ritual, or they go by different names. But the essence of those techniques is what I find most interesting.

MOYERS: And what is the essence?

ORNISH: The essence consists of tools for quieting the mind and body, and also focusing it. When the mind quiets down, an individual can begin to experience more of an inner sense of peace, contentment, and well-being—health, if you will.

MOYERS: Just exactly what is the mind? When you talk about your body, I can see it there, sitting in front of me. When you move your body, I see what you're moving. But when you're talking about your mind, what are you talking about?

ORNISH: Philosophers have wrestled for centuries with the question of whether the brain and the mind are the same thing. I tend to view the mind as one's consciousness, what defines us as separate people. The brain is simply the organ that processes that. But we're more than just a collection of neurons and synapses. I think that consciousness really goes beyond that.

MOYERS: In your lecture you referred to consciousness as another form of energy.

ORNISH: I think, ultimately, everything is a different form of energy. Even matter that seems solid as a rock is energy. We know from Einstein that energy and matter are interconvertible. Now, what I find interesting is that when you can focus energy, you gain more power, for better and for worse. For example, if your mind is focused, then its effect on the body becomes enhanced, also for better and for worse. Unfortunately, in our culture we tend to have our minds most focused when we're angry, upset, afraid, or worried. You know, someone once said that anger wonderfully concentrates the mind. That's really true, but that form of concentration can have a negative effect. Your heart rate goes up, your blood pressure goes up, the arteries in your heart may begin to constrict, and the blood may clot. But we can use that same principle in a healing direction rather than in a harmful one by learning to concentrate mental energy.

I am coming to believe that anything that promotes isolation leads to chronic stress and, in turn, may lead to illnesses like heart disease. Anything that promotes a sense of intimacy, community, and connection can be healing. Most of us have had moments when we felt as if we were part of something larger than ourselves. Some describe this in a religious context as "God," and others in a more secular context as "consciousness." On one level, of course, we are separate: you're you, and I'm me. But on another level we are part of something larger. Sometimes people describe this as the light behind the images projected in a movie theater. The ancient yogis and swamis and priests and rabbis didn't develop yoga, meditation, and prayer just

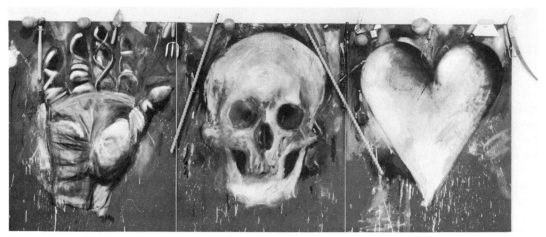

Jim Dine, *The Room in Blue,* 1985

to lower cholesterol or blood pressure or to unclog arteries; these are tools for transformation, for giving people the direct experience of this consciousness.

MOYERS: Is stress the primary condition that mind/body alternatives address?

ORNISH: It depends on how you define stress. We tend to think that we have a choice between being productive in an interesting but stressful world, or retiring to sit under a tree and watch our life go by. Maybe we live longer—or maybe we're so bored that it seems as if we're living longer. But that really isn't the choice, because stress comes not simply from what we do, but, more important, from how we react to what we do. So then you could ask, "Why do we react in ways that are stressful?" It's not because the world is suddenly a more stressful place than it once was. People tend to think about modern culture as somehow more stressful because we have fax machines and cellular phones, and because modern life is so much more fast-paced. But our ancestors had to wonder whether the crops were going to come in, or whether their children were going to die of polio before they reached the age of thirteen. Clearly, that has to be as stressful as whether the fax has come in on time.

But something has changed. What is different now is that cultural isolation is so pervasive in our culture. We used to have extended families, and at the church or synagogue or workplace or in the neighborhood we felt a sense of safety and community. We often don't have that now. Two-parent households are the exceptions rather than the rule. There aren't many places where people can feel safe enough just to be who they are without having to create a mask or a facade to experience the intimacy and the community that we are all looking for.

MOYERS: Is that why you decided to make group therapy part of your program?

ORNISH: It's not group therapy in the usual psychiatric sense. We are not trying to work on people's childhood issues and psychodynamics and so on. It began as a support group to help people stay on the diet, to encourage the exchange of recipes, to share shopping tips, and so on. But it evolved into something else: we created a community. I have had the rare opportunity of working with the same relatively small group of people very intensively over several years. As a result, we have gotten to know each other very well, and I have gained some insights that I might not otherwise have had the chance to do. One of them has to do with how important it is to address these deeper issues of isolation and loneliness. There is a real yearning for community in our culture. I think that is one of the reasons you see so many different types of support groups, such as AA, Overeaters Anonymous, or our cardiac support group. It's too bad that in our culture you often have to have an illness or an addiction before you can become part of a community. But if you talk with people, the community really helps keep them on a program like this—because it fulfills that deeper need.

MOYERS: Researchers have told me that participating in a group and sharing feelings is good not just for the person who's doing the sharing, but also for the other people taking part. In a way, it's a gift. There's something that happens in a group that is healing.

ORNISH: That's true. The root of the word "heal" is "to make whole," to bring together. And that bringing together is what many of us, to one degree or another, are looking for. As an individual rather than as a scientist or educator, what I find most interesting about doing this work is how the pain of having a heart attack, and being depressed, can be a catalyst not only for transforming behaviors like diet and exercise, but also for becoming aware of the more fundamental issues that underlie those behaviors.

MOYERS: But science doesn't tell us how to deal with these other issues, does it?

ORNISH: Well, we're learning. A number of studies have shown that people who feel isolated have three to five times the mortality, not only from cardiovascular disease, but from all causes, when compared to people who don't feel isolated. What is also interesting is that this mortality rate is usually independent of their blood cholesterol level, their blood pressure, and even whether or not they smoke. Now those are powerful figures, especially when contrasted to studies of cholesterol-lowering drugs, or antihypertension drugs, which tend not to change overall mortality, and all of which have side effects. So if we don't deal with the cause of the problem, all too often we end up substituting one set of problems for another without changing the overall picture.

It may seem hard for people to believe that such simple ideas as sharing feelings or eating a low fat vegetarian diet or doing meditation or walking could have such powerful effects, but they seem to do that. It is especially hard for people in this culture to believe, because we tend to think of a breakthrough in medicine as being something like a new surgical technique or a new drug. We have a hard time believing that these simple, ancient, inexpensive approaches can be so powerful. But we're finding that they often are.

MOYERS: What do you say to the individual who is constitutionally unable to accept the intimacy involved in being part of a group? I've seen people who are frightened and simply find it impossible to take part in a group.

ORNISH: Most people, including me, are frightened to take part in a group. It is not easy to talk about your feelings, to share yourself, and to let walls down. At some time or another, most of us have been betrayed and hurt very badly, and we have learned to build defenses, which, at some stage of our life, were essential to our survival. And sharing your feelings with a group doesn't mean that the walls and defenses should never be there. If you are going for a job interview, you don't want to start talking about your demons and your inner secrets.

MOYERS: My father had a hard time sharing his feelings with a group. What would you say to someone like him, or to someone who thinks that what you're doing is the kind of touchy-feely encounter group associated with the sixties?

ORNISH: We are not replicating encounter groups. We're not asking people to say whatever comes to their mind, or to yell and scream at each other, and get out their feelings that way. What we're trying to do is to create a place that feels safe enough for people to let down their defenses and share more of who they really are and not be socially isolated. The same walls and defenses that protect us can also profoundly isolate us if the walls are always up, if we have no one or nowhere that feels safe enough to let them down.

MOYERS: I'm not sure I grasp what you mean by socially isolated, because in talking to some of your patients, I didn't find any of them who led socially isolated lives. There's a cardiologist with a busy practice, and an export-importer who travels often to Asia, and most of the others are at the center of institutions or businesses. They're not socially isolated.

ORNISH: There's a difference between aloneness and loneliness. You can be alone by choice, and not feel isolated. You can be the head of a large company, you can be the center of your world, and still feel very isolated. By isolation I mean not feeling a real sense of intimate connection with other people. Many people with a lot of friends and family will say to themselves, "There are parts of me that no one really knows—and if they did know, then they'd be out of here, they'd leave me." To a degree, we all put our best foot forward, and we create facades, some more than others.

One of my patients pretended to be very successful and wealthy and drove an expensive car and wore two-thousand-dollar suits. And yet, after a period of time, he was able to confide in the group that he had been bankrupt for years. No one else really knew that. Another patient pretended to be heterosexual, but he was gay, and he was afraid that if he told people in the group, they would reject him. After a time, he said, "I appreciate the fact that you all like me, but there's something you need to know. I'm gay." Someone else then said, "Well, you know, I used to beat up gay people for fun." Now, that's not something he went around telling people. The group provided a safe place for them to learn to love the ways they were similar and to respect their differences.

You see, people who make this leap find their lives transformed in ways that go beyond just opening the arteries. Of course, we can view illness as a mechanical problem that needs to be fixed. If I break my leg, I want a good orthopedic surgeon to fix it. In some ways, even heart disease is a mechanical problem that needs to be fixed. But it's also more than that. There is an emotional heart disease, if you will, and there is a spiritual heart disease, if you will. And Susan Sontag notwithstanding, there is a metaphorical basis to heart disease. It's not just because we don't know enough about it to understand the physical basis, as she might say. In fact, the more we learn about it, the more we see how multilayered it is.

MOYERS: Are you talking about emotional heart surgery?

ORNISH: Well, you could say it's a different kind of open heart surgery. We are asking people to open their heart in ways that go beyond just splitting open their chest.

MOYERS: People are going to say, "Yeah, that's where he gets off science and into psychology."

ORNISH: Well, that may be true. But I am not sure that science and psychology are mutually exclusive. It is true, though, that if I give a lecture, some cardiologists will say, "Your lecture was really good until you got to all the touchy-feely stuff." And I have noticed that if I tell a joke or show a funny slide in my lecture, most people will laugh, except the physicians. I think, on the whole, we doctors are a very depressed group of people. We have one of the highest rates of drug addiction and suicide of any professional group. A recent survey revealed that a majority of physicians would not recommend medicine as a career for their sons or daughters. Practicing medicine is not much fun if you only write prescriptions and don't have the time to get to know your patients.

I got interested in this work out of my own depression, when I was a freshman in college and doing very well, but feeling that somehow I was merely pretending to be a smart person. And now that I was in a school where there were a lot of smart people, it was just a question of time before they found out how stupid I really was, and then they would reject me, and I would be all alone. Of course, then, I would never get into medical school, I would never fulfill my dream of being a doctor, I'd be a loser, I'd be isolated, and life wouldn't be worth living.

But then I had a spiritual revelation—or crisis, depending on how you want to look at it—where I realized that even if I got into medical school, and even if I got all the things that I had been taught would bring me a sense of happiness and peace and well-being and love, and even if I got fame and fortune, it really would not bring me the sense of intimacy that I think, ultimately, all of us are really yearning for. I became so depressed, I came very close to committing suicide. Surviving that experience taught me things that I probably would not have learned any other way, although I don't recommend it as a learning tool. But the point is that many people who suffer heart disease are going through that same process.

MOYERS: Did you turn to diet, meditation, and exercise?

ORNISH: Well, as it turned out, I did. My older sister, who was a college student at the time, was studying yoga with Swami Satchidananda. My parents decided that yoga had

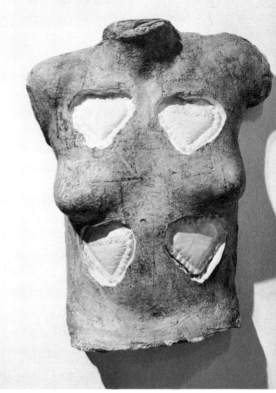

Irina Nakova, untitled, 1992

helped her, and they wanted to support her interest in it, so when the swami came to Dallas, they decided to have a cocktail party for him. This was 1971, in North Dallas—I guess, being from Texas, you can appreciate what that would be like. The swami gave a lecture in our living room which began with the statement, "Nothing can bring you lasting happiness and inner peace." Well, I had figured that out already, and I was miserable. But he went on to say something which for many people now may sound like a New Age cliché, but which, at the time, turned my life around. He said, "Nothing can bring you lasting happiness and inner peace—but you have it already if you just quiet down your mind and body enough to experience it."

The irony here is that when we are not aware of that truth—as I certainly wasn't—we end up running after things that we think will bring us peace, like getting into medical school. In the process, we end up disturbing our inner sense of peace and contentment.

Now, you can find that idea in all cultures, in one form or another. For me, it happened to come in this particular form. So I decided that I would try it, and I could always kill myself if it didn't work. I began eating a vegetarian diet. I began doing yoga, and meditation, and exercise, and got glimpses of what it meant to feel at peace, and to realize that it came not from doing but from undoing. When we work the with heart patients in our study, at the end of a yoga class or a meditation, when they feel that same sense of peace and well-being, we point out that their sense of peace didn't come from getting something they were lacking, but, rather, that they simply quieted down enough to experience what they already have.

That may seem like a simple idea, but it has powerful implications. I still make the same mistakes. I think, "Oh, gee, if only I can write a best-selling book, or if only Bill Moyers would interview me, you know, then I'll be okay, and then I can relax and be happy." When that happens, I start to get anxious and stressed. If I had heart disease, which I don't, maybe I would get some chest pain. But I could use that pain as a teacher, reminding me that I am looking in the wrong places, instead of seeing it as some kind of punishment or bad genes or bad fate or bad luck. I can make other choices.

MOYERS: But by sharing your weakness, you've acknowledged a strength which, perversely, your critics use against you. Critics say, "Dean Ornish does really good work, but only because he's such a good therapist. What he does won't work anywhere else because we can't clone him."

ORNISH: While I listen to critics and try to learn from them, they don't bother me as much as they used to. People have power over you only to the degree that you think you need something from them. If you are more inwardly defined, then you need less, because you are empowered from within. It's a kind of paradox. You have worked a lot with presidents and very powerful public figures, so you've observed people who are often acutely aware of what other people think of them, and in many ways lose a lot of their power and peace because of that. Doing this work helps me learn who I am. I want to do my best to help people and to enjoy my own life.

When I first began planning this study, we had a great deal of difficulty getting funding from the National Institutes of Health or the American Heart Association or major foundations, because they said, "It is impossible to reverse heart disease. And even if you could, you would have to use drugs, and a year is not long enough, and no one can change their life-style anyway and stick with it." So I would respond, "Well, let's find out. That is what science is all about." And they would answer back, "No, we know it can't be done, so we won't even bother."

So we raised our original funds from some Texas developers like Gerald Hines and bankers and energy companies and airlines—just wherever we could. It was an unusual way to go about doing a study, but we were in a catch-22 situation. Nobody would give us the funding until we proved it could be done; and until we got the funding, we couldn't do that. So we raised the money as we went along.

Now we have demonstrated that we had only one dropout from our study even though our subjects were people who were recruited at the hospital because they had just had an angiogram, not because they were terribly interested in our approach. And we showed that many people will make and maintain these changes, and that if they do, they often show some degree of reversal of their arterial blockages.

So now some critics may say, "Okay, we'll agree that heart disease can be reversed—but only your patients would do this kind of program. Ours wouldn't do it." The reason I wrote *Reversing Heart Disease* was to make this approach generally available to people. I have letters from people all over the world who have done it just on the basis of reading the book. My favorite is from a man from China, who addressed his letter, "Dear Onions." How he got a copy of the book I don't even know. One of the people here today, on the basis of reading the book, did it on his own, and his thallium scan showed a 50 percent improvement. And I have many calls and letters from physicians and other health professionals who are using my book with their patients and finding similar results. They find working with their patients in this way to be extraordinarily gratifying for both them and their patients.

MOYERS: So people out there can do this themselves?

ORNISH: Some can. It is not for everyone. But more people are willing to make these changes than we might think. The reason many doctors don't offer it to their patients is that first, it is easier just to write a prescription. And second, we don't get reimbursed for it. If I were qualified to do bypass surgery, the insurance company would pay $30,000 or $40,000 without blinking. If I did an angioplasty, it would be $10,000 dollars. If I wrote a prescription for cholesterol-lowering drugs, they may cost $1500 a year, but the insurance company pays for most of that. But if I tell a heart patient, "I want to teach you how to change

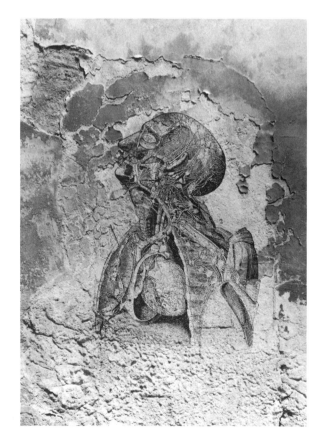

Doug Prince, untitled, 1991

your life-style," maybe they will pay me $50. And if you don't yet have an illness, and I want to try to keep you healthy, the insurance company won't pay anything at all.

The insurance industry is really the major determinant of health care in this country—not science and not clinical experience, but what third party will pay for. Now, I think that is going to change, especially in the area of cardiovascular disease, because health care costs have gotten so high that people are looking at alternatives. But most of the alternatives that they are looking at don't really deal with the fundamental question of why people get heart disease in the first place, or why we get sick. So we just end up with a different kind of health care rationing, no matter what we call it.

MOYERS: What do you mean by "health care rationing"?

ORNISH: The current health care system, which is really a disease care system, has de facto rationing: if you don't have insurance or a lot of money, you don't get very good access to medical care. If we adopted the Canadian or British national health insurance type of system, we still wouldn't have the resources to do bypass surgery or angioplasty on everyone. And so we would end up just substituting one kind of rationing for another.

Now, if it could be shown that for every dollar you spend on life-style changes, you would save three or four or five in health care costs, we might begin to have viable alternatives to our rationed health care system. There is a real window of opportunity now because the easy answers to the medical cost crisis have not worked. Shortening hospital stays has not done very much, and shifting to outpatient surgery really has not slowed the escalation in costs, and whereas in the past, insurance companies would just pass along the premiums, these premiums are now so high that people are rebelling. Many companies are becoming self-insured and are not using the carriers.

MOYERS: Some people say that gene therapy, not life-style changes, will make the most difference to the health of the next century.

ORNISH: Gene therapy will play an important role, just as drugs have played an important role in this century, but I don't think that's the answer because it, too, doesn't really address the more fundamental issues. It is more fundamental than what we are doing so far, but when you start tinkering around with a genome, you never quite know what you are going to end up with. That seems to be our basic pattern—to get a quick fix, we will try to do anything, and yet, at the same time, we will avoid looking at our own behaviors and at what underlies these behaviors. But if we want the most powerful healing, we will have to begin addressing the deeper issues.

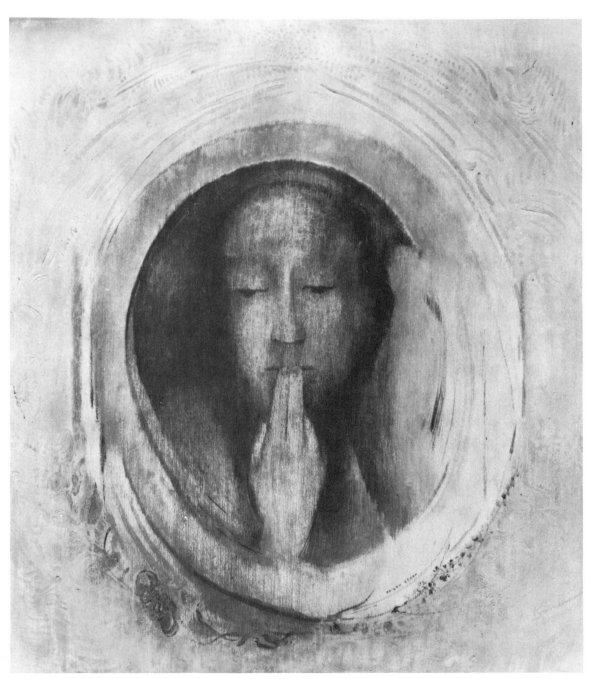

Odilon Redon, *Silence,* 1911

MEDITATION

Jon Kabat-Zinn

Jon Kabat-Zinn, Ph.D., is founder and Director of the Stress Reduction Clinic at the University of Massachusetts Medical Center and Associate Professor of Medicine in the Division of Preventative and Behavioral Medicine at the University of Massachusetts Medical School. Internationally known for his work using mindfulness meditation to help medical patients suffering from chronic pain and stress-related medical disorders, Dr. Kabat-Zinn is the author of *Full Catastrophe Living: Using the Wisdom of Your Body and Mind to Face Stress, Pain, and Illness.*

MOYERS: How do your new patients react when you begin to talk with them about meditation?

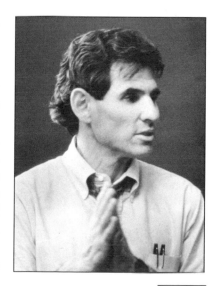

KABAT-ZINN: One of the questions we had to answer right from the beginning was: would this be so weird that nobody would be interested in doing it? People might say, "What are you talking about? Meditation? Yoga? Give me a break!" Meditation had never been tried before in a medical center, so we had no idea whether mainstream Americans would accept a clinic whose foundation was intensive training in meditative disciplines. Doctors refer patients to us for all sorts of very real problems. These people are not at all interested in meditation, or yoga, or swamis, or gurus, or Zen masters, or enlightenment. They're suffering, and they come because they want some relief from their suffering, and they want to reduce their stress. But we discovered that people take to our program like ducks to water. One reason is that it's completely demystified. It's not anything exotic. Meditation just has to do with paying attention in a particular way. That's something we're all capable of doing.

MOYERS: I wonder if it would have been as successful if you'd called it "Courses in Meditation" instead of "Stress Reduction Clinic."

KABAT-ZINN: Oh, I can guarantee you that it wouldn't have been. Who would have wanted to go to a meditation class? But when people walk down the halls in this hospital, and they see signs saying "Stress Reduction and Relaxation," they respond, "Ah, I could use that." Then doing meditation and yoga in the stress reduction clinic seems to make sense to people because we're trying to penetrate to the core of what it means to work with the agitated mind by going into deep states of relaxation.

MOYERS: That makes me wonder whether you may have tapped into the power of the placebo here. People think it will work for them, so they feel better even though they're not sure what is happening.

KABAT-ZINN: Why not? I'll take transformational change any way it comes. One way to look at meditation is as a kind of intrapsychic technology that's been developed over a couple of thousand years by traditions that know a lot about the mind/body connection. To call what happens "the placebo effect" is just to give a name to something we don't understand. If people have very strong expectations that something might happen, that expectation itself might be useful to them. We're going to ask people to do a lot of hard work, so we hope they will start out with a positive attitude even if that might be thought of as a placebo. But actually, very often people start out with more of a negative attitude. We ask them just to try to suspend judgment and not to become either true believers or skeptics so hard to convince that they can't listen to their own breathing or observe their own minds.

MOYERS: What do your hard-nosed colleagues, the cardiologists and brain surgeons, for example, think of you and this little crowd down here in the corner?

KABAT-ZINN: We get patients from all of them, and many of them come themselves. You know, when you identify too strongly with your discipline, you can often forget your humanness. Here we focus on who you are as a human being, and never mind what coat or hat you're wearing. I think that my hard-nosed colleagues, if you care to call them that, feel that the proof is in the pudding, and that what we really need to do is to study this stuff a lot more in as effective a way as we can. Our contribution is just one small brick in a wall that's being built by lots of people all around the world who have become newly interested in this very old perspective—that the mind and body are actually different sides of the same coin.

MOYERS: It goes all the way back to Hippocrates.

KABAT-ZINN: Yes, it goes all the way back to the origins of medicine. For most of its history, the practice of medicine was not separated from other aspects of human activity.

MOYERS: Is that why you begin with something as common and simple as eating a raisin?

KABAT-ZINN: Yes. The point of that is to respond to all the baggage people carry about what meditation is. We want to dispel those notions right away. So we say, "Look, the first meditation exercise we'll do isn't breathing, it isn't sitting in the full lotus posture and pretending you're in a fine arts museum, or standing on your head, or some weird thing. We're just going to eat a raisin—but to eat that raisin mindfully, with awareness." You look at the raisin, feel it, smell it, and with awareness bring it to the mouth gradually, and see that the saliva starts to get secreted by the salivary glands just as you bring it up. Then you take the raisin into the mouth, and you begin to taste this thing that we usually eat automatically.

MOYERS: And usually a handful at a time.

KABAT-ZINN: Yes, and you're on to the next handful before you've finished chewing this one. In this exercise, people realize, "My goodness, I never taste raisins. I'm so busy eating them that I don't actually taste them." From there, it's a very short jump to realize that you may actually not be in touch with many of the moments of your life, because you're so busy rushing someplace else that you aren't in the present moment. Your life is the sum of your present moments, so if you're missing lots of them, you may actually miss much of your children's infancy and youth, or beautiful sunsets, or the beauty of your own body. You may be tuning out all sorts of inner and outer experiences simply because you're too preoccupied with where you want to get, what you want to have happen, and what you don't want to happen. From the meditative perspective, the normal mind state is considered to be extremely suboptimal.

MOYERS: So in giving them the raisin, you're giving the mind one thing to keep track of.

KABAT-ZINN: Yes, although when you look at eating, it turns out to involve lots of different things: there's the chewing, the tasting, the functioning of the tongue—but it all has to do with concentrating on the experience of eating in the present moment.

MOYERS: And do you bring people back to their breathing for the same reason—just to give the mind one thing to concentrate on?

KABAT-ZINN: Yes, exactly. Once we do the raisin exercise, people begin to realize that there's nothing magical about mindfulness. When you're eating, for example, just eat. Be completely with the eating and the tasting.

Now most of us do a lot of different things at the same time when we're eating. There's eating and reading the newspaper. There's eating and having a conversation. There's eating and watching television. And sometimes there's eating so fast that you're out of touch with it completely. Slowing it down and really tasting helps bring you into the present moment.

Then we transfer mindfulness from eating to the breath and say, "Now, taste your breath in the same way." We use the word "taste" because we usually don't think about the breath, just as we usually don't think about how our food tastes. Some people say, "You're telling me to pay attention to my breathing, but why should I? It's so uninteresting." And I say, "Well, if it's so uninteresting to you, try this experiment: clamp your thumb and forefinger over your nose like this, and keep your lips closed. Then see how long it takes for breathing to become really interesting." It turns out it's not very long.

We don't appreciate some of the things that are most valuable and rich in our lives. Breathing is central to every aspect of meditation training. It's a wonderful place to focus in training the mind to be calm and concentrated. As we experience the flow of the breath, the same reaction often comes up in relation to breathing as came up when we ate a raisin with mindfulness: "Wow, I didn't realize a breath is such a rich experience."

MOYERS: Are you suggesting that my mind shouldn't be wandering, or fleeing, or that it shouldn't be distracted?

KABAT-ZINN: No, I'm not. A wandering mind is the normal state of affairs. But from the meditative perspective, the normal state of mind is severely suboptimal. It's more asleep than awake. The mind is someplace else, and the body is here. In that state, you can't function at your best. Any athlete will tell you that. If you're on top of a 40-foot diving board, you want your mind and your body to be right there together. You don't want the mind to be thinking about how you're going to look on television or whether you're going to hit your head on the board. You have to be completely calm and present, and focused in the moment.

You can train yourself to focus in the present moment the same way you train yourself to jump off the board, or lift weights, or do anything else. The mind that has not been developed or trained is very scattered. That's the normal state of affairs, but it leaves us out of touch with a great deal in life, including our bodies. Many people really feel frightened by their bodies, and don't even like them very much, or they may be upset about the aging process. All of this is usually happening below the surface of awareness, which means that our unconscious thoughts are creating a kind of prison for us which regulates a lot of our behavior. A thought comes up and you'll say, "Oh, I've got to do this," and you run to do that. Then the next thought comes, and you say, "Oh, I've got to do that," and you run to do it. Very often, you are just not in the present moment.

MOYERS: What does that have to do with pain, depression, anger, and stress?

KABAT-ZINN: These are mind states, just like many others that come up. Pain is something that can be worked with, although it's a lot easier to work with a raisin or with your breathing than it is to work with intense pain. But from a meditative perspective, pain can be a profound experience that you can move into. You don't have to recoil, or run away, or try to suppress it.

MOYERS: You mean I should concentrate on my pain? Isn't that accentuating the negative?

KABAT-ZINN: Well, you can call it negative, but if you look at it carefully, you'll see a sensory component to the pain which is just sensation. It can be very, very intense, and the mind will habitually interpret it as noxious. But if you understand it, you may be able to tolerate it better. Let's say you have a pain, and you don't know its origin. That can be very frightening. Sometimes people feel comforted when a pain is given a diagnosis or a name. But often—as with back pain, for instance—no precise physical cause for the pain may be found. Sometimes, you have to learn to live with certain kinds of pain. Pain is the source of enormous disability in our society. It costs 40 or 50 billion dollars a year just to deal with the problem of chronic pain in the U.S.

MOYERS: But how does meditation help deal with pain?

KABAT-ZINN: It allows you to learn from your own inner experience that pain is something you can work with, and that you can actually use pain to grow. Sometimes you have to learn how to work around the edges of your pain and to live with it. The pain itself will teach you how to do that if you listen to it and work with it mindfully.

MOYERS: "Mindfully," meaning—

KABAT-ZINN: Meaning that when pain comes up in the body, instead of focusing on the breath, you just start breathing with the pain. See if you can ride the waves of the sensation. As you watch the sensations come and go, very often they will change, and you begin to realize that the pain has a life of its own. You learn how to work with the pain, to befriend it, to listen to it, and in some way to honor it. In the process of doing that, you wind up seeing that it's possible to feel differently about your pain. Sometimes, when you focus on this, the sensations actually go away.

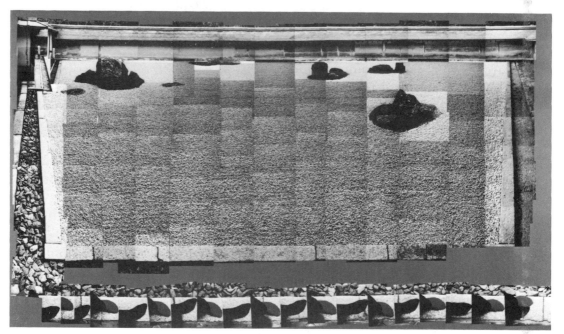

David Hockney, *Walking in the Zen Garden in the Ryoanji Temple, Kyoto, Feb. 21st, 1983,* 1983

MOYERS: Doesn't that suggest that by focusing on breathing you're simply not thinking any longer about your pain but shifting your focus to something else?

KABAT-ZINN: Actually, the instructions are exactly the opposite. I don't say, "Well, just fantasize something that will be so interesting that you'll forget about your body." I say, "Go *into* the body, go *into* the shoulder, go *into* the lower back, breathe with it, and try to penetrate the pain with your awareness and with your breathing." So it's the opposite of distraction.

Laboratory studies of induced pain suggest that distraction is a very good strategy for tolerating pain up to a certain level, but beyond that level it's not as effective as mindfulness, as actually attending to the sensations themselves and then noticing that you can uncouple the sensations from your thoughts about them. You might be thinking, "This is killing me, it's going to last forever, and there's nothing I'll be able to do about it." You learn to realize those are just thoughts. You ask yourself, "Is this killing me right now, in this moment?" The answer is usually, "No, it's not." But then you might think, "My God, if I have to live with this for thirty years—" But at that point you say, "Wait a minute, the idea is to just be in the present moment. Let's just experience it as it is now and let go of our alarmist furture thinking." In this way, over a period of time, people learn to relate differently to their pain.

MOYERS: And physiologically, does that reduce stress?

KABAT-ZINN: It certainly does. Stress is the response to the demands placed on your body and mind. The more you are in distress from pain or anxiety, the worse you'll feel, and that will have physiological consequences. If you can learn to be comfortable within the pain or anxiety, the experience will be completely changed. But you're not trying to make the pain go away. This is a fundamental point that people sometimes misunderstand at first. They'll come to the stress clinic thinking we'll make all their stress go away. But we actually move into the stress or pain and begin to look at it, and to notice the mind's reactions, and to let go of that reactivity. And then you find that there is inner stillness and peace *within* some of the most difficult life situations. It's right in this breath, and it's right in this experience. You don't have to run away to get it someplace else.

MOYERS: When you said to your patients this morning, "Your mind has a life of its own," was that just a figure of speech?

KABAT-ZINN: No, that refers to mindfulness. If you spend a lot of time observing your thoughts and feelings, you begin to realize that your thought process is very chaotic—it's here and there and everywhere else. And when you try to focus your attention on one thing, say, your breathing, or the experience of your body, very often the mind doesn't want to stay focused on it for very long, and it will go off and think about this or that. So when I say your mind has a life of its own, I mean that it has a certain kind of energy that likes to go different places and that it's very hard to concentrate and reach a state of calmness.

MOYERS: When you told them to bring their minds back, I thought, "Well, there is an 'I' that is independent of the mind and that can stand aside like the rider of a horse."

KABAT-ZINN: We often call it "I" and then don't think very much more about it. We don't ask, "Who is it that says 'I'?" The way we usually talk about it leads us to the conclusion that "I" am not my body. Whoever that "I" is has the body. Now when Freud was translated into English, he referred to what we call the "ego" as "das Ich," meaning simply "the I." "The I" got translated into this highfalutin idea of "ego," which we then made into a separate thing.

We don't know what the "I" is, but we do know that human beings have a capacity for awareness and self-observation. That is really what meditation is all about—cultivating and developing the capacity to attend from moment to moment. If you ask, "Well, who's doing the attending?"—the answer is, "Who knows?" In some ways we don't have a vocabulary for talking about that, except in paradoxical language. That's why Zen practice requires you not simply to answer questions in language but to demonstrate your understanding, because, as the saying goes, if you open your mouth, you'll be wrong. So it would be wrong to say, "I am the observer."

On the other hand, there is no denying that observing is going on. But when we put the pronoun "I" on it, then we identify with that "I" in a certain way, and that can be the cause of a lot of problems in our lives. For instance, if you have cancer and say, "I have cancer," you may begin to think of yourself as the cancer. The identification may then take over so much of your life that if you're not careful to see the cancer as a process that's happening in a larger field, you may lose the opportunity for a certain kind of meaning.

Often we do what's called "selfing," where something comes up that we identify with so strongly that we think, "That's me." It takes many forms: "I'm a failure, I'm no good, I'm inadequate, I'm unworthy." Feeling unworthy is not a problem; unworthiness is a common human feeling. But as soon as you connect "I" to it, you ossify it, and it becomes much more real, more concrete. Then you've got a real problem.

We often work with people who have panic attacks and extreme anxiety. If you have panic disorder, and you say, "I'm afraid," and the "I" function, the observing function, identifies with the content in the mind that is fearful, then the fear takes on a reality of its own and begins to take over your life. Usually, at that point, you have to reach outside yourself for some kind of drug to help you reestablish control. But if you step back, and just look at the fear, and notice that fear usually takes the form of thoughts and feelings in the mind, and then if you don't make the leap of identifying with this mental content, all of a sudden you become the observer: "Oh, there's that thought coming up in the mind. The content of it is fear, and it has a heavy-duty charge, but I don't have to get sucked into it."

A lot of the people you saw today have learned how to step back from their own thought processes to the point where they're no longer making strong, unconscious identifications with "I, me, and mine."

MOYERS: Is that what you meant when you said to them, "I want each of you to become the scientist of your own mind and body?"

KABAT-ZINN: Exactly. To know about it from the inside. To become so familiar with its workings that when something comes up, you actually observe it, and you can say, "Wow, I haven't seen this one before." For instance, there was a woman here who has a disregulated hypothalamic condition, which is quite unusual. Doctors think it might be due to a brain tumor, although they haven't yet finished diagnosing it. Because of the condition, this woman sweats profusely. By playing around with the yoga and meditation, she discovered on her own that if she just did the yoga, she would sweat profusely, but if she calmed herself down in the meditation practice and then did the yoga with the same level of intensity, she would not sweat. This is an example of becoming the scientist of one's own mind/body connection—

MOYERS: —by observing and drawing conclusions and then acting on the conclusions. But then, what about people like me who are "Strangeloves"? If I tried to become the scientist in my own body, I would probably blow the field apart.

KABAT-ZINN: Being the scientist of your own mind/body connection doesn't mean you have to control it. In my book, I quoted Lewis Thomas, who said he'd rather be at the controls of a 747 trying to land than in control of his liver for thirty seconds. I completely agree with that. It's not as if we're trying to get hold of our superphysiological control knobs and then tune up our immune system, and tune down something else, and regulate our heart rate, or anything like that. What we're learning is a new kind of science. It's an inner science that marries the subjective and the objective, in which you become more familiar with the workings of your own body. That doesn't mean that you could write a scientific treatise about it. What it means is that you'll live more intelligently. You'll make decisions that are more apt to bring you in touch with the way things work for you in the world.

MOYERS: Is there a scientific basis for the work you're doing with meditation?

KABAT-ZINN: We're trying as best we can to deliver this intervention based on intensive training and mindfulness, without, of course, the Buddhist framework or terminology. At the same time, we're attempting, as best we can, to study it scientifically. Now that's a very difficult thing to do because you're wearing two hats, and when you're doing science, you have to be very careful that your inner biases don't wind up influencing the way you see things or interpret what you see. But what we've found in attempting to study our patients as best we can, first from a descriptive point of view and then over the years with more intensive, randomized types of trials, is that there seems to be remarkable symptom reduction over the eight-week course. This symptom reduction is both physical and psychological, and it tends to persist over time.

MOYERS: What do you mean by "symptom reduction"?

KABAT-ZINN: At the beginning of the program we give people a list of 140 symptoms such as headaches and high blood pressure, and ask them to check off the symptoms they've experienced in the past month. Then we give them the same list at the end of the stress reduction program, and we find a sharp reduction in the reported symptoms. Now that's descriptive, of course. We don't have randomized controls that would tell us whether symptom reduction would be happening in some other group. First we need to establish scientifically that something is changing before we try to see what it is that is changing and carefully control for it.

At this point we do know that people report reduction in psychological and physical symptoms, including pain. What's even more interesting is that when we give them questionnaires having to do with personality variables such as coherence and stress hardiness, and with variables having to do with their relationship with the world and how they see the world, we find that these also change over the course of the program. The interesting thing is that these measures are not really supposed to change in people. They're supposed to be relatively stable traits.

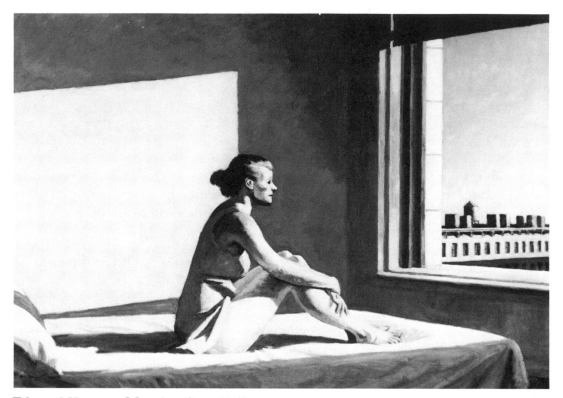

Edward Hopper, *Morning Sun*, 1952

MOYERS: What does that suggest?

KABAT-ZINN: It suggests to me that people may be changing on a much more profound level over the course of these eight weeks than simply having the head-aches disappear, or living with their back pain better, or watching their blood pressure go down. They may be undergoing some kind of a rotation in consciousness that allows them to have a different relationship with their body and with their mental activities, as well as with the outside world, in terms of the pressures and stresses that they're under.

MOYERS: Are these changes physical or mental?

KABAT-ZINN: Well, here we go again. Some of these changes are seen in the body, and other changes are seen in the mind and in behavior.

MOYERS: But you can't have a change in behavior unless you have a change in the body.

KABAT-ZINN: In some ways, absolutely. You might say, "Well, everything is the body then, because if there are changes in behavior, at some level there has to be physical change, or you wouldn't see it." But that's somewhat reductionistic.

MOYERS: But we know something happens.

KABAT-ZINN: Yes, we know something happens, but we don't know what. Let me give you a concrete example. People come to the clinic with panic disorders, which are usually treated with medication. These people come into the program, where they're with all sorts of other people with different kinds of problems. We don't address their panic or fear directly, we just teach them mindfulness, and they practice that over the course of the eight weeks. And when we plot their levels of anxiety and panic, they drop dramatically over the course of the eight weeks and then stay down for a three-month period, and, according to our later study, for at least three years. How do you explain that?

MOYERS: Yes, that's a good question, Doctor, how do you explain that?

KABAT-ZINN: Something is going on here that reaches the organism as a whole. So let's not talk reductionistically about the mind or the body. Let's encounter each person as a person and offer these people some tools that they can work with to try to know themselves better.

MOYERS: Can you be more specific about what you mean when you say you want the person to be a person?

KABAT-ZINN: The trouble is that language is always limiting here. But let me give you an example by walking you through what we do to bring about change in these people who have panic disorder. You see, we believed that this change would happen. We predicted it. What it involves is basically training people to watch their thought process as a flow and to step back from it in the way that we were talking about before and not immediately hook the "I" onto it. So people start off following their breath and doing a body scan and doing yoga, forty-five minutes a day, six days a week. That's a major investment of time and energy for everybody in the program. Now the people with panic disorder may or may not be experiencing fear at any given moment while they're practicing, because the mind is constantly changing and coming up with this or that. They're simply asked to observe, to be mindful, to stay in the body, and to watch what's going on in the mind, learning neither to reject things nor to pursue things, but just to let them be and let them go. But gradually their mindfulness practice starts to spill over into the rest of their lives because we're cultivating a certain way of being and of seeing the activity of the mind.

So, for instance, imagine a woman who is frightened of elevators and hasn't gone on an elevator for twenty-five years. The elevator phobia has hampered her life in many, many different ways. Now the woman comes out of this seventh-floor class that she's walked seven flights up to, and she has this idea: "I think maybe I could go down in the elevator and stay with my breathing all the way to the bottom. And then when thoughts of panic come up, I'll notice that they're just thoughts and come back to my breathing." So she walks into the elevator and goes down, for the first time in twenty-five years.

Now that's an example of phobia, but the same thing applies to panic. You may not know what's causing it, but you can realize, "Right now, in this moment, I'm having these feelings." Because you've been training yourself in the meditation practice to stay in the present moment, and calmly to watch these events in the field of your consciousness, like waves coming up in the mind, you don't get so hooked by the emotional content, and you aren't sucked into terror. You realize, "Well, those are thoughts, too," and you come back to your belly and back to your breathing. In that way, you begin to experience what I mean when I say "your wholeness." You realize that you are more than a body. You are more than the thoughts that go through your mind. And you begin to realize that you're an elaborate universe that's very hard to describe or understand, but that is quite miraculous. If you feel comfortable within it, even if you don't understand it, then you can live your life with a greater sense of control, especially in relation to situations that previously might have sent you spinning out of control.

MOYERS: Yes, but you do have a technique, which is to bring people back to their breathing.

KABAT-ZINN: That's right, that is a technique, and there are lots of techniques in meditation. But if you just stay at the level of technique, then this way of being doesn't develop. Also, the stress reduction program will probably not have the profound effects on the body and on life-style that it would if you made that jump from just doing some kind of technique to doing it from the inside as a way of being.

MOYERS: See, here's the problem: A lot of people watching are going to think, "Well, why don't I just relax on the couch instead of doing this exotic, un-American kind of thing? All that mumbo-jumbo about mindfulness—I mean, what in the world is going on?"

KABAT-ZINN: When you're lying down on the couch, and taking it easy, if you watch what's going on in your mind and body, you may discover that it's far from relaxing. You may be doing a lot of thinking, or daydreaming, or worrying, or fantasizing, or whatever.

MOYERS: Well, my mind constantly chatters.

KABAT-ZINN: Meditation is really about learning how to recognize that. Most people don't realize that the mind constantly chatters. And yet, that chatter winds up being the force that drives us much of the day, in terms of what we do, what we react to, and how we feel. Meditation is a way of looking deeply into the chatter of the mind and body and becoming more aware of its patterns. By observing it, you free yourself from much of it. And then the chatter will calm down.

When you start focusing on your breathing, for instance, you're giving the mind one thing to do: just ride the waves of the in-breath, then ride the waves of the out-breath. There's nothing magical about it. But as you continue to ride the wave of the breath in, and ride the wave of the breath out, you'll begin realizing that it doesn't take long before the mind wants to go someplace else. It doesn't want to just stay with the breath. It doesn't want to just experience one thing. It wants to go to a lot of other places, and it wants to think about the future and the past.

Meditation is a discipline for training the mind to develop greater calm and then to use that calm to bring penetrative insight into our own experience in the moment. From that insight comes greater understanding and, therefore, greater freedom to conduct our lives the way we feel would lead to the greatest wisdom and happiness.

Now that sounds like a big mouthful, but it turns out that it's a very practical thing to do. It's not at all un-American. In fact, Thoreau went off to Walden Pond, as he said, "to live intentionally, to live deliberately," so that when death came, he wouldn't discover that he hadn't lived. Much of the time we run around so much on automatic pilot, and we have so much chatter going on, and we're so busy, we hardly know who's doing the doing. Meditation is a way of slowing down enough so that we get in touch with who we are, and then we can inform the doing with a greater level of awareness and consciousness. Does that make any sense to you?

MOYERS: I would prefer you to describe it in the first person singular. What happens to your mind when you, Jon Kabat-Zinn, are meditating? You talk about being in the present moment. What do you mean by that, in your own experience?

KABAT-ZINN: When I focus on my breathing, I feel the breath moving into my body and out of my body. It's a feeling. It's not thinking about breathing or what breathing is doing. It's just feeling the breath. And then I ask myself to stay on the breath, to ride the waves, much as if I were lying on a rubber raft on the ocean and the waves were picking me up and taking me down. I'm just feeling the lifting and the falling away. Lifting and falling away. I carve out a period of time to just stay with that feeling of the breath. While I'm doing that, my mind will sometimes go off and start thinking about what I need to do later.

MOYERS: Then you're not meditating, are you?

KABAT-ZINN: It depends on how you handle it. It's the bringing back that's the essence of the meditation, not the staying on the breath.

MOYERS: You have to lasso it and bring it back.

KABAT-ZINN: It's the willingness to lasso it gently and kindly, and to escort it back to your belly or to wherever you're feeling the breath moving in and out. So if the mind wanders a million times, you just bring it back a million times.

MOYERS: But you have to think to do that. And you said to your patients this morning, "Don't think."

KABAT-ZINN: By that I'm referring to the pursuit of a line of thought. Meditation is the direct observation that the attention is not on the breath at a certain point, usually because you're pulled into thinking. Then at the point you notice it, the thought may come up, "Aha, I'm not on the breath." That's a thought, true. But that's a thought that ends the stream of automatic thinking and brings you back to the present moment. Now when you cultivate this over some period of time, you begin to feel that when you are in the present moment, time slows down and can even stop, because at those moments you're in a now that's continually unfolding.

MOYERS: But we all know that time doesn't stop. Time is a ceaseless flow of seconds.

KABAT-ZINN: But our perception of time varies. Time can slow down for people facing death under fire so that their entire lives can seem to flash before their eyes. In meditation practice, your experience of the flow of time is very different. Some people say that we measure inward time by the space between two thoughts. But if you're slowing the thought process down by calming the entire mind down, then you have fewer thoughts, and you feel much more in the present moment.

MOYERS: Is the purpose of meditation to slow the mind down?

KABAT-ZINN: I would say that there is no purpose in meditation. As soon as you assign a purpose to meditation, you've made it just another activity to try to get someplace or reach some goal.

MOYERS: But third-party insurance companies are not underwriting the cost of your patients being here for no purpose.

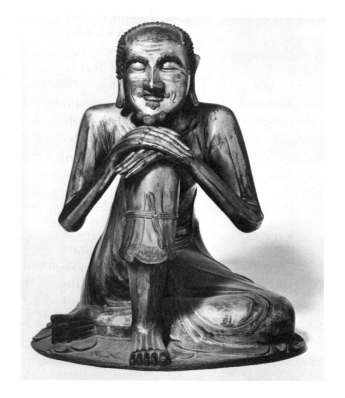

Monk Seated in Meditation, late Ming, 17th c.

KABAT-ZINN: That's true. The people in the program are all here for a purpose. They were all referred by their doctors in order to achieve some kind of improvement in their condition. But paradoxically, they are likely to make the most progress in this domain if they let go of trying to get anywhere and just learn through the practice of meditation to experience their moments as they unfold.

MOYERS: What does that have to do with stress and healing, which is why they're here and why they're reimbursed?

KABAT-ZINN: It may turn out that the deep physiological relaxation that accompanies meditation is, in itself, healing.

MOYERS: What's your experience with meditation and healing?

KABAT-ZINN: The science of meditation and its physiological and psychological effects is in its infancy. When I set up this program back in 1979, the idea was to explore the possibility of creating a clinical service in a major medical center that would catch people who were falling through the cracks of the health care system and to challenge them to do something for themselves as a complement to whatever their medical treatments were. The idea would be not to cure them, but to help them to access their deep inner resources for healing, calming the mind, and operating more effectively in the world and to help them develop strategies and resources for making sensible, adaptive choices under pressure, coping with stress, feeling better about their bodies, and feeling more engaged in life. We wanted to see whether these inner resources would have any effect on their chronic medical conditions—and it turned out that they did, and that people improved in many ways.

Measuring the effects of what we did is a different story. We have decades worth of science left to do in order to get to the bottom of what it means to go into deep states of relaxation and to change one's relationship to one's own body in terms of the actual felt experiences of it. Feeling more comfortable with one's body must have physiological effects, and we are currently studying what these are.

MOYERS: The very word "meditation" suggests something about healing. It's not very far from the word "medicine" or "medication."

KABAT-ZINN: Yes, they actually share the same root. I learned this from a physicist named David Bohm, who wrote a very interesting book, *Wholeness and the Implicate Order*, in which he looks at wholeness as a property of the physical, material world. Bohm points out that the root in Latin means "to cure," but that its deepest root means "to measure." The question is: what does medicine or meditation have to do with measure? It has to do with the platonic notion that every shape, every being, every thing, has its right inward measure. In other words, a tree has its own quality of wholeness that gives it particular properties. And a human being has an individual right inward measure, when everything is balanced and physiologically homeostatic—that's the totality of the individual at that point in time.

Medicine is the science and art of restoring right inward measure when it is thrown off balance. And meditation is the direct perceiving of right inward measure. From the meditative perspective, and from the perspective of the new mind/body medicine, we would say that health was not some kind of static thing that you grab and run with to the goal line. Health is a dynamic energy flow that changes over a lifetime. In fact, health and illness very often coexist together. The body is constantly being catabolized, broken down, and built back up. That's one of the reasons we eat and breathe. Another kind of example: mothers sometimes take their children to be exposed to chicken pox so that the child builds up an immunity to something that might be much more dangerous if contracted later in life. If we start thinking in these terms about the mind and the body and health and illness, then we'll begin to develop a more sophisticated perspective of right inward measure, in which psycho-social influences, thoughts, belief systems, and emotions would be seen to play a role in the health of the body. We're moving in the direction of mind/body medicine today.

MOYERS: How would you define mind/body medicine to me?

KABAT-ZINN: Over the past several hundred years we've tended to look at disease as being more or less a function of the physical body, and to look at thoughts, feelings, emotions, and social interactions as being in the domain of the mind. For the most part, we've thought that the disease process is independent of mind. If, for example, you get a bacterial infection, how you feel about that infection is not going to make a difference—but penicillin will make a big difference. In this model you diagnose what's the matter with the body, treat it, and then get on with your life. You set the broken bone, and then it heals. You diagnose the infection, treat it, and then it heals.

But as we begin looking at chronic illnesses like cancer and heart disease, which aren't infectious, we see more and more evidence that how we live our lives and, in fact, how we think and feel over a lifetime can influence the kinds of illnesses that we have. So the mind/body connection really has to do with understanding that the mind and the body are only artificially separate, that they've always been together, and that they have an interactive influence on each other.

MOYERS: Is there a short way of describing how feelings are expressed in the body?

KABAT-ZINN: Yes—for instance, we say that we have a broken heart, or we speak of gut feelings. These are linguistic ways of expressing the mind/body connection. "Mind" and "body" are really different ways of talking about the same thing.

MOYERS: Is this really a new idea? I picked up a book from your library shelf over there, and in the introduction the editor talks about Socrates coming back from military service and reporting to his Greek countrymen "that in one respect the barbarian Thracians were in advance of Greek civilization. They knew that the body could not be cured without the mind."

KABAT-ZINN: No, this idea is not new—it's as old as medicine. It's as old as humanity. I think what's new is the introducing of it into modern Western medicine. The Cartesian split between the mind and the body in the early seventeenth century resulted in science emphasizing the body and medicine going in the direction of science.

MOYERS: Why the reunion now?

KABAT-ZINN: To a large extent, it's because some very interesting developments have been happening in science that have forced us to look again at this division. Also, we've reached certain limits in terms of what medicine can do. Americans tend to expect medicine to cure everything—but medicine is capable of doing far less than we expect. We also expect to understand everything—but we don't even know what a thought is, although we know we have them.

Another reason for the new emphasis in Western medicine on the connection between mind and body is that current research points to connections between the nervous system and the immune system, for example. Now it stands to reason that there would be such a connection because the body is one interconnected whole. But traditionally, we have split it into organ systems and have emphasized this splitting off through our language and habits of thought. For the longest time no one paid any attention to how the nervous system might regulate the immune system. We thought of it just as a kind of independent, functioning organ system for defense.

MOYERS: Is that why your class begins with a body scan—to make people aware of the whole body?

KABAT-ZINN: That's one reason. The body scan is a kind of Greyhound bus tour through the body that takes forty-five minutes. People think, "My God, how could I possibly stay with my body for forty-five minutes?" But when you let go of your other agendas and make time just for being, it's an absolute pleasure to be in your body. It's better than the best television. It's really wonderful.

MOYERS: What exactly is happening during the body scan?

KABAT-ZINN: I don't know what's happening physiologically because we haven't wired up people and watched them go through this. But the chances are that they're learning how to relax and dwell in the present moment. In the body scan, you lie on the floor, and without moving begin by directing the focus of your atten-

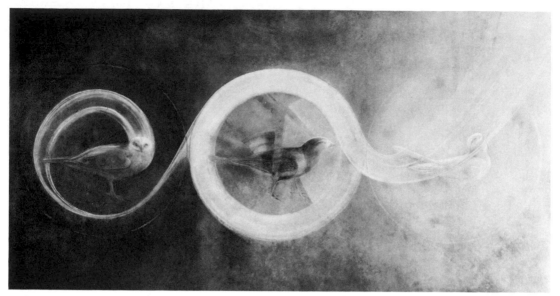

Morris Graves, *Waking, Walking, Singing in the Next Dimension?*, 1979

tion to the toes of your left foot, and then, gradually, up through your leg, and over to the other toes, and the other leg, and eventually through the whole body. After forty-five minutes you're often in a state of deep relaxation, and you have a sense of profound well-being. You're in the present moment. In fact, forty-five minutes could feel like no time at all.

MOYERS: That actually happened to me both times that I experienced the body scan with you. The first time I'd been up all the previous night, and this morning I had flown ten hours the day before to get here, so I came to both sessions really dragging my body like a sack of potatoes. But something happened during the body scan. I don't know what to call it, because physically, I haven't really had that kind of experience before. Perversely, during the sitting meditation, I got agitated, and I had to get up and leave. That's happened to me in meditation before. The body scan worked for me, but the meditation didn't.

KABAT-ZINN: Well, you see, I would throw out your whole formulation. You think that the body scan worked because you had a feeling you liked. And you think the sitting meditation didn't work because you had feelings you didn't like, such as agitation, impatience, and so forth. I would say that the sitting meditation was at least as valuable a teaching for you because it showed you how difficult it is to just be still and watch all the various mind states and body states that will come up.

MOYERS: But I didn't get those agitated feelings during the body scan.

KABAT-ZINN: Right, but all these various methods are one laboratory in which to learn more about the mind/body connection. And so if our goal was to just put you into a fantastic state of inner peace or deep relaxation, we could do that extremely well and extremely reliably. But then, when the proverbial stuff hit the proverbial fan in your life, and you didn't have forty-five minutes to lie down and get into deep relaxation, but you had to be right here in this moment and to handle things with clarity and a sense of calmness—well, how would you do that? What kind of resources would you draw on?

We're trying to cultivate the soil of those inner resources in people and help them to realize—that is, make real in their lives—that they can bring mindfulness, concentration, calmness, and clear seeing into the moment-to-moment stuff of life. Now if they just had good experiences in this training, then they wouldn't be prepared to handle what hit them in daily life.

MOYERS: Or when you're not around—because I thought the explanation for the difference I experienced was that you've got a good bedside manner, and during the body scan, your gentle, soothing voice was a friendly ally in my descent into the body. But in the sitting meditation, you withdrew, and left me sitting there by myself.

KABAT-ZINN: Well, you thought I withdrew myself, but actually I was present— I just wasn't speaking. You see, the people in my class had been practicing meditation for weeks, and so for them I wasn't withdrawing, I was giving them permission to be with themselves without hearing me yakking. When a bunch of people are sitting in a room, doing some variation of this, it looks like nothing is happening, but actually there's an elaborate structure to this nondoing. People are working really hard to fine-tune into the awareness of moment-to-moment experience and to bring the mind back when it's wandering. Whether they're meditating lying down or sitting or standing on their head is immaterial. The question is the quality of mind that you bring to each moment.

Now had you brought your mind back to the moment in the sitting meditation, for instance, you would have noticed, "My God, I'm sitting here, and I'm supposed to feel relaxed." First wrong idea. "All I'm feeling is this horrible stuff." Second wrong idea. In other words, you're saying that what you're feeling is horrible. Actually, what you're feeling is just what you're feeling. It turns out that you have an agenda. You want something to happen, and it's not happening, so your response is "Come on, get with it." That's why we teach meditation as a course rather than simply meeting you for fifteen minutes to give you the magic instructions so that you can go off and do it and solve all your life problems. You need to work on this over a period of days and weeks and months and years to begin to realize that all your mind states are okay. All your body states are okay. And when you've realized that all the states are okay, you can choose to work with them in various ways. Impatience, for instance, is a wonderful state to work with; boredom is another. Like the exercise of tasting the raisin, looking at how much the mind gets into judging, disliking, and discarding is an opportunity for moment-to-moment experience.

Meanwhile, there's no agenda, no place to go, and nothing to do. Just be here, hanging out with yourself.

MOYERS: But do you mean that the insurance companies will reimburse you for teaching people to hang out with themselves that way?

KABAT-ZINN: Well, if it's therapeutic, why not? It's a hell of a lot cheaper than opening up their chests. If one person is saved one major operation by learning how to self-regulate using these mind/body techniques, we've paid for most of the other patients in the clinic for an entire year.

Medicine is reaching the point of increasing expenses with diminishing returns. Part of the problem is that a very profound element is missing in medicine: the active participation of the patient. That's where optimizing the mind/body connection really becomes critical. And cheap. If it's possible to teach people how to self-regulate so that, for instance, they don't go into panic so much, and their blood pressure doesn't escalate so often under stress, and they can handle their musculoskeletal pain in such a way that they don't constantly have to go to the emergency rooms, or be medicated because of it, can you imagine how much money that would save the system? So it's totally in the interest of the health care providers and insurance companies to support this kind of thing.

Actually, I think it's a misnomer to call what we have a "health care system." It's really a "disease care system." But we need to create a health care system. Many of the clinics that are developing along these lines are challenging patients to see what they can do for themselves as a complement to their medical treatments. These clinics are at the forefront of a new area of medicine called "behavioral medicine," which emphasizes moving towards greater levels of health rather than more and more disintegration. I've seen people in their nineties who are healthy as hell, and other people in their thirties who are an absolute mess. If you had some kind of inner control over that, you could save the system an awful lot of money and save yourself an awful lot of grief.

MOYERS: And by behavioral medicine you mean medicine that enables me to take charge of my own behavior and conduct myself so as to live more healthily.

KABAT-ZINN: Right, and your doctor can never do this for you, Bill. If you smoke, your doctor can't make you stop smoking. If your doctor gives you medication for high blood pressure, you still have to take it. If you don't understand what's in your own best interest, you may not comply with what the doctors tell you to do. I think one of the reasons clinics like this one, which focus on the mind/body connection, have such high levels of patient satisfaction and compliance is that we make this stuff fun. Meditation becomes so compelling that you don't want to stop. You wouldn't want to go through this eight weeks and then give it up. That may be one reason why people like Dean Ornish—who trains people in yoga and meditation at the same time that he asks them to make radical changes in diet—get such good results. People stay on their diets because the diet is seen in a larger framework. It's part of working on oneself to develop one's inner capacity to be whole.

There's something about the discipline associated with these mind/body techniques that empowers individuals and, at the same time, deepens and broadens their perspective on the value of having a body and of taking care of it and nourishing it in a certain way. I think that any doctor would give his or her right arm, so to speak, to have patients who have this perspective because it would help the doctor to care for patients as best he or she could.

MOYERS: True. But when you say you want it to be fun, you also say it requires discipline, and discipline is hard and not always fun.

KABAT-ZINN: Well, this is one of the problems in America—the word "discipline" has gotten a bad rap. But any athlete who wants to go to the Olympics doesn't think discipline is a bad thing. Anybody who wants to develop powerful biceps has to do a lot of weight lifting that is potentially very boring. How different is that from attending to the breath coming in and the breath going out?

MOYERS: But what about the people like me, who have a negative experience with meditation?

KABAT-ZINN: Part of it depends on the context in which you first experience it. Very often people can be turned off by the trappings. If meditation is done in a foreign idiom, for instance, if it's Buddhist or Hindu, people will often be turned off. What we've tried to do is capture what we believe to be the essence of what are often called "consciousness disciplines"—meditation, yoga, and so forth. The essence of these disciplines is universal and really has to do with cultivating awareness and a deep understanding of what it means to be human. Now there are few people who couldn't benefit from a greater dose of awareness. If we were more in touch with the present moment, almost everything would become more vivid and alive.

MOYERS: Yes, but what if that present moment is one of physical pain? A friend of mine who read your book said to me, "You know, he says that we should relax into physical discomfort. I don't want to relax into physical discomfort. I don't want any discomfort."

KABAT-ZINN: Well, maybe medicine will come up with some magic pill that will make your friend's discomfort go away completely so that he can just continue to live his life. But the people that we see in the clinic have been that route, and they haven't gotten satisfaction. So then the question becomes: What other possibilities are there? What do I do now?

MOYERS: What do you do with that physical discomfort? Do you really just say, "Relax into it"?

KABAT-ZINN: If you pull that out of context and say, "Jon Kabat-Zinn says to relax into physical discomfort," it can sound insane. But this is said as part of a program that requires you to roll up your sleeves and go to work. Part of the commitment patients make to the program is to suspend judgment. We tell them they don't have to like the program, they just have to do it. Then, at the end of the eight-week period, they can tell us whether it was full of baloney. But while they're in it, they just do the whole thing and watch what's happening as a dispassionate observer.

You might ask, "Is this for everybody? Aren't there all sorts of people that aren't willing to go to the line with themselves?" Perhaps. A lot of people think the last place they want to look into is their own minds. Someone with that attitude might not be the best person for the doctor to refer to the stress clinic. But very often the person's spouse might take the stress reduction program and get deeply into meditation, and it will have a profound effect. A wife, for example, might start to change the way she relates to her husband as a result of her meditation practice. She might be more in the present, more calm, less reactive. There might be fewer fights in the family, or the fights would have different outcomes, so to speak. The husband might begin to think, "Wow, you're really behaving differently. You're not taking things so personally. You're not attacking me so much. You seem calmer. Maybe there is something to that meditation stuff. Maybe I should get myself down there to the hospital."

From a public health point of view, mind/body medicine is not going to be seen immediately as the thing to do. For instance, most Americans are not going to start doing yoga and body scans, or carve out forty-five minutes a day to sit in a full lotus posture. That is not what our program is going to bring at all. But a number of people will experience profound effects from these disciplines, and as soon as they feel it in themselves or see it in other persons, they will want to continue feeling at home in their own skin.

That doesn't mean that if you meditate, you'll always be relaxed. At times it may be appropriate to be tense—but the question is, at these times do you know you're tense? Can you feel it? Can you work with it? Or is it going to end up "doing" you and giving you all sorts of symptoms, and pain, or translate into anger and create more pain and suffering?

MOYERS: One aspect of your meditation disciplines is yoga. What does the word "yoga" mean?

KABAT-ZINN: The word "yoga" comes from the ancient Indian Sanskrit language, and it means "yoke." Yoga is a form of meditation whose aim is to realize that the individual self and the totality of the universe are no different. When you experience that, you experience unity. In other words, you experience yourself not as a separated, individual billiard ball bouncing around with all these other billiard balls, but as part of a larger whole and, at the same time, whole yourself. "Yoga" refers to yoking together the individual mind and the totality of the universe.

Now, the practice of yoga has a lot of different aspects to it. What we do is hatha yoga, which is a form of body yoga that allows you to feel the body, perhaps as you've never felt it before.

MOYERS: So there's a physiological response that is influenced by, or influences, the mind and the emotions.

KABAT-ZINN: In all of this work, it's back and forth that way between the mind and the body, or physiology and psychology. We use yoga in part because many Americans never do anything with their bodies. They sit all day long at work, they drive a lot, and then they sit for hours in front of a television. When the body is not being used, it tends to develop disuse atrophy, where the joints and muscles gradually get flabby and are much more apt to be injured. As the physical therapist put it, "If you don't use it, you lose it." A lot of people just don't use it. So yoga is a very wonderful and gentle way to take people who are in pain or who have not used their body for thirty or forty years, and to get them down on the floor and to start appreciating that the old body still does a few things.

If you do this for any period of time, lo and behold, you'll find the real value of yoga: to work at your limits nonjudgmentally. So, for instance, if you're sitting on the floor, and you're trying to bring your head to your knee, and you can bring it down only a little way, you might see that the person next to you has brought the head all the way to the floor. You might say, "Holy cow!" and then realize, "Wait a minute, I'm not supposed to be competing with somebody else, or comparing myself to somebody else. I'm supposed to just stay here at my limit and breathe with it and feel my body like this." So you do that. And if you do that over a period of days and weeks, you'll find that before you know it, and without realizing how it happened, your head is down to the floor. And you realize, "My God, the body is more capable of change than I had thought. Just because I'm sixty years old, I'm not washed up."

A lot of people swear by the yoga—they love that more than anything else we do. It's just another form of mindfulness, but you're giving the body something to do, and it has the added benefit of reversing disuse atrophy and really toning the body. It's a full-body, musculoskeletal strengthening and conditioning exercise.

MOYERS: So, in effect, by changing my body you're changing my attitudes and feelings.

KABAT-ZINN: Exactly—starting with your attitudes and feelings towards your own body.

MOYERS: And the impact on health and healing?

KABAT-ZINN: The same as with the meditation, except that there are added benefits for people with spine or back or shoulder problems. Again, the science of yoga in the West is in its infancy, unfortunately.

MOYERS: What's the significance of the constantly shifting poses in yoga?

KABAT-ZINN: For one thing, it provides something to do for people who can't stand being still. That's very important, because we want everybody in our classes to taste some profound sense of inner stillness. And yoga is a very powerful way to do that.

The essence of the practice is that you're putting your body into various postures, and then you're experiencing the feelings, the sensations, and the breath in that posture. You're holding the posture, but you're also relaxing into it, so it's not a big effort. Then you go back to lying down on the floor. So it's a sequence of lying on the floor, doing something, and going back onto the floor. And lying on the floor isn't merely breaks. It's a continuous stream of mindfulness, moment-to-moment awareness. If the mind wanders, you bring it back.

Now every attitude that the body takes, whether you're standing on your head, which we don't do with our patients, or something much simpler, like drawing your

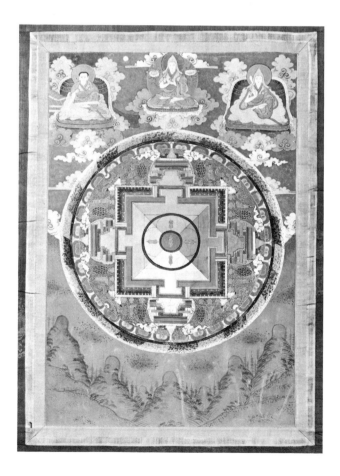

knee up to your chest, has an associated feeling state. Very often we're driving so hard, we're out of touch with our bodies. This gives us a chance to get back in touch with our bodies and to feel our mood states and feelings. You can experience this just by curling up the corners of your mouth into a half-smile the next time you're feeling low.

MOYERS: Smiling is good for you?

KABAT-ZINN: Smiling is in fact good for you. You can experience for yourself how body positions influence your feelings. For example, make a fist, and feel the energy that's associated with that. When you have a really strong fist, notice how your arms feel. Then unclench

Mandala, Mongolia, 19th c.

your fist and put your hands together in the traditional position of prayer. Can you feel the difference? The next time you're really angry, just try putting your hands together like this, and see how long you can hold on to your anger.

MOYERS: What does that do for healing?

KABAT-ZINN: It redirects the energy flow in your body and your mind. That's what yoga does as well. But what it does for healing, I don't know. If your heart is incredibly angry, and you were to do this every time anger came up, it might heal the anger in your heart, which would be phenomenal. But the point is that it would be an experiment that you'd have to do for yourself.

When you use yoga as a door into awareness of the body, it can teach you all sorts of things. For example, it can teach you what kinds of limits you have to watch out for in the morning if you wake up with a stiff back. You get to know your body on a totally intimate level. After I practice yoga in the morning, I'm ready to go out and face the world because I know how my body is. If I have chronic pain, some days are going to be a lot worse than others. But if I've worked with the body, I can take the edge off my bad days and shift the balance to the better days. That's helpful, whether I'm dealing with pain or anxiety or any other kind of disability.

MOYERS: During one of the yoga sessions, a patient began to cry. Is that common? And is it good?

KABAT-ZINN: I don't project onto her crying either "good" or "bad." It just happened, so I assumed that it was important that it happened. Whether she laughs or cries is fine with me.

When you're practicing yoga, you're releasing tension, and the tension isn't always in the body, it can also be in the heart, in the mind, or in feeling states. Release of that tension can put you back in touch with yourself on a very deep level. For instance, you may have grieving to do that you haven't done because you've been out of touch with yourself for so long. It's an inner experience of coming home. Very often we feel so alienated from our bodies that we may not have had a positive experience of being in our body since we were five years old. If that happened for her during that session, she might have been crying with a combination of joy over the experience and grief over the fact that it had been a long time since she had had that kind of experience. I don't know. People get in touch with all sorts of feelings, doing this work.

MOYERS: In your sixth class you asked one of the patients to run at you as hard as he could. What was that about?

KABAT-ZINN: These are pushing exercises that we do to act out and embody different kinds of emotional states that are often involved in reacting to stressful situations or relationships. So when somebody throws some negativity at you, or attacks you, or when you're in a very stressful situation, you can respond with mindfulness rather than reacting automatically.

Very often we get into situations where a particular stimulus pushes our buttons, and we react in a certain way. Your children know best how to push your buttons, but work situations will do it, too. A lot of our patients want to learn to cope better with the stresses in their lives. These pushing exercises model the possibility of doing things differently. The person running at me is embodying a stressful situation. One option I have is just to get knocked to smithereens by it. When I allow this to happen, I ask the patient how he or she feels, and I talk about how I feel. Then the next time I'll duck out of the way, which models being very passive—whenever somebody comes at you, you're just not there. Then there's engagement, which uses the energy of somebody's irrational attack on you to turn things in such a way that without harming the other person you insure that you're not being harmed either.

You know, much of our stress comes up in communications with other people. Just look at the amount of domestic violence we have. We can get stuck in ruts where nothing ever gets solved by the expression of the anger. Also, hostility and anger seem to be statistically associated with a higher probability of heart disease, all other things being equal. On the other hand, suppressing anger or emotions seems to be associated with a higher statistical probability of cancer. Emotions have a great deal to do with our state of well-being in terms of health or illness. Suppressing anger, for example, is not a particularly healthy thing to do, but neither is acting out anger, like a bull in a china shop. Finding a middle path allows you to use your emotions in such a way that you create a good interaction with a useful outcome.

Emotions are not bad—they're just what you're feeling. The point is to get out of the same old emotional ruts. Meditation can wake you up to the fact that in the present moment there may be new options, and new ways of relating to old situations. We've found people who were very dissatisfied in their relationships with their bosses or their spouses or children, who were able to encounter these people in a totally new way. Even if a lot of negativity is coming at them, they can learn to breathe with it and find a new kind of response that completely changes the ground on which everybody's standing.

MOYERS: Of course, the other side of what you're doing here is that you're spending eight weeks with these people. Most doctors spend ten minutes a month with them, if that. So isn't there a form of TLC, tender loving care, in all this? Isn't there something of the bedside manner of the doctor who pays attention, and in paying attention, so humors, or flatters, or encourages, or nurtures a patient that there is a response?

KABAT-ZINN: Of course there is. That's one of the domains that really needs to be carefully controlled when we do the science. But our major purpose in setting up this clinic was not to study the science but to see if we could even set up such a clinic

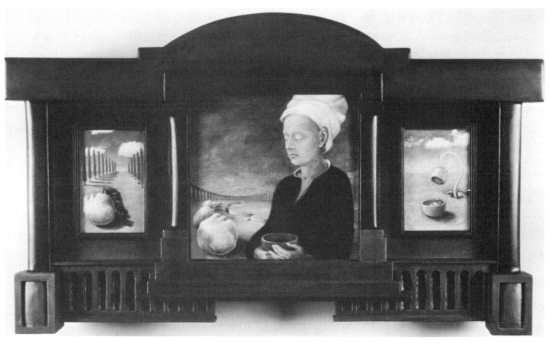

Holly Lane, *Valetudinarian Aided by the Labors of Plants and Bugs,* 1991

in a major medical center like this. If we had wanted it to fail, we could have thought of a thousand ways to set it up to fail. One would be to be completely cold, hard, and clinical, and not give any TLC—not to be a human being yourself.

MOYERS: But isn't there a scientific basis to tender loving care?

KABAT-ZINN: There may be a scientific basis to tender loving care. We just don't know. And we don't know how much of the therapeutic benefit of this program is due to the TLC, how much of it is due to the group interaction, and how much of it is due to the intensive meditation training. These patients practice on their own, at home. Forty-five minutes a day, six days a week. It's a very intensive and demanding program.

MOYERS: Sometimes it seems to me that what you're doing is group psychotherapy. Is that right?

KABAT-ZINN: No, we don't see it as group psychotherapy at all. In fact, we see it as intensive training in meditative practices. But we do it in a group because it's much more effective when done in a group. For one thing, it's cost effective and time effective, because you're working with twenty or thirty people at a time rather than one-on-one. But the other thing is that in a group, people get to see what each other's problems are with the meditation practice, and they learn a lot by listening to and talking with each other. It's different from group psychotherapy in that we're not aiming at developing profound emotional bonds between people, or having people tell each other about their feelings or their personal history or their current dilemmas and so forth. In the stress reduction program we focus on what's right with people. We simply try to help people develop the capacity to go into deep states of relaxation, calmness, stability of mind, and mindfulness, and we let what's wrong with them take care of itself.

MOYERS: Are you practicing medicine or religion?

KABAT-ZINN: It depends on what you mean by medicine and what you mean by religion. Medicine is changing profoundly, and its borders are blurring as it recognizes that in order to deal with the totality of the organism, it has to take into account belief systems, expectations, world view—

MOYERS: —philosophy, faith.

KABAT-ZINN: Yes—and whether this is religion depends on what you mean by religion. The word "religion" actually means to link together. So fundamentally, it's no different from "yoga," which means yoking together. Religion binds together what is fragmented, the self, with the totality—God, or whatever you want to call it. But meditation practice simply has to do with understanding what it means to be human. Medicine, too, has something to do with human experience, when it comes to health and illness. But health comes from a root associated with "whole" and "holy" as well as "heal," so there's already a tie-in between religion and medicine. We've separated the two simply for the sake of defining narrowly what medicine is and what religion is. But these domains are becoming more blurred.

MOYERS: Does meditation eventually become just another Band-Aid, something I do when I start to feel bad?

KABAT-ZINN: A lot of people think that's what meditation is all about. I'll learn a little meditation technique, and then when things get too stressful, I'll use my little technique and relax. But meditation is definitely not a Band-Aid, although in our culture we can tend to treat it that way. When we're feeling a certain way we don't like, we take a drug—maybe caffeine, maybe nicotine, maybe one of the many prescription drugs—so that we feel better. Many people think that's what meditation is about—something to be used when you need it.

Actually, meditation is best described as a way of being. It's like weaving a parachute. You don't want to start weaving the parachute when you're about to jump out of the plane. You want to have been weaving the parachute morning, noon, and night, day in, and day out, so that when you need it, it will actually hold you. You have to carve out some time every day that's your time for just being. And then when stressful situations come up, and you feel like doing more, you have a framework in which to do it and a reservoir of inner calmness and stability and insight.

MOYERS: But you're expecting a lot of Americans if you expect them to do nothing in order to get better.

KABAT-ZINN: Nondoing is not the same as doing nothing. Americans are capable of a lot—that's why we have people practice the meditation forty-five minutes a day at one stretch rather than ten or fifteen minutes. We're not asking people to do nothing, but to practice nondoing. In this culture we are busy doing all the time, and most of it is pretty automatic and unconscious. I'm suggesting that if we focused a little more on present-moment experience and the domain of being, we could develop a far broader and deeper repertoire of what it means to be human.

A lot of people are running around on the planet, trying to get somewhere, and they're very unhappy and relatively unhealthy. But you could actually feel comfortable in your body right now, just the way it is, whether you had heart disease, or cancer, or, for that matter, even AIDS or an HIV diagnosis. The only time that any of us have to grow or change or feel or learn anything is in the present moment. But we're continually missing our present moments, almost willfully, by not paying attention. Instead of being on automatic pilot, we can explore what's possible if we start to kindle the flame of being fully alive.

MOYERS: I never thought I would be hearing this kind of talk in a major American hospital.

KABAT-ZINN: Well, times are changing. If we hope to understand what it means to be a human being, we have to take seriously the efforts that people have made for thousands of years to look inward. For the most part, except for a few deviants like Thoreau, the West has been directed outward, studying nature and then paving over it, or controlling it for our own purposes. Whereas in the East, the emphasis has traditionally been on understanding how to live in harmony.

Now the planet has gotten incredibly small. There is no East, and there is no West, and the human race needs all the wisdom it can get. We need to take what's most valuable from all the various consciousness traditions, integrate them into Western behavioral science and mainstream medicine, and study them as best we can in terms of the most sophisticated and stringent scientific methodologies. We need to ask: what is it about these ancient traditions that tells us something valuable about healing and the mind?

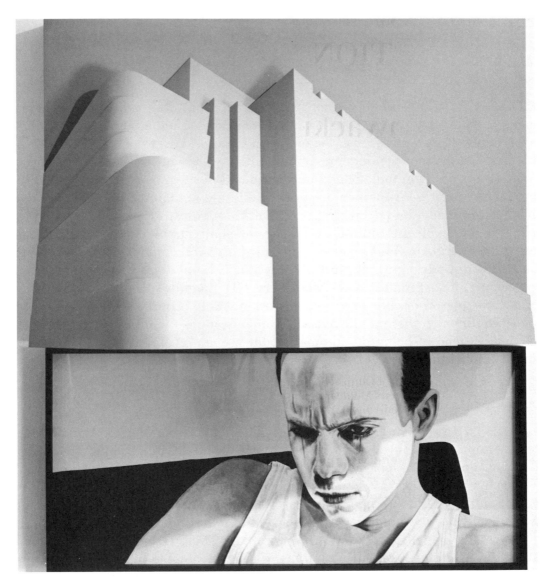

Robert Longo, *Pressure,* 1982

STRESS
REDUCTION

John Zawacki

JOHN ZAWACKI, M.D., is Director of Clinical Services in the Division of Digestive Disease and Nutrition at the University of Massachusetts Medical Center in Worcester, Massachusetts. In addition he is an award-winning Professor of Medicine at the University of Massachusetts Medical School.

MOYERS: Why do you send your patients to the stress reduction clinic?

ZAWACKI: Often, it's out of a sense of frustration. When physicians refer patients to other people, they've often reached the end of the road in terms of the things they can do for the patient, and they're looking for help.

MOYERS: You used to be the end of the line. The other doctors would send these patients to you because you were the last resort. And now you call in Jon Kabat-Zinn.

ZAWACKI: Yes, now Jon's the end of the line.

MOYERS: What kinds of problems do these patients have?

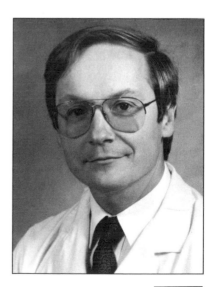

ZAWACKI: While there are many types of problems that might lead me to refer someone to the stress reduction clinic, the main problem is pain. Some patients have pain they can't control. When we don't know what causes that pain, and pain medication hasn't worked, and the pain clinic hasn't worked, we have sent patients to the stress clinic to learn how to live with their pain and sometimes to overcome it.

MOYERS: So these are not patients to whom you can give Tagamet for curing an ulcer. Their problems are more complex.

ZAWACKI: That's correct. They're often people with abdominal pain that they do not understand or people with chronic diarrhea. They can't go anyplace without having pain and diarrhea, and there's no obvious colitis or any inflammation I can give a medicine for.

MOYERS: They come to you wanting you to heal them, and sometimes you have to say, "I can't."

ZAWACKI: That's right. I was thinking just recently of a patient I went to see. I dreaded walking in the door because I knew I couldn't help this patient. I didn't have an answer. And like many physicians, I often think the answer has to lie with me, that I have to do something. But Jon's course has helped us see that patients can empower themselves and that we physicians don't have to have all the answers. Patients can learn more about themselves and learn how to change their life-styles and handle the emotional component of conditions like irritable bowel syndrome.

MOYERS: So Jon is not dealing simply with emotions but with serious physical illnesses, even though the cause of these illnesses may be emotional.

ZAWACKI: That's correct. He deals with the toughest ones. That's one reason I admire him so and why I think most of the physicians do—because he takes the people we can't help.

MOYERS: Can you remember the most difficult referral you ever made to Jon?

ZAWACKI: I can't remember the one, but I know the category—people who are so overwhelmed by anxiety that they can't even sit still.

MOYERS: And their pain is the result of this anxiety?

ZAWACKI: It is related to their intestinal complaints, which in turn is related to anxiety and often to a history of physical abuse. One of the amazing, devastating statistics in the United States right now is the number of people with chronic pain, especially abdominal pain, who have been physically and sexually abused. It's an epidemic that's rampant in this country but that people don't talk about. It devastates people for a lifetime—they never totally recover. But I've seen Jon enable that group of people to adapt to daily life, even though they're among the toughest cases. I remember one woman whose case history filled twenty-four volumes. That body of hers was just being overcome by physical pain all the time. What allowed this lady to survive and have a life was what she learned from Jon. And then the beauty of that was that this wounded woman would go help other people and tell her story and be part of that healing process. Even as her body disintegrated, her emotions and who she was as a person just glowed. She became a magnificent person.

MOYERS: How do you tell your patients that you're going to prescribe meditation for them? Do you have to be sensitive to the idea that most people think meditation is something difficult and exotic?

ZAWACKI: I usually try to prepare them a little bit for it. I tell them, "You know, sometimes when people have a gnawing toothache, it affects them emotionally and it's difficult for people to be around them." Most people can relate to that. Then I show them that it can also work in reverse, that just as physical pain can affect emotions, emotions can affect physical pain. I say, "Why don't you do something simple, like just walk slowly, and see what effect that has. Exercise a little." I start telling them to do these little things, and to call me back to tell me how they're working. Then, when they call back, I say, "Now that little thing has helped you. Let me tell you about where you can go and really learn about this."

I was just doing that tonight, before I came over to talk with you. A woman said, "Gee, the things you told me to do, like slowing things down—it's really helping me with my digestion and my bloating and discomfort. And you asked me to look at my life and what was going on in my relationships. I realize a lot of things that are going on are really crazy. I see that there are some issues there."

Then I said, "How would you like to learn how to be able to deal with those things in a better way?"

MOYERS: So you didn't quite use the word "meditation."

ZAWACKI: Sometimes I use the word "meditation," and sometimes I say "stress reduction." I don't have a planned approach, and I don't do it the same way every time. But eventually I tell them about the course and that it's been very effective for many of my patients.

MOYERS: When you tell your patients you're going to refer them to a meditation course, how do they react?

ZAWACKI: In a variety of ways. Most express a little bit of surprise or fear, and some simply say, "Not for me." Some people are afraid that anything in your mind that affects you physically is related to mental illness.

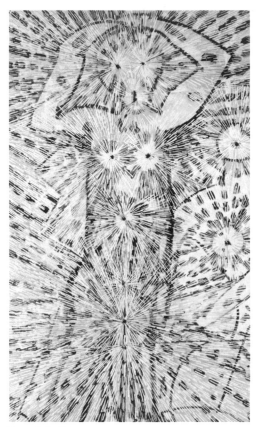

Lee Mullican,
Cosmicon #1, 1990

MOYERS: The instinctive reaction is that if it's in my mind, the doctor must think I'm crazy.

ZAWACKI: No question. But when people say, "Not for me," I tell them, "What have you got to lose? It may be the only door you have. I've tried it myself. I haven't been able to do it, but I've tried, and I use some of the things I learned in the course, and it helps. It might offer you a lot of benefit."

MOYERS: You've tried meditation?

ZAWACKI: Well, I took a course Jon offered for physicians. He takes you through these exercises to help you become aware of the moment. In one, you just eat a peanut, and in another you roll over, ever so slowly, taking what seems like a decade just to roll over. Then you get into breathing. On the meditation retreat, when I had nothing else to do in my life, I did very well. For example, I went to church on the Sunday morning of the weekend of that course, and I listened to the organist, who always plays terribly, and I turned to my wife and said, "This is the best organ music I've heard from this lady." She was still hitting wrong notes, as always, but I heard it differently. I went to Jon and said, "Gee, this is wonderful." He just smiled knowingly. Then I went to work the next day, Monday, and had ten phone calls in fifteen minutes. Because I was mindful of things, I saw how crazy my life was. The heightened awareness of how stressful my life was made it even more stressful.

MOYERS: So you learned your life was crazy, but you didn't do anything about it.

ZAWACKI: I didn't do much about it. I tried the meditation each morning, but I found I wasn't as disciplined as I thought I was. I wasn't very successful.

MOYERS: What happens to you when you're trying to meditate?

ZAWACKI: I have a tendency to hold on to ideas that float by my mind. Jon says, "Don't hold on to them too long. Just let them go." But I grab them and look at them and turn them around every which way, and I have a hard time letting go of them. Concentrating on my breathing was also very difficult for me. But I have learned to be mindful of some of the things that I do. For example, as I walk down the corridor of the hospital, I think whether I am feeling my foot, and that mindfulness slows me down. Or when I'm in the midst of a difficult procedure that's not going well, I immediately go to my breathing, and that helps.

MOYERS: Why do you think meditation works for your patients?

ZAWACKI: I think they tap into some portion of themselves that they didn't know they had and that we probably all have.

MOYERS: What do you think it is?

ZAWACKI: I don't know what that source is, but I think it's partly learning to love oneself. I started to understand that I have abilities and talents that I never knew I had, and that I have people around me I never knew I had. Just slowing down and being aware of what you do have, even within, is very healing. People learning to love themselves and to accept themselves for what they are has amazing healing power.

MOYERS: What changes do you see in patients after the eight-week course?

ZAWACKI: They have come to an understanding that they can adapt, and that they can carry out their daily activities despite discomforts, and that they can enjoy life more.

MOYERS: They still have their pain.

ZAWACKI: Yes, frequently they still have pain off and on. But they can deal with it in ways that don't interfere with their daily activity, so that's a major advance.

MOYERS: How do you know they're better?

ZAWACKI: I see it in their faces. They don't call as much. They come less often, they require fewer medicines, and they're happier in their whole demeanor. It's wonderful to see.

MOYERS: To what extent do you think it works because the people you send to the stress reduction clinic want it to work? You haven't been able to fix them, and they're desperate and have nowhere else to turn. If this doesn't work, they're really up that creek without a paddle.

ZAWACKI: I've seen people with that attitude who walk in, wanting it to work, and it wouldn't work, because sometimes wanting it is not the right thing.

MOYERS: So it's not just a placebo effect.

ZAWACKI: I don't think so. Wanting it can be a barrier.

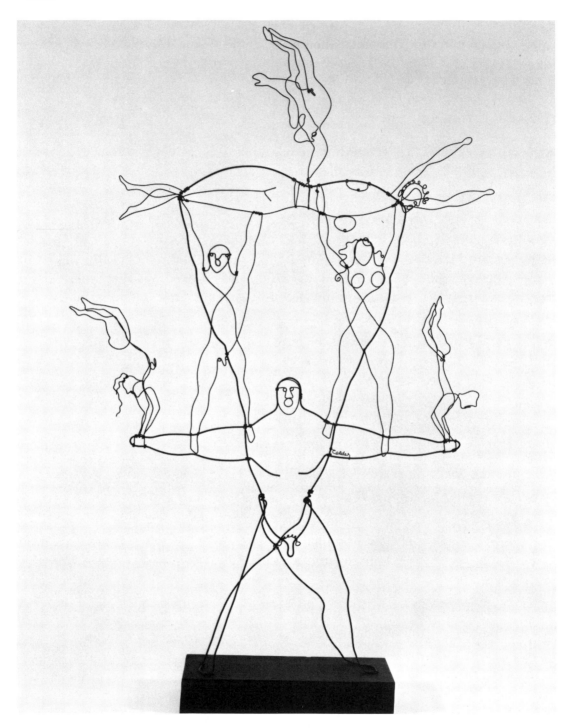

Alexander Calder, *The Brass Family*, 1927

MOYERS: Maybe simple caring is part of the healing. I was struck that Jon will spend hours with these patients when economics and other considerations make it likely that many doctors will spend no more than ten minutes with them.

ZAWACKI: Yes, as physicians, we need to make more time for people. Jon is an example of how giving time to people can help empower them and educate them to help heal themselves.

MOYERS: Yes, you could tell that the people in Jon's course were learning a lot of techniques that were foreign to them when they came. But do you think that what he does is basically just tender loving care? Or is it more than that?

ZAWACKI: Oh, he's a professional; but he is also caring in his own very professional way, and he creates an environment of caring, which is really the essence of healing. It's that deep respect. You walk into Jon's stress reduction class, and you are immediately respected as a person.

MOYERS: But if I came to you, the gastroenterologist, and said, "I have an ulcer," I'd want you to cure my ulcer. I wouldn't necessarily care whether you had a deep respect for me.

ZAWACKI: I can take care of you on the level of your ulcer. But if I have a basic respect for you when you walk in, I can listen to you better, and I can really understand some of the things that are causing your ulcer and perhaps do more for you than just give you a pill and say good-bye.

MOYERS: Do you see the doctor in our society as a healer?

ZAWACKI: You can categorize doctors in different ways. Doctors can simply be health care providers who say, "So you have an ulcer? Here's a pill," and you're on your way. You got a service, and you're satisfied. A doctor can also be a professional in the sense that you may come in with a more complex problem. The doctor may listen and analyze in a more detailed way and use the very latest techniques and technologies. But the real physician is a healer, perhaps with a natural talent or gift of healing.

MOYERS: Is Jon a healer?

ZAWACKI: No doubt. No doubt.

MOYERS: That leads to one criticism of the stress reduction clinic—that Jon does very well with the patients you and the others at the hospital send him, but since we can't clone Jon Kabat-Zinn, we can't get these techniques to the masses.

ZAWACKI: I don't think there's just one Jon Kabat-Zinn out there. I think there are many Jon Kabat-Zinns who haven't been discovered yet but who are excited

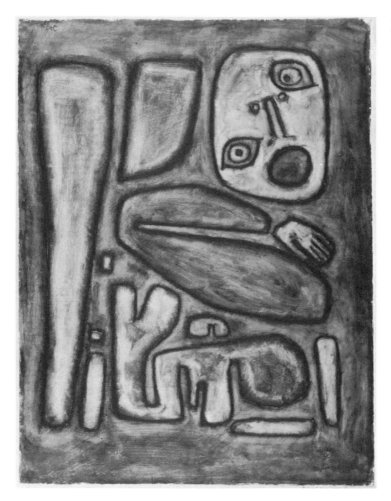

Paul Klee,
Outbreak of Fear,
1939

about this, and who could teach it to other people. And other people have this healing gift. For example, when physicians affirm people, they start to create a healing process.

MOYERS: Is the stress reduction clinic just tolerated, or is it looked upon as integral to the mission of the hospital?

ZAWACKI: That's a very good question. Certainly, in my mind it is. I can't speak for the policy of the medical center, but I know that practicing physicians see the clinic as an absolutely essential element of the center.

MOYERS: So how would you describe to a layman the place of the stress reduction clinic in the setting of the modern hospital?

ZAWACKI: It's an integral portion of a medical center that claims to be a home of healers. If all you can do is the physical technology, you're a limited institution. If you bring in the emotions and the mind/body relationship, you're adding another essential piece to that healing process. I would like to see scientific research applied to understanding the connection between the two.

MOYERS: That's what's beginning to happen now, isn't it?

ZAWACKI: That's correct, especially in the field of the immune system and its relation to the emotions.

MOYERS: Is this the medical center of the future?

ZAWACKI: I hope so. I think medical centers should be about healing and understanding healing on a scientific basis, no matter where healing comes from. So if there's an emotional component in healing, we should understand that. People have physical, emotional, and spiritual aspects—and so those are all aspects of healing, too, and they overlap. If you're treating somebody with alcoholism, you're treating a ravaged liver and other parts of the body that may be damaged. But that's driven by emotional aspects such as deep hurt, or emptiness and pain. As a physician, you can create an environment in which patients have an opportunity to discuss their pain honestly. Illness breaks barriers, and patients will tell you things they can't tell anyone else. Sometimes you're the confessor.

MOYERS: And here's Jon, who tells patients that he wants them to become mindful of the preciousness of the moment. Now that's what a priest and a poet used to say—but it's being said right here in a big Massachusetts hospital and paid for by medical insurance. Somebody's going to walk in and say, "What's the world coming to?"

ZAWACKI: I would just say, why don't you ask the people who take the course what it has done for them? And why don't you talk to the patients who have learned how to tolerate their pain and are excited about learning how to care for themselves and to deal with difficult issues in their lives? Just judge by the results.

MOYERS: In the meantime, you're not advocating that we do away with all these wonderful technological gadgets you folks have brought us, are you?

ZAWACKI: Oh, no, I think you embrace those and make them available to everybody. That's the challenge of our medical society and our health care system—making our technology available to everybody.

MOYERS: Including these mind/body techniques.

ZAWACKI: Absolutely. I just sat with a man who is out of work, an alcoholic. He had been a woodcutter—"in the wood trade," as he put it. He talked about how lonely he was and that he was homeless and didn't have any money. I just sat and listened to him talk about how the pain in his life drove him to drink. Listening to people, and empowering them, and giving them a sense of worth is directly related to healing.

MOYERS: What have you learned in your twenty-three years as a physician about the role of the mind in healing?

ZAWACKI: I'm amazed what happens to people when they start to believe in what they can do for themselves and start to like themselves. There's an awful lot of emotional pain, and it has a tremendous effect on the body. For example, under stressful conditions people will often be in chronic intestinal pain. When they learn that the pain is a physical manifestation of their anxiety, they see how the mind plays a role in their bodily condition and how finding some way to relieve the anxiety can have a salutary effect.

MOYERS: So what have you learned about the physician as healer?

ZAWACKI: Help the patients heal themselves. Be an instrument. Bring medicine, bring technology, bring understanding, bring caring, bring knowledge, and put it all out on the table. Then share an experience, and listen. In a way, all that is healing.

MOYERS: And the physician is not doing the healing?

ZAWACKI: In some cases, we are. For example, a surgeon removes diseased organs and replaces arteries, and so forth. That's physical healing. But there are

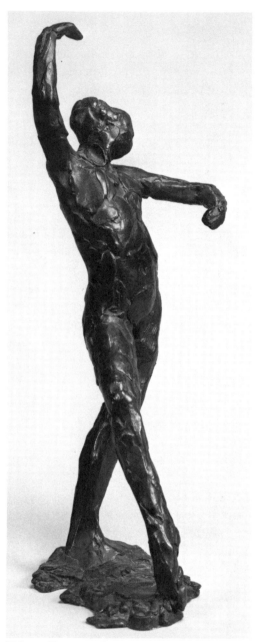

Edgar Degas, *Spanish Dance*, 1896–1911

other, emotional healings that are just as important and that last longer. I can tell you stories of patients who didn't want to leave the room because they've never been affirmed in their life or acknowledged for the difficulty they've had. So physicians play multiple roles. The key is to find out what is needed, and to create an honest and caring environment.

MOYERS: If you're around another twenty-three years, do you think you'll see medicine change because of these mind/body healing techniques?

ZAWACKI: I hope so. I hope we become more open and less fearful of the mind. When you talk about the mind and the psychiatric implications, many doctors get uncomfortable. The real healers understand that connection and know how critical it is. We need to integrate our magnificent technological advances with techniques that empower people to mindfulness, as Jon would say.

MOYERS: Did they teach any of this to you in medical school?

ZAWACKI: No, I learned it as I went along, and I had learned it earlier from my father, who was a physician and a psychiatrist. I didn't learn it from what he said but from observing how he lived and how he was with people.

MOYERS: Well, that raises an interesting point. We've known for thousands of years that the mind influences the body. But something seems to be different about our attitude now. What is it?

ZAWACKI: I hope it's an openness for people to investigate what happens physiologically when the mind becomes peaceful, and what happens when it becomes anxious. And what effect does that have over a short period of time or over a long period of time? If we're open to investigating that, we can begin to understand how the body heals itself.

Some people say that the body has all it needs to live for maybe a hundred years. We have it all within us—the ability to fight infections, kill tumors, what have you. But what we expose ourselves to in the environment, and what we eat, and what we do to ourselves emotionally—all these things cut down our years of life.

The body is a magnificent instrument. If we'll open our minds to study how emotions influence health, then maybe we'll eventually open our minds toward the spiritual dimensions of health.

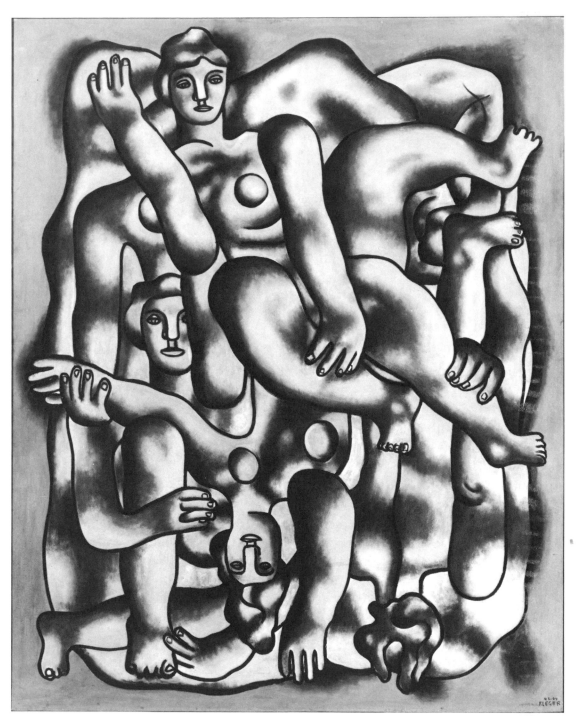

Fernand Léger, *Les Acrobats en Gris*, 1942

THERAPEUTIC SUPPORT GROUPS

David Spiegel

DAVID SPIEGEL, M.D., is Professor of Psychiatry and Behavioral Sciences and Director of the Psychosocial Treatment Laboratory at Stanford University School of Medicine. In 1989 Dr. Spiegel published a landmark study on the effect of psychosocial treatment on patients with metastatic breast cancer. Also known for his work in hypnosis as treatment for pain, he is coauthor, with his father, Dr. Herbert Spiegel, of *Trance and Treatment: Clinical Uses of Hypnosis.*

MOYERS: When I read about your study, it just seemed so commonsensical that people who get their feelings out in the open, who have the support of loving friends and family, who are able to distract themselves from pain, and who know that they're not unique in suffering or alone in dying are going to be happier and more hopeful, and therefore better able to cope with disease. I can certainly see that psychologically, but I have a hard time understanding what it means physically, and, therefore, how it helps to prolong life.

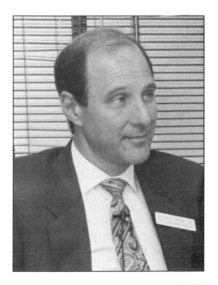

SPIEGEL: We don't know the answer, physically. But if thinking about death elicits a kind of fight-or-flight reaction, and you're in a chronic, unmodulated state of discomfort, your body is busy handling all these signals, and it becomes stressed. Whereas, if you get to the point where you can say, "I don't like the idea of dying, and it will sadden me that I can't do what I've done in the world, and that I will not be with the people I love and care about"—then you're more in control of your mental state, and your body is not responding in that same helpless, aroused way. We think that may have some impact on how the resources of the body are available to do what it has to do to fight disease. Now that's only a theory at this point, but we think that may be what's going on.

MOYERS: So my mind is summoning my body to a different response than it might have given on its own without the conscious effort on my part.

SPIEGEL: That's a good way to put it. If you can't control whether or not you die, you can at least control how you live and how your body is handling the stressors that you're facing.

MOYERS: How important is self-hypnosis in all of this?

SPIEGEL: Self-hypnosis is very important as one highly structured way of regulating your inner states. As part of the treatment, we end each group with a self-hypnosis exercise. Hypnosis is really just a state of focused concentration. It's like being so absorbed in a good novel that you forget that you're reading a book, and you just get caught up in the story. We couple that with learning to control the way your body responds. So, for example, right now, you have sensations in the part of your back that is touching the chair, but until I mentioned it, you probably weren't aware of it. We call that "dissociation." You've put those sensations out of your conscious awareness. If you can do that with the chair, you can do it with pain. So people who are focused on one thing in hypnosis can often filter out many uncomfortable sensations. They can learn to transform the feeling into some other feeling, or just pay attention to a different part of their body. And they can also learn to face a problem that worries them without having their body react so much to it. For example, we teach them to imagine that their bodies are floating in a hot tub or floating in space, feeling comfortable, while on an imaginary screen they're dealing with some issue that concerns them.

MOYERS: So hypnosis is not a form of black magic.

SPIEGEL: Absolutely not. It's an everyday form of highly focused concentration.

MOYERS: Is it like meditation?

SPIEGEL: There's some overlap with meditation. The meditators would say that in meditation you concentrate on nothing, and in hypnosis you focus on something. There's also a difference in the ceremonial ritual that surrounds it. But anything that gets you into a state where you're mentally alert while physically relaxed has elements of a hypnotic or trancelike state to it.

MOYERS: Even though it's hypnosis, it'a conscious effort to control part of what's happening, right?

SPIEGEL: Yes, absolutely.

MOYERS: It increases my control even though I'm a victim of disease.

SPIEGEL: One of the misconceptions about hypnosis is that it's a state where you lose all control. It is true that in a hypnotic state you may be more receptive to input from other people. But hypnosis is really a means of heightening the way you control and regulate your inner states. You can put aside distracting sounds or feelings and enhance your ability to focus on what you want to at the moment. After focusing on something for a set period of time, you're able to put it aside. The ability to put something aside is as helpful as the ability to focus while you're in the hypnotic state.

MOYERS: Did the women in the control group, who didn't get special treatment, report more pain than the others?

SPIEGEL: Yes. We had all the women rate their pain at intervals every four months. Over the initial year, women in the control sample reported that their pain had doubled—from a two to a four on the ten-point scale. But the group that was trained in self-hypnosis reported a slight decrease in pain, so that by the end of the year their average pain ratings were less than two.

MOYERS: What's really going on in self-hypnosis? How does it work?

SPIEGEL: Hypnosis seems to be a way of filtering out information you really don't want to have. We've done some research with a mild electric shock in which we've told a hypnotized subject, "Your hand is in ice water." In that condition the brain does not respond as much to the electric signal as it would if you were simply paying attention to it. In fact, when hypnotized people are told that the electric shock is a really pleasant, interesting sensation, the brain exhibits a stronger response to the signal than it would ordinarily.

Hypnosis is like an amplifier. You have the same signal coming in from your compact disc player, but if you turn the volume up, you'll hear a lot more sound than if you turn it down. Hypnosis seems to help people gain greater control over whether their brain amplifies signals like pain.

MOYERS: So you turn down the amplifiers that are bringing in the unwanted noise.

SPIEGEL: That's right. You have to pay attention to pain for it to hurt. You can lessen the pain either by turning down the pain input or by turning up the attention that you pay to other signals in your body or other thoughts or images.

MOYERS: Can anyone learn how to do this—even a journalist?

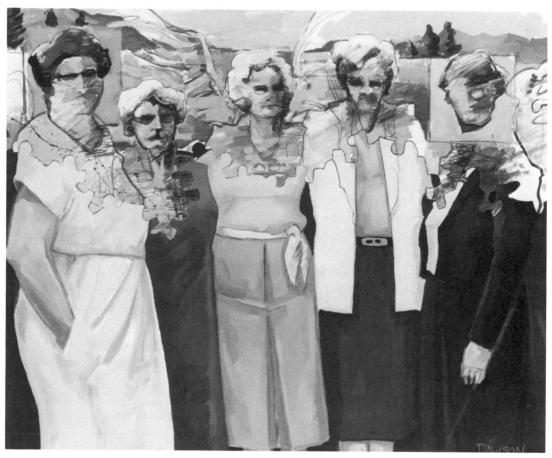

John Dawson, *Patron Saints No. 2,* 1985

SPIEGEL: Even a journalist like you could learn it, but you would have to suspend some of that critical judgment you use so well. Probably eighty percent of the general population is capable of using hypnosis to some degree. About ten percent can use it to a rather profound extreme. There are even some patients with very severe pain who can learn to control that pain primarily with constant use of self-hypnosis.

MOYERS: Listening to you makes me think I might be able to do something like self-hypnosis and be able to face pain better than I thought I could—or even death. But what have you learned about the importance of the doctor and patient relationship in all this?

SPIEGEL: It has deepened my appreciation for what it means to be a doctor and for what patients need. In our medical training we tend to focus exclusively on the technical aspects of what we do—surgery, chemotherapy, and so on. But I feel more strongly than ever that the doctor's role is to help patients cope with all aspects of what it means to be sick and to face limitations in life. The best medical care must always involve attention not only to the physical treatments, but also to the way the patient is coping with them. We must help patients understand what's happening to them and help them mobilize support from family and friends. Just a little bit of caring goes a long way. It doesn't have to be an elaborate thing. Just saying, "I'm really sorry this happened to you, and if you need help, I'll always be there to help you" makes a tremendous difference to patients. Doctors need to know that.

MOYERS: Ironically, your skill in caring can be seen as a flaw in your study. People could say, "David Spiegel is such a good psychiatrist and such a good leader of this group. But, unfortunately, there are not a lot like him." You may be raising hopes that other people can benefit from this kind of group support when in fact you can't replicate the man who makes the program work.

SPIEGEL: Well, I'm honored, but I really don't think it depends on me. It's the combination of the approach that we take, which is teachable and learnable, and what the patients do for one another. I simply try to provide a setting in which I show my caring for the patients, and I help structure what they talk about. I didn't run all the groups in our study—and there were no differences in survival time for the groups that were run by other health professionals. I don't have any corner on the market of human caring. There are lots of very good, caring professionals who can learn to do this if they're willing to unlearn certain parts of their medical training. A lot of doctors, for example, think that crying should be treated like bleeding—just stop it at all costs. But I tell the medical students at Stanford that if you see somebody crying, don't just do something, stand there. Be with them for a few minutes, and let them know that you're open to their discomfort. It doesn't take a lot of sophistication, it just takes knowing what to do in a difficult situation.

MOYERS: But why do you use psychotherapy? Why not offer a simple support group?

SPIEGEL: While I'm a great believer in self-help groups, the kind of support that someone who's dealing with a serious illness needs goes beyond a general sense of "I like you, and you like me, and here's the latest treatment" for this or that. It means being able to tolerate the very strong feelings that arise when people have to give up their ability to do things. Grieving for people you have cared about who have died, and facing your own fears of dying, and handling pain—those kinds of issues require focused attention. They require a serious effort to allow people to share what they're feeling inside so that they feel comfort and supported when they do. That goes beyond the usual notion of support groups.

MOYERS: You're doing this at Stanford Medical School, a fine institution of medical training. Are people out there going to think, "Well, that's wonderful for a select group of people, but I'll never have access to this"?

SPIEGEL: I certainly hope that's not the case. You know, from the perspective of health care costs and implementation, group support is ridiculously inexpensive. It costs virtually nothing. You have to pay a professional salary, and you need a meeting room, and that's it. If you compare the cost of that to even a minor surgical procedure, it's trivial. So what we need to do is to get ourselves back in balance so that helping a patient deal with illness through a support group of one kind or another is considered a routine, necessary part of health care, just like all the other aspects of health care. I can assure you that support groups are far easier to do and far less expensive than many things that we do in health care today.

MOYERS: I believe that, but when you have a group of strangers who have in common only their inevitable encounter with death as a result of cancer, it must be hard to get them to open up to each other. How do you do it?

SPIEGEL: Actually, it's not as difficult as you might think, because we're providing for them something that they know they desperately need. I've been struck by

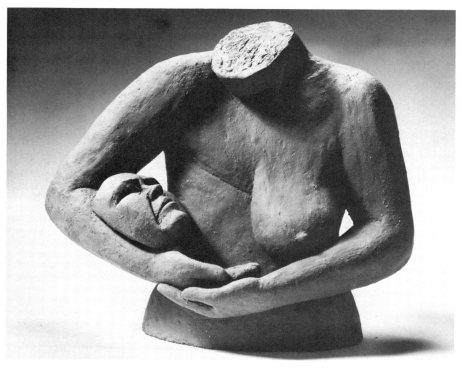

Nancy Fried,
*Cradling Her
Sorrow,* 1989

the fact that if you simply keep the focus on the important issues, these people quickly come to care about one another very deeply. For example, one woman in one of the groups had to go in for a major surgical procedure, and one of the women she'd met in the support group just a few weeks before came to see her in the hospital. When the patient returned to our group, she said to the woman who'd come to see her, "Your visit meant more to me than all the other visits I had. You really know what I'm going through." That sense of being in the same boat is really a very powerful thing when you're dealing with something that's difficult, so I find that it's a lot easier than you might think to get people like this to open up to one another.

MOYERS: When the women come together, exactly what are you trying to make happen?

SPIEGEL: I'm trying to create an atmosphere in which we talk about the hard stuff, not the easy stuff. I'm looking for signs of emotion, for someone beginning to look like she wants to cry, or someone who is feeling worried about something but not quite able yet to talk about it. I try to set it up so that the deeper concerns are the ones that we focus on in the group. And I also try to keep the discussion focused on what's going on in the room. It's very tempting to go into an interesting story about what happened to so-and-so, or whatever. But when that happens, the emotions drain out of the room. I try to keep the focus of attention on what's going on right now: what issues are you dealing with right here, and how can we help you deal with them?

MOYERS: These are women who, in many cases, probably haven't had psychotherapy. They're facing death, they're grieving, they're in pain, and they're feeling isolated. It can't be an easy thing to try to get them to open up and express their feelings to strangers.

SPIEGEL: At first, of course, there's the usual reticence to talk about something that you haven't talked about with anyone else, in a room with people you don't know well. So I try to focus on their common experience, the things that bring them together rather than separate them.

MOYERS: Like what?

SPIEGEL: Like the difficulty some of the women have talking with their husbands about how scared they are. They'll tell their husbands, "You know, I'm really frightened about this physical exam that I have coming up." And the husband will say, "Oh, don't make yourself sad, because you'll just let the cancer get worse," or something like that. The woman takes it as a message that her husband doesn't want to deal with it anymore. Then another woman in the room will say, "You know, my husband was the same way, but I said to him one day, 'Well, you're going to hear me

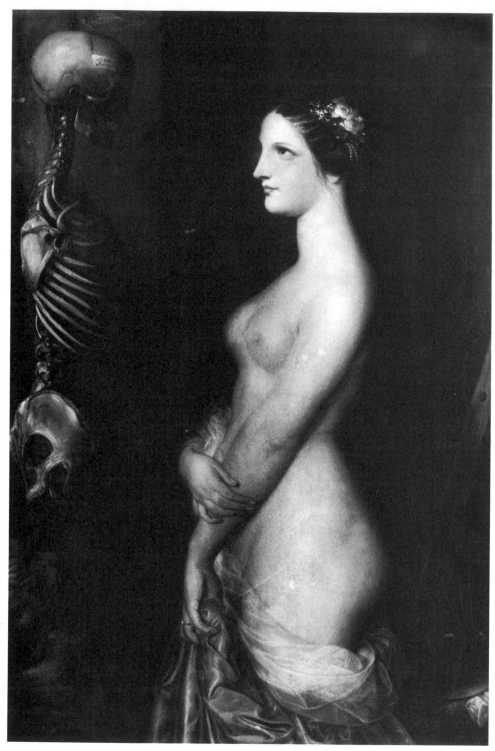

Antoine-Joseph Wiertz, *La Belle Rosine*, 1847

worry whether you like it or not.' " And the first woman will say, "Maybe I ought to try that," or, "I don't know if I can get away with it, but . . ." You begin to get the sense that it isn't "your" problem, it's "our" problem. That happens when people feel that they can take the risk of talking about what they're really scared about.

I'm also very careful to make sure that they get responded to when they do talk. If they say, "I was really scared when I woke up this morning and realized I had to have another bone scan," you respond to it: "You must have felt really terrible. What do you do to help yourself handle those fears?"

MOYERS: What does responding in that way do for them?

SPIEGEL: First of all, it normalizes the reaction. People sometimes tell themselves, "Well, a normal person would handle this fine. I'm the only one who's really scared like this. I'm being silly. It's just a procedure." But expressing their fear in the group helps them feel that their strong emotional reaction to a tough situation is a perfectly normal thing. It also reminds them that they're not the only person in the world who has this kind of suffering. When you get seriously ill, you tend to think there's this normal, healthy, happy world out there, and everybody else is just trotting along, doing their thing, and here I am, miserable and scared to death. They find out that other members of the group are fighting their own demons as well. And seeing that becomes a way of not feeling so removed from the course of human life.

MOYERS: Do you have a strategy for making this happen, or do you improvise?

SPIEGEL: The strategy is basically to try to draw as many people as possible into discussing the common theme and sharing parallel experiences so that the problem becomes a group problem rather than an isolated individual problem.

MOYERS: What do you do about the woman who wants to deny the experience of illness and who just wants to get fixed and go home?

SPIEGEL: I gently, and sometimes not so gently, challenge the denial. Usually, if somebody really wants to deny her illness, the issues don't come up. If they bring up issues, they're usually saying, "I'm struggling with this internally, and part of me wants not to deal with it, and part of me knows that I have to." So when they say, "Oh, there's no point talking about this," I'll try to find some hook: "Well, look, it may seem that this isn't very helpful, but you mentioned that it's been on your mind for the last week, and you've had trouble doing your work because you keep thinking about this. So maybe that's your way of telling yourself you've got to do something about it." I'll try to find a way to suggest that they need to deal with it in a more direct fashion.

There was a woman in the group who was rather reluctant to tell other people that she had cancer. That was her way of making it not real—you know, if other

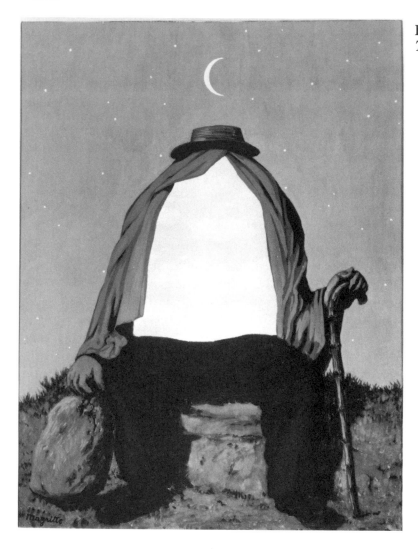

René Magritte, *The Therapist,* 1937

people don't know about it, somehow it isn't really happening. But as she talked, it came out that most people probably already knew she had cancer. What she was really doing was saying to those people, "I can't talk about this with you." I told her, "Look, they know about it. You're just telling them not to discuss it with you." So she began to let the barriers down and to talk a little more about what was going on. When she did, she discovered that it was easier for her to talk with her friends, not harder, if she said, "Okay, this is something we can discuss openly."

MOYERS: You allowed her to let the barriers down—but don't you sometimes have to tear down their defenses?

SPIEGEL: Well, I'm a great respecter of defenses. I'm quite willing to say directly, "Look, I don't see it this way. It sounds to me like so-and-so knows you've got cancer even though you're not talking about it." Now they're free to disagree with me. I can't make people do anything, but I can give them a push in a direction. Also, what really helps in the group is that I'm not the only one saying, "Handle this differently." I can turn to someone else in the group and ask, "What happened when you did this?" You get the shared experience of the group. Also, when I turn to members of the group and say, "I feel so much closer to you now, knowing what you've been going through," that's very immediate. It's not preaching at them, it's a kind of understanding and caring we can feel in the room. And that can be a powerful way of teaching.

MOYERS: How do you know when the group is coming together and beginning to work?

SPIEGEL: The first thing I notice is that there's more going on than I can figure out. When a good group is really rolling, there are a number of very important issues, and I can't quite manage them all. Secondly, the discussion is more or less evenly distributed around the room. It isn't one or two people giving a monologue, it's everybody chiming in with some experience. Third, there's a lot of emotion in the room. People may be crying, or they may be laughing, but there isn't a flat, stiff, empty kind of feeling. Fourth, there's almost a palpable sense of caring. You just have a sense of being together in an intimate way, in which you really care about what happens to the people in the room, and they seem to care about you. That caring grows over time as people share what they're going through and develop a history of helping one another.

In the beginning, a group can be somewhat formal. People tend to overrepresent their resources and how well they're coping. They say, "Well, you know, I don't like having cancer, but so-and-so comes and cooks meals, and so-and-so else comes and takes me out for a walk, and everything is really just wonderful. I've got more support than I know what to do with," and so on. They present themselves as though they had it in hand, and there weren't any big problems, really. But over time they begin to admit that they need help dealing with this illness. They don't quite have it all in hand as much as they said they did in the beginning.

MOYERS: I've known men for whom bravado is the chief resource they call on when they hear this kind of news.

SPIEGEL: Absolutely. Some men, when they start having chest pains with a heart attack, get down on the floor and do push-ups to prove to themselves that it's not happening.

MOYERS: A member of your group, Debbie, recently died. How did the other women react?

SPIEGEL: I think there were a number of complex things going on. They were frightened. No doubt one part of what they were feeling was "There but for the grace of God go I. We have the same illness. She died, and I'm going to die." At one level it was very upsetting. They missed her, and they felt unfinished. They were sort of angry—"Why didn't I say this to her? Why didn't I say that to her?" Also, they were valuing what they had gotten from her. I think it forced some of them to reorder priorities in their own lives, to say, "You never know when it can happen, so if I'm going to do something that I want to do, I'd better do it now, while I can."

MOYERS: What happened to the group as a group after Debbie died?

SPIEGEL: I think the group began to become a much more coherent unit. We were people with a common history, and part of that history was that we had lost Debbie, and we had grieved her loss together. There was a sense that it was very important to be informed right away because we were members of a unit who all deserved to know what was happening with any member of it. The group came to feel much more strongly that there was an understood commitment and caring among them.

Ironically, there's something reassuring about grieving losses. When we spend time mourning the death of someone we knew and cared about, it's also a message to us that when our time comes, we will not slip away unnoticed, but that we, too, will be grieved and cared about and missed. That's reassuring because many of us have an anxious fantasy, as we think about our own nonexistence, that the world will roll on just fine without us. Somebody will throw a flower on our grave, and then we'll be ignored. That can make us very frightened about the prospect of dying. But seeing that what we do is appreciated and cherished by the people we care about makes dying less frightening than it otherwise would be.

MOYERS: You bring the patient's family in when you can. Why do you do that? Isn't this hard on them?

SPIEGEL: What's hard on them is that someone they love has cancer. We do have monthly family meetings at which the spouses, children, and parents of the patients come in and talk about their side of it. John, Debbie's husband, actually put it very beautifully. He said, "You know, at first I hated the cancer. I was angry at it. And then I realized that if I hated the cancer, I hated Debbie, because she had cancer, and part of what she was was that." Many of the members in the room were a little shaken because their own denial was punctured by the fact that one of the members had died. They came to feel that to really be close to the person who had cancer, they had to allow themselves to feel all the discomfort that comes with knowing what

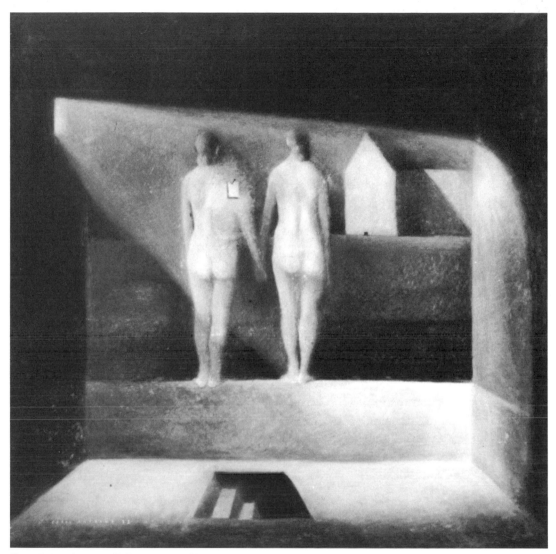

Carol Anthony, *Pilgrimage II,* 1983

cancer is and what it can do. One husband left the meeting saying, "I've been putting off that discussion with my wife about what this means, and I'm going to go do it now." Dying is terrible, but dying alone is worse. And to allow the cancer to interfere with the caring you have for one another is really tragic and unnecessary.

MOYERS: How common is breast cancer in this country?

SPIEGEL: Breast cancer is distressingly common. One in nine women will get breast cancer at some point in their lives. One way to think of it is that a 747 full of women get breast cancer every day in the United States. And a 747 full of women die of breast cancer every third day.

MOYERS: What's the difference between breast cancer and metastatic breast cancer?

SPIEGEL: Breast cancer is a very treatable illness, and the earlier it's caught, the more treatable it is. If the cancer has not spread to other parts of the body, the odds are quite good that it may never do so, and the women will live to die of something else. But once the cancer has spread to some other part of the body, which is what we call metastatic breast cancer, then the problem shifts, and the question is not whether one will die of the cancer, but when.

MOYERS: How long do these women with metastatic breast cancer have to live?

SPIEGEL: After the cancer has returned, the average survival time is two years, although some people survive a long time, even with metastatic breast cancer.

MOYERS: So when you work with these women, you know you're not going to save them.

SPIEGEL: Yes, that's clear. But what I find very rewarding is getting to know them and trying to help them live as richly as they can with the time they have, because the issue that we deal with in the groups and the issue in all of our lives is really quality, not quantity. It's how you live your life, and how fully you use your own resources, and do what you want to do in the world, and make and cherish relationships that are important. Some people do that in two months, and some people never do it in a lifetime. I find it a privilege to help these women live the lives they have as fully as possible.

MOYERS: If the findings of your study are replicated, what do you think it means for medicine?

SPIEGEL: It will be very exciting, because if they're replicated, what it means is that we have to change the definition of what health care is. We have to add to the surgical and medical interventions—which we're doing with increasing skill—a standard component of treatment that involves helping the person who has the disease deal with it and feel supported through it. It means that health care is more than just physical intervention. It's support from a caring physician and health care team and some kind of group intervention to help people who are seriously ill learn how to cope with it as fully as possible. That would be a wonderful change in the direction of health care and a cost-effective addition to helping people live better and perhaps live longer.

III

THE MIND/BODY CONNECTION

*"What is mind? No matter. What is matter?
Never mind."*
— THOMAS HEWITT KEY

"Recite the Gettysburg Address," she says.

We are at the Rainbow Babies and Childrens Hospital in Cleveland. Dr. Karen Olness has attached me to a biofeedback machine to demonstrate how she helps children cope with the pain of migraine headaches. Her request mystifies me, but . . . no problem, I tell myself confidently. My high school speech teacher, Julia Garrett, made me memorize Lincoln's famous speech before she would consider me for the senior play, and I've never failed her since.

I close my eyes and begin: "Fourscore and seven years ago, our fathers brought forth on this continent a new nation, conceived in liberty and dedicated to the proposition that all men are . . . created . . . equal. That all . . ." My mind goes blank. I open my eyes. The little white line measuring my heart rate on the screen is bouncing up and down.

"You were groping," Dr. Olness says, looking at the screen. "And your heart rate jumped." I don't tell her it was because of fear of failure or embarrassment.

She suggests a different approach. "I would like to ask if you would mind closing your eyes and thinking about something that is a very comfortable place for you, something that's very relaxing, perhaps someplace where you'd like to be or have been. And just focus on enjoying that feeling for a couple of minutes."

I close my eyes again. In my mind I am standing on a peak near the western slopes of the Rockies. I have been to this spot only once, a dozen years ago, but the experience is as immediate and exhilarating now, in my mind's eye, as it was that day, when my friend and I paused to catch our breath and found ourselves silently, slowly turning in a circle, a complete circle—Black Elk's Great Hoop—and seeing, as far as one could see, nothing but sky and clouds and mountains, a 360-degree prospect, as pure as Eden, as peaceful as a baby's breath.

"That's very nice," Dr. Olness says. She is watching the screen. "Nice and steady. Just look at that pattern for a minute."

I look. The little white line moves serenely across the screen, like a sailboat on the waveless horizon.

"You obviously are even more stable than your normal pattern when you think of that place," Dr. Olness says.

"I'll have to go back one day," I reply.

"You just did," she says.

It came as no surprise to me that biofeedback could demonstrate that what we think and feel indeed influences the response of our bodies. But paradoxically, I also knew as I began this journey that for hundreds of years philosophers and scientists separated mind from body. We owe great advances in medical science to that sharp distinction. Scientists analyzed organs, tissues, and cells independently of mind, and learned how to explain disease in terms of germs or wayward genes. They didn't invoke the mind to explain sickness. It wasn't necessary. Infectious diseases such as smallpox and polio succumbed to a medical model that leaves mind out.

As we researched this series, we found that scientists now have begun to challenge this fundamental assumption. They say we are on the verge of a medical revolution that is bringing mind into the equation.

I found striking examples in the work of two men at the University of Rochester. Scientists had long thought that the immune system, our bulwark against disease, operated alone, making us better or worse on its own, without the mind's influence. But neuroscientist David Felten has traced the nerve threads that run like wires between the human nervous system and the immune system. The mind and the immune system "talk to one another," as he puts it. What he has found leads him to say that "we can no longer pretend that the patient's perceptions don't matter. And we can't pretend that healing is something doctors do *to* a patient." His colleague Dr. Robert Ader, an experimental psychologist, provided a practical demonstration of the link between the nervous system and the immune system in his work with laboratory animals. In an experiment based on classic conditioning techniques, Ader found that rats could learn to suppress their own immune system.

Other scientists have been exploring the chemical links between mind and body. Candace Pert, former chief of the Brain Biochemistry Section of the National Institute of Mental Health, says that molecules called neuropeptides provide the crucial connection. Strung together like a strand of pearls, the neuropeptides act as messengers, traveling through the body and linking with specific receptor molecules as if guided by antennas tuned to the brain. Because their activity fluctuates with our states of mind, Pert refers to these peptides as "the biochemical units of emotion," translating emotions into bodily events.

Traditionally, we have thought of the brain as the mind's home. Pert believes that the mind resides in the body as well as the brain. "Indeed," she argues, "the more we know about neuropeptides, the harder it is to think in the traditional terms of a mind and a body. It makes more and more sense to speak of a single integrated entity, a body-mind."

If, as it now appears, mind and body are intimately connected, I wonder whether scientists can tell us precisely how that affects our health. "That's what we're still working on," says Margaret Kemeny, a psychologist and researcher at UCLA. We know that "when we feel happy, or sad, or angry, or fearful, there are very clear changes taking place in regions of the brain which cascade down through the body, but just how our immune system or our cardiovascular system is changed by specific emotional states is still the subject of much debate.'' Kemeny makes it very clear that the popular notion that happiness is good for our health while sadness is bad for us has no scientific basis. Her own research seems to suggest that the most harmful state of mind is chronic depression—as distinguished from sadness or grief. But she warns that scientists are still gathering the evidence.

I listen to these men and women, each of whom is tentative, cautious, suggestive rather than emphatic about conclusions, and believe them when they say we are a long way from understanding the manifold connections between mind and body. But even the journalist, himself wary of excessive claims in a field where dashed hopes are legion, can sense the importance of their work. If someday we do understand these connections, we will have redefined human physiology and gained the basis for expanding the frontiers of healing.

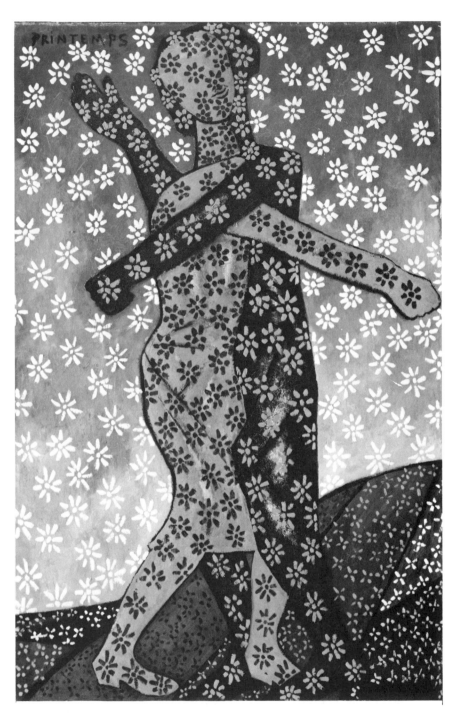

Francis Picabia, *Printemps,* 1937–38

THE CHEMICAL COMMUNICATORS

Candace Pert

CANDACE PERT, Ph.D., is Visiting Professor at the Center for Molecular and Behavioral Neuroscience, Rutgers University, and a consultant in Peptide Research in Rockville, Maryland. She was formerly Chief of the Section on Brain Biochemistry of the Clinical Neuroscience Branch at the National Institute of Mental Health. She discovered the opiate receptor and many other peptide receptors in the brain and in the body, which led to an understanding of the chemicals that travel between the mind and the body.

MOYERS: As a research scientist, how did you get interested in the connection of mind and body?

PERT: Well, I started out being a very basic molecular biologist working on the receptors of psychoactive drugs, particularly the receptors for the opiates—you know, opium, heroin, codeine, Demerol. There's a chemical in your brain, almost like a keyhole, that receives all of these opiates, and that's called the "opiate receptor." As a student, I developed ways to measure these receptors, which had been hypothetical up until that time. That led to the discovery that the brain makes its own morphine, and that emotional states are created by the release of the chemicals called endorphins, which is shorthand for "endogenous morphines."

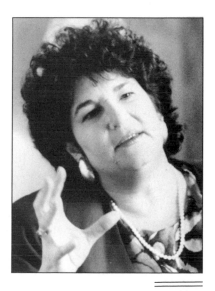

In the beginning, like many other neuroscientists I was secretly interested in consciousness, and thought that by studying the brain I would learn about the mind and consciousness. And so for most of my early research I concentrated from the neck up. But the astounding revelation is that these endorphins and other chemicals like them are found not just in the brain, but in the immune system, the endocrine system, and throughout the body. These molecules are involved in a psychosomatic communication network.

MOYERS: "Psychosomatic communication network"?

PERT: Information is flowing. These molecules are being released from one place, they're diffusing all over the body, and they're tickling the receptors that are on the surface of every cell in your body.

MOYERS: Are the receptors like satellite dishes?

PERT: Very much so. That's a good image of it if you can imagine millions of satellite dishes all over one cell. The cells are being told whether they should divide or not divide, whether they should make more of this protein or that protein, whether they should turn on this gene or that gene. Everything in your body is being run by these messenger molecules, many of which are peptides. A peptide is made up of amino acids, which are the building blocks of proteins. There are about twenty-three different amino acids. Peptides are amino acids strung together, very much like pearls strung along in a necklace. If you can imagine twenty-three different-colored pearls, you can see how you could have information capable of making infinite numbers of peptides. Some peptide strings are quite short. For example, the peptide enkephalin, which is the brain's own morphine, is only five amino acids long. Others, like insulin, are a couple of hundred amino acids long.

MOYERS: Where are they?

PERT: They're everywhere and that's what really shook everybody up. After the brain's own morphine turned out to be a peptide, many scientists began searching to see which peptides they had known in other contexts could be found in the brain. The answer was, just about all of them. And then in the eighties we began to find peptides in the immune system and everywhere else.

MOYERS: Why are they important?

PERT: They seem to be extremely important because they appear to mediate intercellular communication throughout the brain and body.

MOYERS: How are they related to emotions?

PERT: We have come to theorize that these neuropeptides and their receptors are the biochemical correlates of emotions.

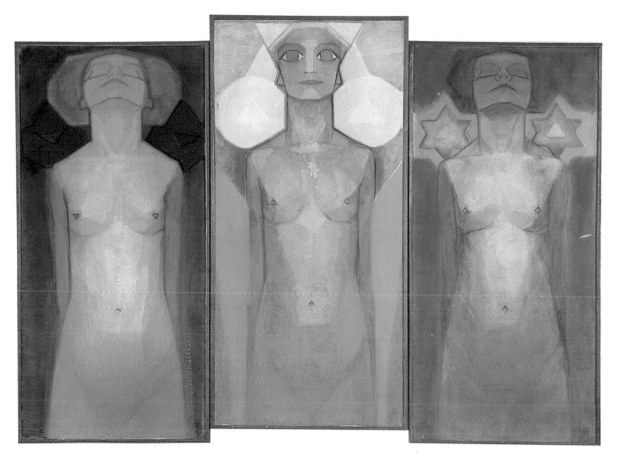

Piet Mondrian, *Evolution*, 1910

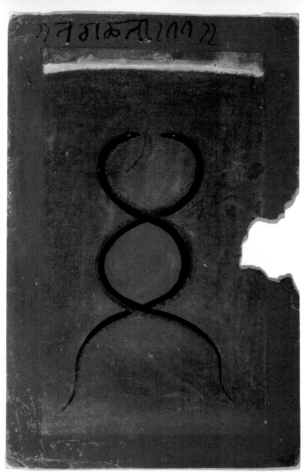

Intertwined Serpents, Indian manuscript, 18th c.

Winthrop Chandler,
Dr. William Glysson, ca. 1780

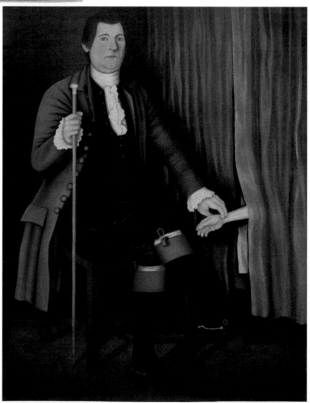

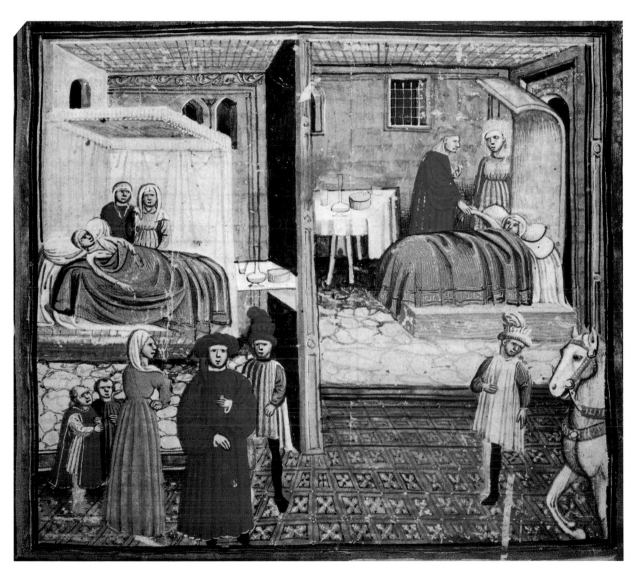

The Doctor Visits, French manuscript, 15th c.

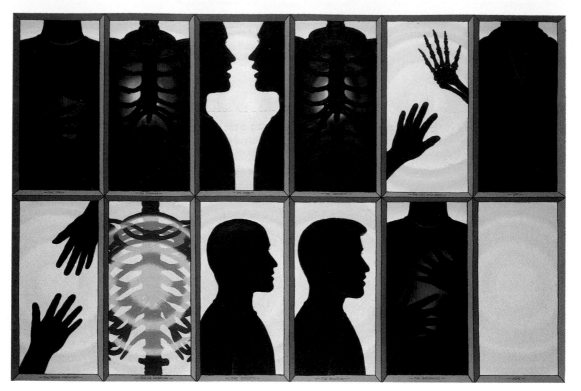

Roger Brown, *Cancer*, 1984

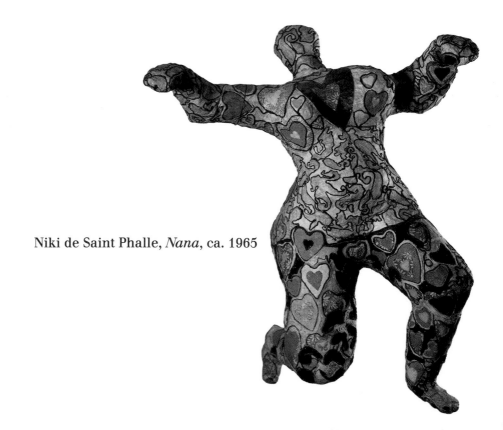

Niki de Saint Phalle, *Nana*, ca. 1965

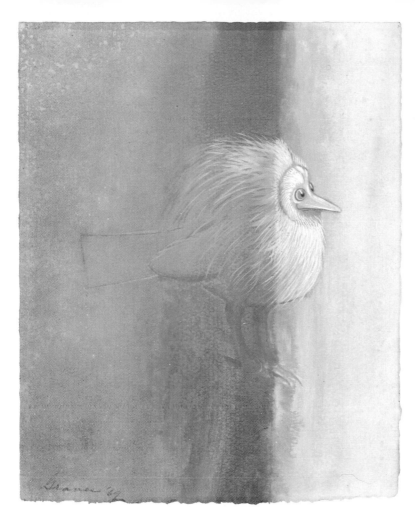

Morris Graves, *Bird Experiencing Light*, 1969

Transformation mask, Haida, 19th c.

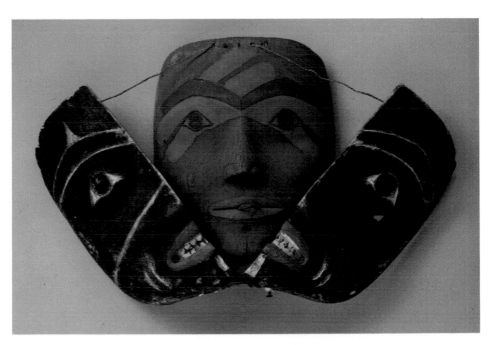

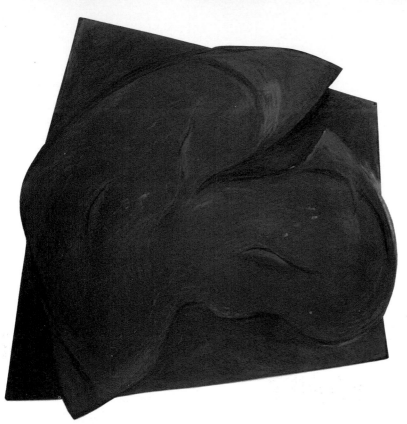

Richard Pousette-Dart,
Call Out into Space, 1991

Joan Grubin, *Heart*, 1990

Pablo Picasso,
Brooding Woman, 1904

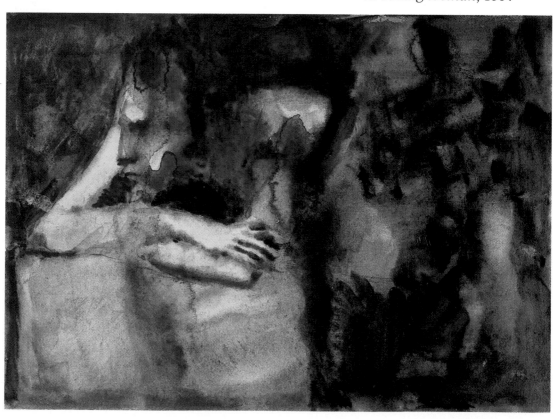

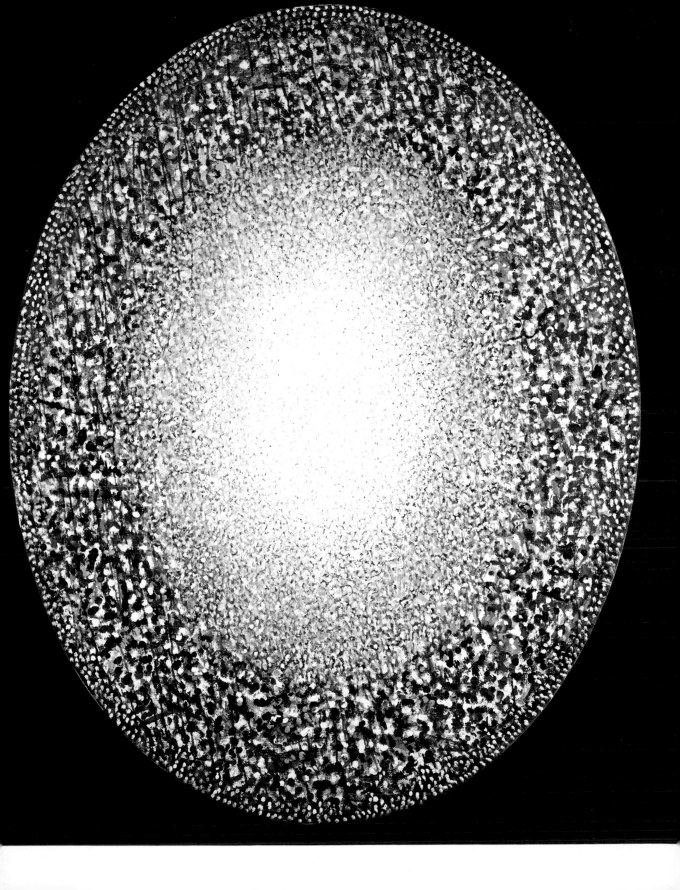

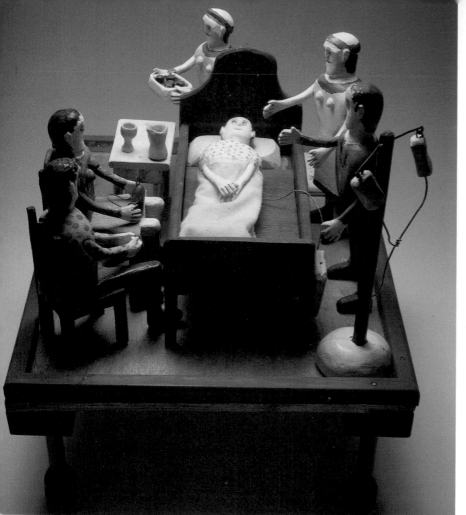

Carleton Garrett,
Visiting Hour, 1989

Alfredo Castañeda,
What Has Happened to You,
Seeker of Treasures? 1985

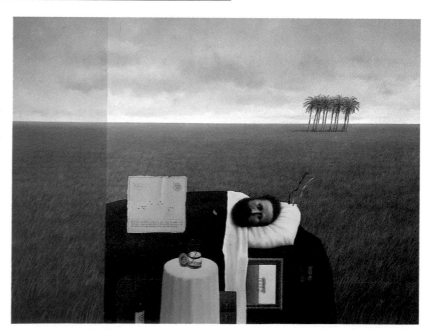

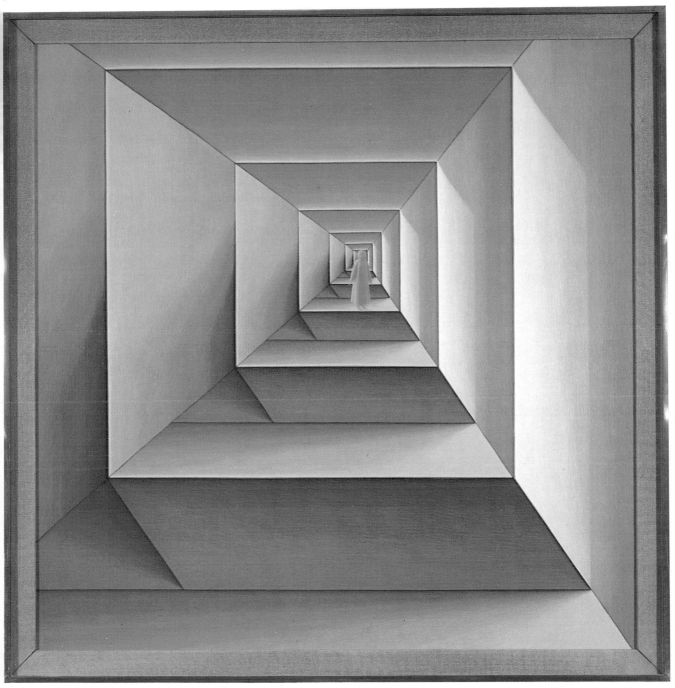

George Tooker, *Farewell*, 1966

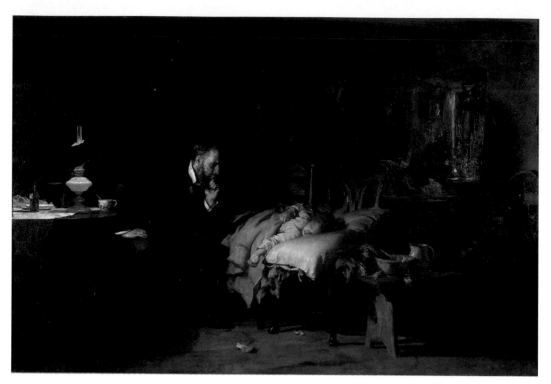

Luke Fildes, *The Doctor*, 1891

René Magritte, *The Future of Statues*, 1937

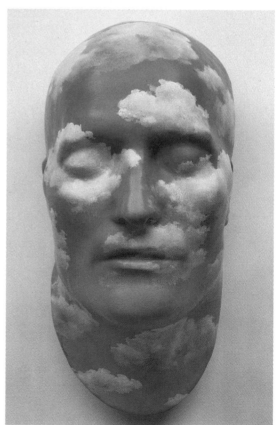

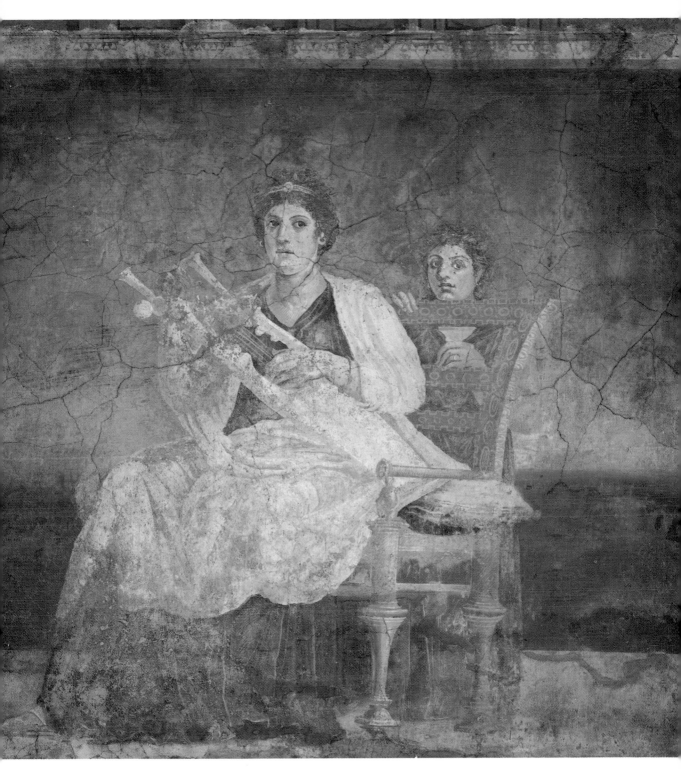

Woman Playing a Kithara, Roman fresco, ca. 50 B.C. (Greek ideas of the therapeutic values of music persisted on into Roman times)

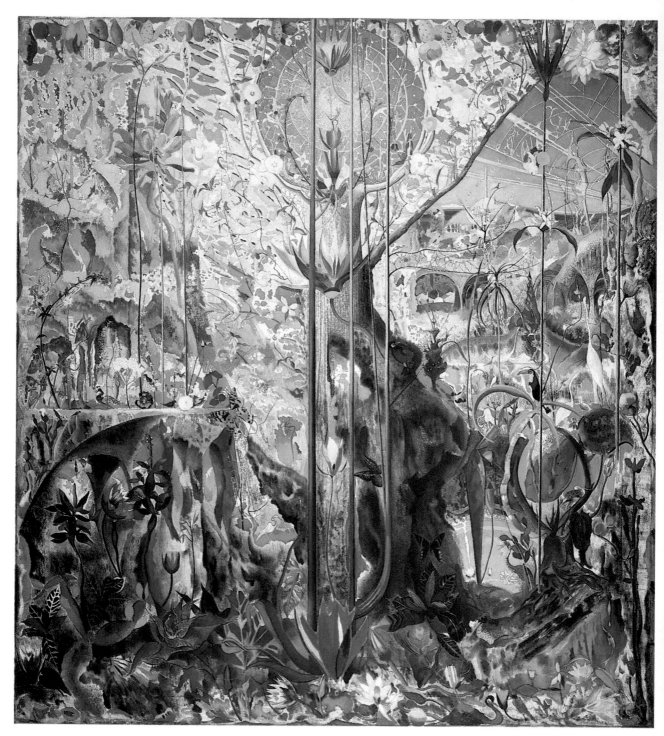

Joseph Stella, *Tree of My Life*, 1919

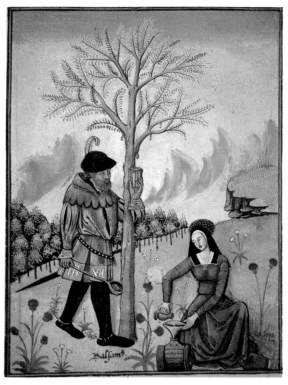

Balsamus (collecting balsam for medicinal use), French manuscript, 1480

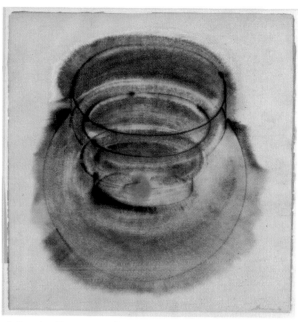

Morris Graves, *Morningstar Kiva*, 1970

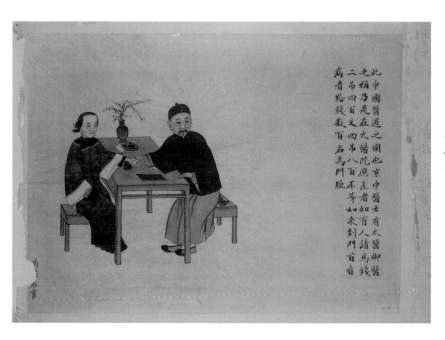

Zhou Pei Qun, *Physician Taking Woman's Pulse*, 19th c.

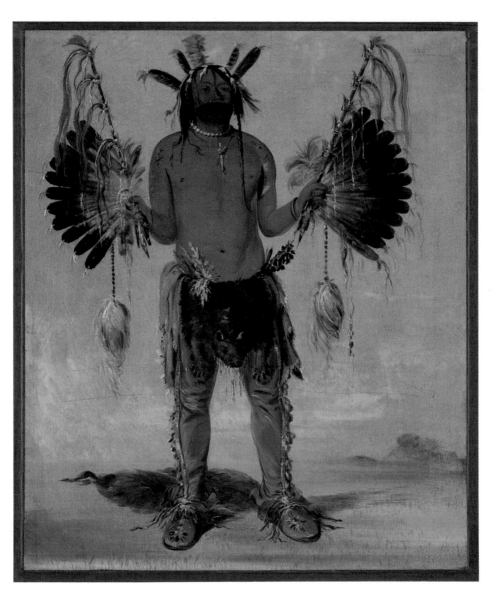

George Catlin, *Old Bear, a Medicine Man*, 1832

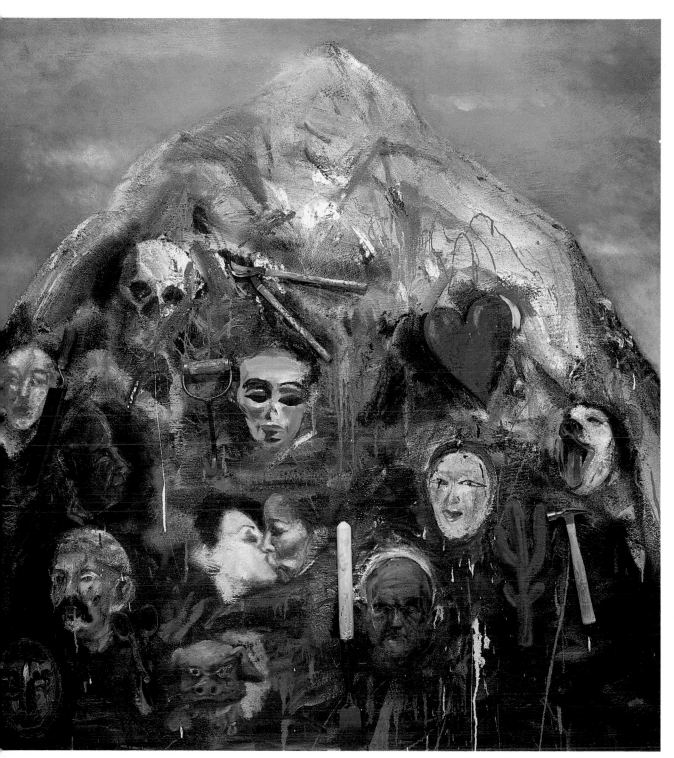

Jim Dine, *The Mountain*, 1991

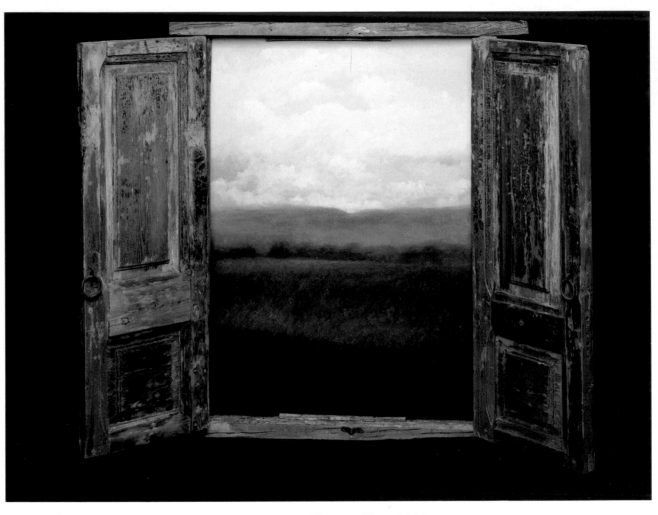

Carol Anthony, *New Mexican Window: A Western View*, 1991

MOYERS: But we think of emotions as psychological.

PERT: Yes, psychological—in the realm of "psyche," or "soul." But I'm saying that we've actually found the material manifestation of emotions in these peptides and their receptors. These receptors floating around on the surface of the cells put out their little antennae and receive what's coming in. There's actually a physical attachment process between the peptide and the receptor. And once that binding process occurs, the receptor, which is a big, complicated molecule, wiggles and changes in such a way that things start to happen. Ions start pouring in, and other changes happen, and eventually the brain receptors perceive what's happening as emotions.

MOYERS: For example, if I'm at a football game and somebody steps on my toe, I first feel pain, and then almost instantly I feel anger. How dare you do that! Is that a neuropeptide saying "Feel angry, buddy!"?

PERT: Well, the pain is conducted along a nerve and all the way up into the brain. Those pain pathways through neurons are extremely well worked out in scientific studies. The anger response is not so well worked out, but we think it involves the release of a neuropeptide somewhere. We don't know which neuropeptide. You notice the anger is a little slower because the neuropeptide has to be released, and there has to be a diffusion to the receptors.

MOYERS: But is the anger mental or is it physical?

PERT: It's both. That's what's so interesting about emotions. They're the bridge between the mental and the physical, or the physical and the mental. It's either way.

MOYERS: So, to carry the metaphor forward, the peptides are sort of like radar coming from the brain, and these receptors are taking them in.

PERT: I like the image of the radar because it starts getting out of the mechanistic model of lock and key that most people use, and it reflects the energy aspect of all of this. We're not locks and keys, and we're not clocks; we're living matter. And living matter is not the same as nonliving matter. Right within the brain itself there are about sixty of these neuropeptides. The endorphins are one.

MOYERS: Are you saying that the mind talks to the body, so to speak, through these neuropeptides?

PERT: Why are you making the mind outside of the body?

MOYERS: It's been knocking around the West a long time—the notion that the mind is somehow distinct from the body.

PERT: Well, that just goes back to a turf deal that Descartes made with the Roman Catholic Church. He got to study science, as we know it, and left the soul, the mind, the emotions, and consciousness to the realm of the church. It's incredible how far Western science has come with that reductionist paradigm. But, unfortunately, more and more things don't quite fit into that paradigm. What's happening now may have to do with the integration of mind and matter.

MOYERS: We journalists are often guilty of missing the answer by posing the wrong question. I asked, "Is the mind talking to the body?" and you caught me on that. So if you were posing the question appropriately from your research, how would you phrase it?

PERT: I would ask, "How are mind and matter related to each other?" But remember, I'm a scientist, not a philosopher, and I get a little frightened if I'm pushed too far out of my realm. I think, though, that we have sufficient scientific evidence to hypothesize that these information molecules, these peptides and receptors, are the biochemicals of emotions. They are found in the parts of the brain that mediate emotion. They control the opening and closing of the blood vessels in your face, for example. They allow the systems of the body to talk to each other.

MOYERS: They're agents of information?

PERT: Exactly. They carry messages within the brain, and from the brain to the body, or from the body to the body, or from the body to the brain. The old barriers between brain and body are breaking down. The way scientists like to work is to have the immunology department over here and the neuroscience department over there. People from these departments don't talk to each other that much unless they're married to each other. But in real life the brain and the immune system use so many of the same molecules to communicate with each other that we're beginning to see that perhaps the brain is not simply "up here," connected by nerves to the rest of the body. It's a much more dynamic process. I once went to a meeting in Rome called "Opiate Endorphins in the Periphery." The "periphery"—that's anything except the head. But the old emphasis on the brain is breaking down now that we're discovering, for example, that cells of the immune system are constantly filtering through the brain and can actually lodge there. We're discovering things that are shocking even me!

When people discovered that there were endorphins in the brain that caused euphoria and pain relief, everybody could handle that. But when they discovered they were in your immune system, too, it just didn't fit, so it was denied for years. The original scientists had to repeat their studies many, many times to be believed. It was just very upsetting to our paradigm to find mood-altering chemicals in the immune system—and not just the chemicals, but the receptors as well.

MOYERS: These messenger molecules you're talking about are also called neuropeptides, are they not?

PERT: Right. I call them neuropeptides because I'm neurocentric. I started as a neuroscientist. But in a way that's a silly word, too, because there's more endorphin in your testes than there is in some parts of your brain. One way to think of neuropeptides is that they direct energy. You can't do everything at every moment. Sometimes the energy needs to go toward digesting food. At other times more blood needs to flow through your spleen. If you've been challenged with a bug that can cause a fever, then you've got to put more energy into your spleen and less energy into digesting your food. Something needs to tell you, "You'd better not eat right now."

MOYERS: Why do you call these neuropeptides "biochemical units of emotion"?

PERT: Well, it took us fifteen years of research before we dared to call them that. But we know that during different emotional states, these neuropeptides are released. It looks like emotion in the broadest sense. Let me give you an example. A peptide called angiotensin is connected with thirst. You can take an animal that's sated with water, but if you inject it with angiotensin, it will just drink and drink. The peptide binding to that receptor makes the animal's mind feel thirst. That same peptide binding to the lung makes the lung conserve water. That same peptide binding to an identical molecular entity in the kidney makes that kidney conserve water. The molecular entity is the same. It's like a brick that can be used in the basement of a house or in the attic of a house—it serves different functions in different locations, but it's the same brick. And overall, there's an integration process affecting the behavior at the whole-animal level so that everything in the animal's mind and body is saying, "I want water, I want to save water, I don't want any water to be lost."

MOYERS: I can see that, but what makes me say "I'm sad" or "I'm happy"?

PERT: It may just be some peptides in your intestine. In other words, it goes both ways. If you accept the premise that the mind is not just in the brain but that the mind is part of a communication network throughout the brain and body, then you can start to see how physiology can affect mental functioning on a moment-to-moment, hour-by-hour, day-to-day basis, much more than we give it credit for.

MOYERS: So instead of saying the mind is talking to the body, you would say "I'm talking to myself," because these neuropeptides are regulating the emotions that I "feel."

PERT: Yes, through receptors in the parts of the brain that we've long known are associated with the experience of emotions. Years ago it was shown that when surgeons electrically stimulated the brains of people undergoing epilepsy surgery, they would laugh or cry or be in ecstasy—in other words, the patients would emote just from electrical stimulation of certain parts of the brain. We now know that those parts of the brain are loaded with virtually all of these peptide-information substances and their receptors.

MOYERS: And so they send these messages like little canoes down into the body, where they find waiting ports of call.

PERT: Well, it gets weirder than that. The message doesn't literally have to go from the brain into the body. It can happen almost spontaneously.

MOYERS: But what's happening?

PERT: We don't know, but I feel that the person who will figure this out is going to be a physicist, because clearly there's another form of energy that we have not yet understood. For example, there's a form of energy that appears to leave the body when the body dies. If we call that another energy that just hasn't been discovered yet, it sounds much less frightening to me than "spirit." Remember, I'm a scientist, and in the Western tradition I don't use the word "spirit." "Soul" is a four-letter word in our tradition. The deal was struck with Descartes. We don't invoke that stuff. And yet too many phenomena can't be explained by thinking of the body in a totally reductionistic fashion.

MOYERS: And by "reductionistic," you mean—

PERT: That it's just chemical and electrical gradients, and that one day everything will be explained without invoking some other energy.

MOYERS: But what you're describing with neuropeptides seems to me essentially a chemical reaction. You call these neuropeptides chemical messengers. As they go from one place in the body to another, the body creates a physical response.

PERT: You're right—and that's what makes it all so fascinating, that emotions are in two realms. They can be in the physical realm, where we're talking about molecules whose molecular weight I can tell you, and whose sequences I can write as formulas. And there's another realm that we experience that's not under the purview of science. There are aspects of mind that have qualities that seem to be outside of matter. Let me give you an example. People with multiple personalities sometimes have extremely clear physical symptoms that vary with each personality. One personality can be allergic to cats while another is not. One personality can be diabetic and another not.

MOYERS: But the multiple personality exists in the same body. The physical matter has not changed from personality to personality.

PERT: But it does. You can measure it. You can show that one personality is making as much insulin as it needs, and the next one, who shows up half an hour later, can't make insulin.

MOYERS: So in the person with multiple personalities, the brain is releasing different messengers.

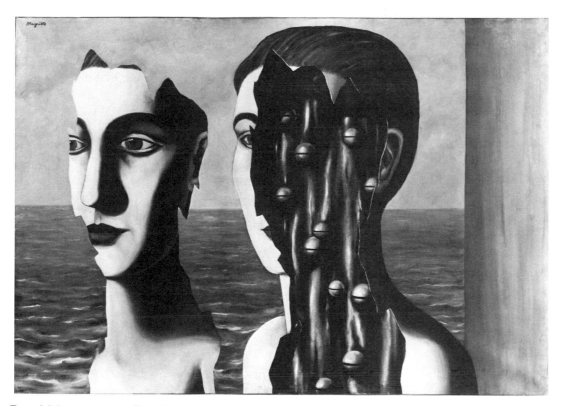

René Magritte, *Le Double Secret,* 1927

PERT: That's one possibility. We just haven't done the research to know that yet.

MOYERS: On the basis of the research you have done, what do you think is going on when I get a "gut reaction"?

PERT: Well, your mind is in every cell of your body. We know that because so many cells of the body contain these molecules that we've been mapping.

MOYERS: So this gut reaction is a mental act?

PERT: Yes, it's a mental act—the wisdom of the body. We don't have to sit here and say, "Okay, stomach, it's time for you to move that food along. Okay, spleen, we need a few more white cells for these viruses." All that is going on beautifully on a subconscious level that we don't need to deal with. Someone stepped on your toe, and before you even thought, "Someone stepped on my toe," you felt anger. Your body was alerting you. These things have survival value.

MOYERS: Just the other day I stepped out into the street, and a cab came down almost on top of me. I immediately stepped back. I didn't tell myself to step back, my body just took me back. After the taxi had passed, I got angry at the driver, and I wanted to curse. All the same thing?

PERT: Sure, that's the wisdom of the body. It's not as if your head is thinking up things and telling your body what to do. Your body is knowing what to do.

MOYERS: The danger was instant and then the anger at the driver was instant. And all of this is physical, chemical?

PERT: Of course. And it's also emotional and in this other mental realm, too.

MOYERS: So you're saying that my emotions are the same as my physical reactions, and that they occur when a particular molecule hits a particular receptor?

PERT: I believe that's true, yes.

MOYERS: You've seen the molecule hit a receptor?

PERT: Absolutely. I've measured it.

MOYERS: But have you seen the emotion it carries with it?

PERT: I've seen animals behave as if they had that emotion. Scientists who study rat and monkey behavior have seen animals behaving and have measured increases and decreases in the amounts of the neuropeptides being released.

MOYERS: You know from scientific research that certain reactions occur when the neuropeptide hits the receptor. But there isn't any way to identify the emotion that emerges from that, is there?

PERT: We're really in the very early stages of being able to figure out which peptide mediates which emotion or whether combinations of peptides are involved. We have a few that we know pretty well because we have psychoactive drugs that give a certain effect. For example, we know that cocaine is a euphoriant, and we know what receptor system it interacts with in the brain.

MOYERS: When you snort cocaine, you immediately get a rush, or a "high," as it's called.

PERT: Right. And the reason you get this high is that the receptors for taking up and inactivating one of the messenger molecules gets blocked by cocaine. It binds to that receptor and interferes with the normal destruction of the chemical that causes euphoria.

MOYERS: But euphoria is a physical response to a drug. Grief is something else, is it not?

PERT: You bet, but I'm sure there are chemicals that mediate grief. If there were a plant that made us feel grief, nobody would have cultured it, and so nobody would know about it today. It might be growing down there in the Amazon right now, but who would know?

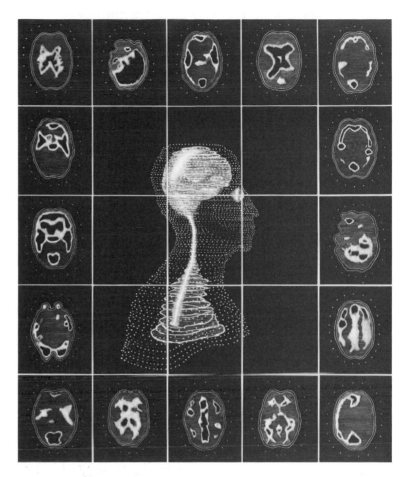

Joshua Simons, *16 States,* 1987

MOYERS: But you haven't identified the grief peptide, have you?

PERT: I haven't, but maybe one of the peptidologists has, and we might know it under another name. We might not realize yet that it causes grief because if we dropped that molecule into a rat's brain, we couldn't tell if the animal was feeling grief.

MOYERS: The existence of peptides is not conjecture, you've seen that.

PERT: Me and ten thousand other scientists.

MOYERS: But isn't it conjecture that from the reaction of peptide to receptor comes an emotion?

PERT: I think we're on firmer ground with some peptides than we are with others. There's a lot of work to be done, and the killer experiment that will link mind to matter, and peptides and receptors to emotion, has not yet been done. But we do know that not all the emotions are up in your head. The chemicals that mediate emotion and the receptors for those chemicals are found in almost every cell in the body. In fact, even one-celled animals have these peptides.

MOYERS: But simple organisms have no critical faculty. My big toe may feel something, but it can't tell whether it's feeling fear or anger or happiness or sadness. My mind has to come into play.

PERT: To say, "I am feeling this," and to analyze that, your brain is of course coming into play. But there are many emotional messages that don't percolate up to your level of knowing them. Even so, they are used to run everything in your body.

MOYERS: Wait a minute. You're saying that my emotions are stored in my body?

PERT: Absolutely. You didn't realize that?

MOYERS: No, I didn't realize it. I'm not even sure what I mean by that. What's down there?

PERT: Peptides, receptors, cells. The receptors are dynamic. They're wiggling, vibrating energy molecules that are not only changing their shape from millisecond to millisecond, but actually changing what they're coupled to. One moment they're coupled up to one protein in the membrane, and the next moment they can couple up to another. It's a very dynamic, fluid system.

MOYERS: And every time they couple, every time they connect, every time they respond one to another, chemical messages are being exchanged. And my body responds differently according to what cell is getting what chemical.

PERT: Absolutely. You got it.

MOYERS: Then are you saying that we're just a circuit of chemicals?

PERT: Well, that gets to be a philosophical question. One way to phrase it would be, can we account for all human phenomena in terms of chemicals? I personally think there are many phenomena that we can't explain without going into energy. As a scientist, I believe that we're going to understand everything one day, but that this understanding will require bringing in a realm we don't understand at all yet. We're going to have to bring in that extra-energy realm, the realm of spirit and soul that Descartes kicked out of Western scientific thought.

MOYERS: But I can't think of information being elsewhere other than in the cells of my body. That's all I can experience.

PERT: Yes, I used to say that neuropeptides and the receptors are the physical substrate of emotions. Then someone yelled at me and said, "What do you mean, 'physical substrate'? That makes it sound as if they're the foundation of emotions. How do you know the foundation isn't in another energy realm? Why don't you say neuropeptides are the biochemical correlate?'' It's tricky. I don't have the right language because I'm not quite sure. I can say that what it looks like to me is that the currency with which mind and matter interconvert might be emotions. Emotions might actually be the link between mind and body—although I hate the word "link," because it's mechanical and Newtonian, and it suggests fences.

MOYERS: But we do know that body events occur when my cells receive these messages from the neuropeptides. So are you saying that it's the body's reaction that creates the emotions?

PERT: The body's and brain's reactions, yes. The body's everyday physiological functions, both normal and pathological, are creating emotions.

MOYERS: So you are not just speaking metaphorically when you say that the mind is in the body?

PERT: Not at all. I think it's physical, and I think it's real. There are hundreds of scientists who've found these molecules in the various parts of the body.

MOYERS: I'll take your word for it that we can see the molecules in the laboratory, but can we see the emotions carried by those molecules?

PERT: Well, that's where we have the problem. Those pesky emotions. They have a nonphysical as well as a physical reality, so they're hard to study in a laboratory. Hypnotherapy, for example, shows that people can re-experience strong emotional states from their past and then experience physical changes in their bodies, such as pain going away.

MOYERS: So like the sperm meeting the egg, you can see the chemical interaction take place, but you can't really see the life in that matter.

PERT: That's right. We can measure the chemical reaction that gives rise to an emotion, but we can't look under a microscope and say, "That's grief." We can say that a particular peptide, for example, can create euphoria not only in humans, but also even in rats and simpler animals. In other words, we can measure behavior. In fact, using the laboratory approach, all we can do is measure behavior. My work has been interesting because the receptor is the interface where behavior meets biochemistry.

MOYERS: What does that have to do with emotion?

PERT: Well, why else do you think you behave? Everything you do is run by your emotions.

MOYERS: And your emotions are in that reaction in the receptor when the molecule arrives with its information?

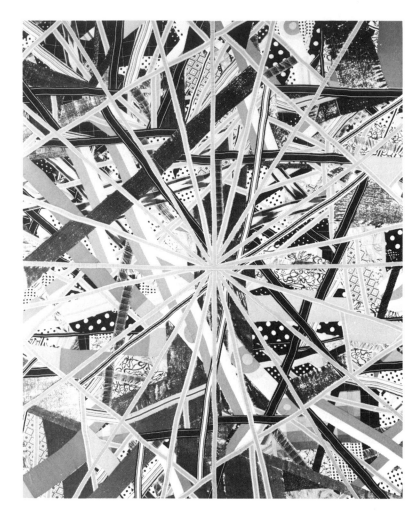

Lucas Samaras,
*Reconstruction
#28,* 1977

PERT: Yes. Remember, though, there are millions of these interactions going on. Like a house made of bricks, your body is made of millions of cells, every one of which is covered with these little satellite dishes.

MOYERS: I understand that in terms of my behavior. For example, if I step into the street, and then I see a car coming, instantly there are messages about danger, and I step back. The brain is talking to me through this reaction in the receptor.

PERT: You're still thinking it's your brain, but it's the wisdom of the body. Intelligence is in every cell of your body. The mind is not confined to the space above the neck. The mind is throughout the brain and body.

MOYERS: So the mind is more than the brain?

PERT: Definitely.

MOYERS: The brain is just three pounds of meat?

PERT: No, the brain is extremely important. It is our window to the outside of the body, through the eyes, the ears, the nose, the mouth.

MOYERS: Then what is the mind?

PERT: What is the mind? Gosh, how frightening! I'm a basic scientist, and I'm having to answer, "What is the mind?" The mind is some kind of enlivening energy in the information realm throughout the brain and body that enables the cells to talk to each other, and the outside to talk to the whole organism.

MOYERS: And what does all of this have to do with my health?

PERT: Everything. Look what's happening to me—I'm becoming a health nut because the implications of this work makes you think more and more about the nature of health and disease. The word "health" itself is so interesting because it comes from a root that means "whole." Part of being a healthy person is being well integrated and at peace, with all of the systems acting together.

MOYERS: Have you changed your notion of health because of your research into peptides and molecules?

PERT: I have changed so much from my research that it's frightening. I've been transformed by my research. For example, when I had my first child, I didn't know that the body makes its own pain relief, its own morphines. When I had my second child, I had learned about these endorphins, and so I thought it was logical that they would play a role in childbirth. Why would they be there? It must be a natural analgesic system. So I went natural with the second child because I had more faith and confidence in my own ability to release the drugs that I needed.

MOYERS: But what about our emotions? Can our moods and attitudes physically affect our organs and our tissues?

PERT: I believe they can, because moods and attitudes that come from the realm of the mind transform themselves into the physical realm through the emotions. You know about voodoo death—in some cultures, if you tell people there's a death hex on them, they'll die.

MOYERS: But what about healing? How does your research help us understand the process of healing?

PERT: Recent discoveries suggest that the surface of the monocyte, which is one of the prime cells in the immune system, is covered with receptors for peptides, these biochemicals of emotion I've been talking about. If you cut your finger, in seconds these monocytes come out of your bone marrow, go right to the site of the injury, and begin to remanufacture and restructure the body fabric.

MOYERS: And that happens instantly?

PERT: It happens all the time. It's happening now. We've probably had five little things happen in the last ten minutes, while we were talking, where monocytes went to the rescue.

MOYERS: I see how these monocytes can help to heal a wound, but I have a hard time seeing how that is connected to the emotions. As a Westerner, I think of illness as being caused by a bacteria or a virus. If I pick up a bacteria, I'm likely to get sick.

PERT: Well, of course your immune system responds— but, just to take one example, viruses use these same receptors to enter into a cell, and depending on how much of the natural juice, or the natural peptide for that receptor is around, the virus will have an easier or a harder time getting into the cell. So our emotional state will affect whether we'll get sick from the same loading dose of a virus. You know the data about how people have more heart attacks on Monday mornings, how death peaks in Christians the day after Christmas, and in Chinese people the day after Chinese New Year. I never get a cold when I'm going skiing. Another example: the AIDS virus uses a receptor that is normally used by a neuropeptide. So whether an AIDS virus will be able to enter a cell or not depends on how much of this natural peptide is around, which, according to this theory, would be a function of what state of emotional expression the organism is in. Emotional fluctuations and emotional status directly influence the probability that the organism will get sick or be well.

MOYERS: That's a kind of conventional wisdom, isn't it? We've known that for a long time.

PERT: Of course it is.

MOYERS: But will we ever be able to put our minds and our bodies in a certain state so that we affect our immune system positively?

PERT: Theoretically, that should be possible, and some people believe they're finding ways to do that. I certainly don't have the answers, though.

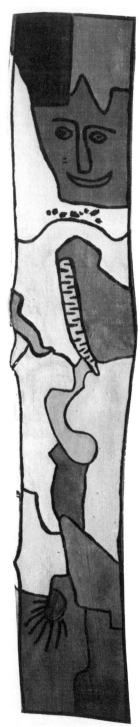

Gaston Chaissac,
Totem, 1959

MOYERS: You're modest in not claiming more than your scientific work allows you to claim, but a lot of people are speculating that the next step will be to try to create the emotion that will help direct our health.

PERT: It's clear to me that emotions must play a key role, and that repressing emotions can only be causative of disease. A common ingredient in the healing practices of native cultures is catharsis, complete release of emotion. Positive thinking is interesting, but if it denies the truth, I can't believe that would be anything except bad.

MOYERS: So a part of health is letting these true emotions of grief and sorrow and anger and fear work their way through to catharsis. Is there anything in your research that suggests that repressing emotions is bad for us?

PERT: Not in my research, because that is on the molecular level. But there is a growing body of literature, much of it European, that suggests that emotional history is extremely important in things like the incidence of cancer. For example, it appears that suppression of grief, and suppression of anger, in particular, is associated with an increased incidence of breast cancer in women. This research is controversial, and there are always methodological issues to address—but it's very interesting.

MOYERS: You've said that we're on the verge of a scientific revolution. What's the nature of that revolution?

PERT: We're well into the revolution, which has to do with incorporating the mind and emotions back into science. The implications for medical practice, of course, are enormous.

MOYERS: So if medicine begins to incorporate mind and emotion, the field might be retrieved from the hucksters, and the charlatans, and the pop psychologists.

PERT: Yes, but just because the hucksters are out there doesn't mean that we should ignore the possibility that there are some very real and valid aspects of what they're doing. We're too presold on the high-tech, highly unemotional approach. Dean Ornish's work has shown that a combination of stress-reduction exercises, meditation, group therapy, and a vegetarian diet can actually reverse damage to the heart muscle. That's very surprising to doctors.

MOYERS: What your research suggests is a physical, biological ground for the effect of emotions on health, right?

PERT: Exactly. The knowledge of these molecules and where they are can provide a possible rationale for the mind and emotions affecting health. Our experiments won't prove that they do, but the rationale is there. Of course, I have to be careful, because I can't be responsible for somebody setting up shop somewhere and saying,

"I'm going to tease your peptides and heal you." But if you want my opinion, I think the pendulum has swung much too far in the other direction. We're sold on high-tech, incredibly expensive medicine that's bankrupting the country. Why not try a little prophylaxis? Let's begin to appreciate simple, less expensive therapies that deal with releasing emotions, and let's get some sound scientific studies to see what works better. For example, the Spiegel study shows that women with breast cancer who met with other women in a support group lived twice as long as women who had the same chemotherapy but didn't get together to talk. I think in Western medicine we've come to the point where we're ignoring what's obvious. I think we need to go back a little.

MOYERS: But researchers and doctors do want to know if there's some physiological basis for this, and that's what your research is trying to suggest. Is your work finding acceptance among your more traditionally minded colleagues?

PERT: They don't disagree with my basic work on any level. Of course, the theoretical ramblings I'm allowing myself here are not really in the scientific literature, so nobody is likely to get me on them.

MOYERS: What would you like me, a layman, to know about healing and the mind?

PERT: Norman Cousins said something to the effect that having the confidence to believe that almost anything is possible can translate into being able to heal. If telling people about my work can provide them with a scientific rationale that gives them greater confidence in themselves, and in their own mind, throughout their body, to heal themselves, then I feel that I'm making a contribution.

MOYERS: But isn't there a danger in that? Now, if I have a cold, I assume it's because a virus entered my body, and so I don't feel guilty. But if I believe that thinking positively can keep me well, then I blame myself for my illness.

PERT: That's part of the tension around this paradigm shift. If it's true that emotions are critical in health and disease, then people shouldn't feel guilt, they should just start to take in this new information. People need to open up and learn not to feel guilty but to learn new ways of being and thinking, new therapies, and new strategies.

MOYERS: What is the research of the nineties? Where is it taking us?

PERT: I think we're going to see more applications to health and disease. Knowing that viruses use the same receptors that we're talking about opens up new forms of specific kinds of antiviral therapies where peptide drugs from the outside can block the ability of viruses to enter cells, and can slow the spread of infection. We're

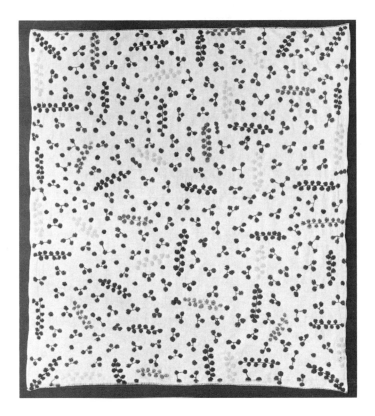

Woman's headcloth,
Guatemala, 1910

going to start using all this theoretical background to come up with new drugs. Parallel to that will be more responsibility for your health using the natural drugs in your own brain. Was it Norman Cousins who said that the biggest and best pharmacopeia is your own brain? It's got every drug in there that you could ever need.

MOYERS: So perhaps in that ancient wisdom there was some real truth—"Physician, heal thyself." Do you really think that we have within us a large capacity for self-healing through our emotions?

PERT: Absolutely.

MOYERS: And you say that as a scientist?

PERT: No, I say that as a human being who's traveling through life and has had some interesting experiences with it.

MOYERS: But where does this trail lead us in regard to emotions and health?

PERT: It leads us to think that the chemicals that are running our body and our brain are the same chemicals that are involved in emotion. And that says to me that we'd better seriously entertain theories about the role of emotions and emotional suppression in disease, and that we'd better pay more attention to emotions with respect to health.

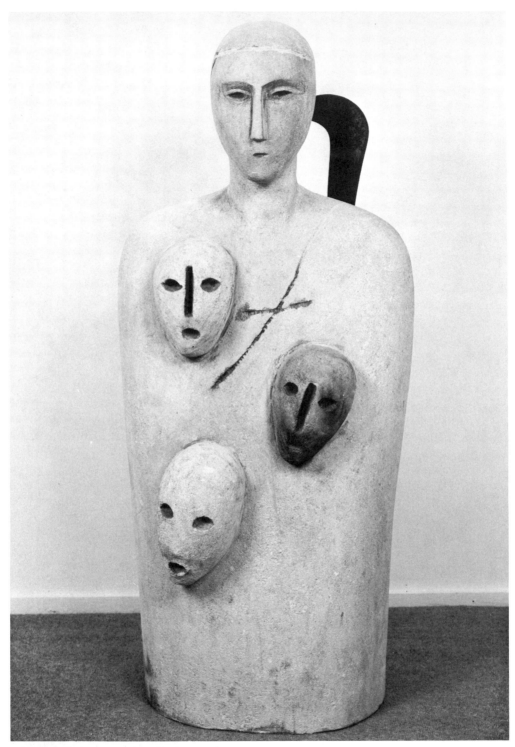

Mimmo Paladino, untitled, 1985

EMOTIONS AND THE IMMUNE SYSTEM

Margaret Kemeny

MARGARET KEMENY, Ph.D., is a psychologist with postgraduate training in immunology and psychoneuroimmunology. She is Assistant Professor in the Department of Psychiatry and Biobehavioral Sciences at the University of California, Los Angeles. Her current research explores the relationship between psychology and the HIV virus.

MOYERS: What are you trying to learn from your work with actors?

KEMENY: The actors study is designed to look at whether short-term emotional changes, such as feeling sad or happy for twenty minutes, affect the immune system.

MOYERS: What led you to use actors for this study?

KEMENY: Well, actors, especially method-trained actors, are perfect for this kind of study because what they do for a living is get themselves into emotional states. They use their own memories and sensations to generate very intense emotional experiences so that when they're on the stage, they can act realistically. If you took one of

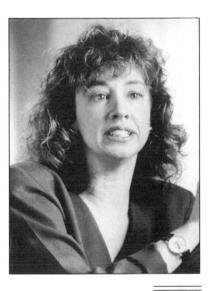

us, for example, and asked us to get very sad right now, we could do it, but not nearly as well as a method-trained actor. So when you're trying to set up an experiment that maximizes the ability of the individual to really experience something intense, one of the best ways is to start with an actor who knows how to do that.

The principal investigator of the study, Dr. Ann Futterman, asked the actors to improvise a monologue based on a standard situation that would elicit sad or happy emotions. Then, when the actor got into that state, we looked for changes in the immune system. For example, we asked each actor to imagine that he had been rejected for a part. He began to feel very intense sad feelings. We found that during the intense sad state there was an increase in the number of natural killer cells in the actor's bloodstream, and that these killer cells were functioning more efficiently than they were when the actor was in a neutral state.

MOYERS: I assume that the natural killer cells are "good" cells—that is, they help us fight off disease.

KEMENY: Yes, in the context of the immune system, natural killer cells are important. They're part of our first line of defense, meaning they can confront foreign organisms without having any prior experience with that organism. They're able to kill cells that have been infected with viruses, and, potentially, they're also able to kill tumor cells. So we need these killer cells, and we need them to be functioning in an optimal way.

MOYERS: What do you mean by "optimal" way?

KEMENY: You need to have them in the right place at the right time, and you need to have them activated so they'll work. And they have to be capable of killing. These cells kill by producing a toxic substance, and they need to be able to do that efficiently.

MOYERS: So when the actor became sad, something healthy happened.

KEMENY: Possibly—at least, it was an increase in the number of these cells and their activity, which potentially is healthy for the individual.

MOYERS: Did this surprise you? Normally, we think that being sad is not good for our health. And here you actually found these killer cells coming prepared to do their job, to defend him against disease.

KEMENY: Right. It was very interesting to us that we found this increase in killer cells with sad feelings—and this was not what we expected. We actually expected the reverse, which would be that with the sad feelings there would be a decrease in the numbers of natural killer cells, and a decrease in their activity.

MOYERS: You also studied each actor as he imagined he got the part and was a big success on opening night. He was exuberant. Did his state of joy have an impact on his immune system?

KEMENY: We found that the effect of the happy state on the immune system was very similar to what we had seen as a result of the sad state. That was very interesting because there really is very little data indicating that happy states have an impact on the immune system. There's a tendency in this field to study negative emotional states rather than happy ones.

MOYERS: Why has science chosen to study negative states?

KEMENY: Well, that's an interesting question that I've always wondered about, too. It may have to do with the fact that medicine is really focused on studying disease processes and not health. The psychiatric model is also focused on pathological emotional states like chronic depression. And it's a very big switch, really, to turn from that model to looking at physically healthy individuals or positive emotional states. When we look at those healthy states, we get a very different picture of how our emotional condition might be related to our biological condition.

MOYERS: Are we discovering that states of emotion, even sad states of emotion, have a positive effect on our bodies?

KEMENY: It's certainly possible. At least these data suggest that when we experience any emotion, there may be similar effects on the immune system, including increases in the number and activity of certain cells circulating in the bloodstream. We've looked only at these two emotional states, but it's very interesting that we find the same immune system outcome for both of them.

MOYERS: What seems certain from your research is that short-term emotions do affect our immune system.

KEMENY: Yes. We saw an increase in killer cells within twenty minutes. And then, once the actor got out of the negative state or the positive state and was sitting quietly for half an hour, the immune system returned to normal. So there was a very brief increase in the number of these cells, and then they returned right back to baseline after the actor stopped experiencing the emotional state.

You know, a lot of research indicates that long-term severe affective states, like depression, influence the immune system. But we really wanted to know what happens in our normal, day-to-day experiences of happiness, sadness, anger, frustration, love. Are those more transitory but important emotional experiences associated with changes in the immune system? And if so, do our emotional states, as we go through the day, have an impact on the development of certain kinds of immunologic diseases, like colds and flu?

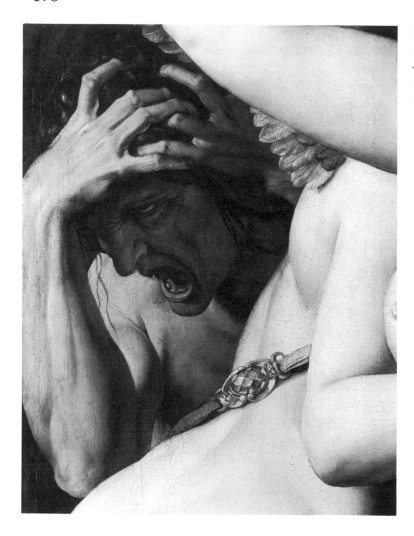

Il Bronzino, *Envy*
(detail from *An
Allegory with
Venus and Cupid*),
ca. 1540

MOYERS: So that if we could learn to alter our emotional states, we might be able to have some positive impact on our body's ability to fight infection?

KEMENY: Right. I think the implication is that there may be a way to use psychological tools and interventions to alter our emotional state in ways that would have positive effects on our immune system. We don't yet know if that is true, although there are some data suggesting that, for example, group therapy has an impact on the immune system. We're only beginning to scratch the surface of that important question.

MOYERS: The possibility that group support could literally have a positive effect on the body in fighting a disease is amazing to me.

KEMENY: Well, it flies in the face of a lot of medical dogma at this moment, which does not put much credence in the psychological condition of the patient. But we have to question that now, because it really does appear that there are linkages between our psychological state and various biological processes. We have not yet taken that important final step, though, which links those changes in biological processes to disease outcomes. We know that the physiology is there—for example, the brain can communicate with the immune system. But we really don't know to what extent that will affect vulnerability to disease. That's why recent scientific work is geared toward trying to make that final link in the chain.

MOYERS: Is there some kind of evolutionary explanation for these physiological changes?

KEMENY: I think a lot of the underlying physiology that explains the relationships between emotions and, for example, the immune system, has to do with promoting the survival of the individual. You're probably familiar with the fight-or-flight response that we generate when something threatens us. You know, we get an adrenaline rush, our pupils dilate, and our heart starts to race. That's adaptive, because it promotes the physiological responses that are required for us to run away or to fight. Emotions are the trigger of the fight-or-flight response.

MOYERS: Do you think that we'll be able to be like the actor and be happy or be sad when we need to affect our immune system?

KEMENY: If you're talking about the ability to control these states and therefore control our physiology, I would point to group therapy as an example of a psychotherapeutic technique designed to help individuals experience feelings more freely. The tendency to suppress feelings is psychologically detrimental.

MOYERS: It could be healthy to grieve, for example.

KEMENY: That's very possible, but again, we're in an area of science that we're really only beginning to understand. It's possible that the experience of feelings per se, whether they're happy or sad, is healthy psychologically and may even be healthy physiologically. Certainly, the actor study suggests that is a possibility. Natural killer-cell activity increased with both positive and negative emotional states. One possible conclusion is that experiencing feelings, even negative feelings, has a positive impact on natural killer-cell activity. And there are some other results that also corroborate that, including one by Dr. Pennebaker of Southern Methodist University, who asked students to write about very traumatic events, and experience the negative feelings that were generated by those events. Pennebaker discovered that when the students dredged up their negative feelings and experienced them, there was actually an enhancement in a particular function in the immune system.

MOYERS: But that seems different from the fight-or-flight response, which happens automatically. My ancestor in the jungle saw the lion and ran. I see the mugger and run. Or I sense the truck come bearing down on me at the intersection, and I run. I don't think about that, I just do it. Why is that?

KEMENY: Well, this is one of the most ancient responses built into us as organisms: that when something threatening appears, we instantaneously experience an emotional reaction, a fear reaction. It's very quick. And we instantaneously experience a cascade of physiological changes that will allow us to mobilize and get out of the situation or deal with it in some way.

MOYERS: But the old dogma used to be that in the fight-or-flight crisis the immune system was unaffected, right?

KEMENY: Yes, it was thought that the immune system played no role in mobilizing the individual to fight or flee, and that it was really an independent process. More recently it was thought that the immune system was a kind of bystander to the fight-or-flight response, so that when you produced all those hormones in response to a threat, a side effect was that the immune system was suppressed. Now there's a third perspective, which is not so well understood, which is that the immune system is part of the fight-or-flight response, and that when you're running away from an animal in the jungle, and you're falling over branches, or whatever, you need a mechanism that will increase the functioning of the first-line-of-defense cells, such as natural killer cells. That way, if you get bitten, or you get a cut, and organisms get into your system, your immune system would be ready to respond and deal with those infections right away. According to this third way of thinking, the mobilization of this first line of defense might actually be a very important part of the fight-or-flight response that enhances the chances of survival.

MOYERS: So this suggests that our emotional responses do enhance our chances of surviving a disease when we're threatened.

KEMENY: Right. While the fight-or-flight response mobilizes your ability to fight or to get away from the threatening animal, the immune system might be protecting you from the other kinds of organisms that are getting into your system as a result of that encounter. Maybe what we're seeing is the emotional reaction to the threatening experience changing all kinds of physiological processes, including the immune system, in an adaptive way.

MOYERS: But you can't say this conclusively yet.

KEMENY: No, this is a theory at the moment, which is supported by our actor study and a couple of other studies, including one we did immediately after the 1987 Los Angeles earthquake. We were interested in finding out whether there would be

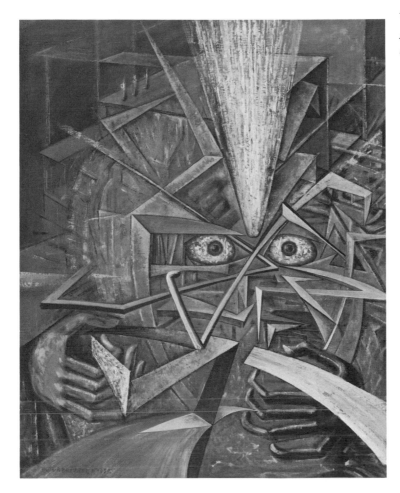

Victor Brauner,
*Breakdown of
Subjectivity*, 1951

any change in the immune system immediately after the earthquake, when people were distressed and afraid and worried that the "big one" might be coming next. We drew blood on nineteen people two to four hours after the earthquake, and then we drew blood on those same individuals over the next year, to establish a kind of baseline. Again, we found that in contrast to what we expected, there was an increase in the number of natural killer cells in the bloodstream immediately after the earthquake. Something about the distress that the individuals experienced appeared to be correlated with an increase in the number of natural killer cells.

MOYERS: What's the significance of that finding?

KEMENY: I think the significance is similar to what we found in the actor study, which is that when we experience an immediate negative emotion like fear, there may actually be a temporary increase in the natural killer cells and their activity. Now if that emotional experience were prolonged for days or weeks, we might see a decrease in these cells and their activity. But if we're looking at that window of time right after the initiation of a negative emotion, or a positive emotion, we see an increase. That finding is very different from the traditional view that negative emotions are associated with decreases in the activity of certain cells.

MOYERS: So if I'm confronted with a situation where I need to fight or flee, I want more killer cells. But what happens if I live with that same fear for a long period of time?

KEMENY: Well, it's possible that if you live with that fear, which many people do, day after day, and month after month, the mechanisms that pump these killer cells into the bloodstream or increase their activity get depleted over time. The same thing is true of the heart. It's very adaptive to have your heart rate increase when you're afraid, because that allows you to run. But if your heart is racing day in and day out, month after month, it may eventually weaken.

MOYERS: So the emotion of fear that is an instant and temporary response to danger could have a positive impact on your immune system. But if you sustain yourself in that state over too much time, it can actually have a negative impact on the immune system.

KEMENY: Exactly. It seems that emotions are important and have their adaptiveness when they are short-term, when you experience them for a number of minutes, or maybe hours. But when you get into situations that provoke emotions over the long term, then you run the risk of ending up with physiological responses that are no longer adaptive.

MOYERS: I've learned that if you lose a loved one, or you suffer a loss in your life, grieving over it is a healthy thing to do. But if you grieve too long, that becomes depression, and that's not good. Is that what you're saying?

KEMENY: It's very important to make fine distinctions between our reactions to events. One reaction to a loss is a grief response that is usually characterized by a lot of sadness. Another reaction to a loss is depression, which isn't really sadness. Often depression is a very empty state that is not characterized by any emotional experience. It's possible that grief has an impact on physiology that's very different from depression.

MOYERS: Does depression have a negative impact simply because it lasts longer?

KEMENY: We don't know yet, but I think it may relate to the idea that being able to respond to the environment emotionally appears to be adaptive psychologically. And as a result of that, there may also be some adaptive physiological consequences to experiencing emotions. States like depression, which don't allow us to experience our emotions fully in response to the environment, may have a different impact. When we're depressed, we often are less responsive to the environment emotionally. There's certainly accumulating data now that chronic depression has negative biological consequences as well as psychological ones.

MOYERS: We hear of people who lose a spouse and then become depressed and die a couple of years later.

KEMENY: There is fairly good data, although it's not consistent, that people who've lost their spouses are at increased risk for dying themselves over the six months to one year after the loss of their spouse. Hypothetically, that's because many of them are experiencing a depression. The loss is extremely significant, and as a result they feel depressed. That depression then may lead to biological changes that make them more vulnerable to heart attacks and other kinds of diseases.

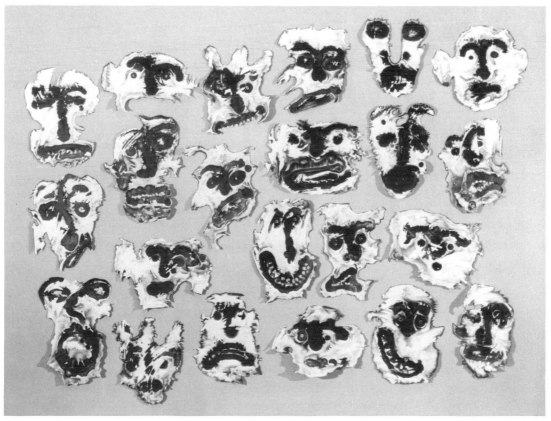

Lucas Samaras, *Head Group No. 3,* 1983

MOYERS: Impairing the immune system.

KEMENY: Yes, there's some evidence now that there is actually an impairment in the immune system of individuals who've recently lost a spouse.

MOYERS: Which means that we're not as able to fight a disease if it occurs in that state?

KEMENY: Now, that's a very important link—but we haven't yet proved it. We haven't yet shown that the immunologic change that is seen with bereavement is the reason for the increase in disease and mortality.

MOYERS: Is grief a mental response to an experience, or is it an emotional response? Is the mind telling the body to grieve, or is the grief just occurring the same automatic way I run if I'm confronted by a lion in the jungle or a truck on the street?

KEMENY: Well, it's interesting to phrase it that way, but the way I look at it—and the way a lot of psychologists look at it—these are simultaneous events. When our mind and our perceptual processes respond to a loss, we respond emotionally to that loss at the same time, and physiological changes are taking place, also, at the same time. When you experience the fight-or-flight response, you feel the emotion of fear, and your heart races, and your pupils dilate, and your muscles tense—all simultaneously. You can imagine the same kind of thing happening with many emotional experiences—for example, with sadness. We don't know so much about it, but there may be an integrated set of mental, emotional, and physiological experiences that take place in response to a loss.

MOYERS: Your own work with AIDS victims seems to bear out some of what you're saying, doesn't it?

KEMENY: Yes, we've been working quite a bit with people infected with the AIDS virus, HIV. Our primary question there is whether or not psychological factors like depression could in any way impact the immune systems of these individuals and increase their risk of developing AIDS.

MOYERS: Any insights yet?

KEMENY: What we've been focusing on is bereavement. We're interested in whether or not men who are infected with the AIDS virus and who are experiencing bereavement, such as the loss of friends or lovers, are more likely to show immune changes. While we've found no relationship between the loss of a close friend and changes in the immune system, we have found that men whose partners died of AIDS did show changes in the immune system after the death of their partners. They're changes that we recognize as negative in terms of the course of the disease, because they suggest that the immune system may be becoming impaired.

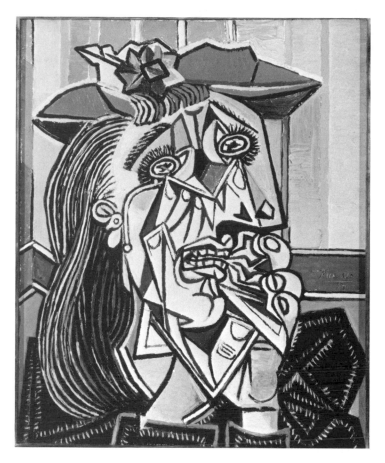

Pablo Picasso, *The Weeping Woman*, 1937

MOYERS: What kind of changes?

KEMENY: We find the immune system becoming more activated. Now, this sounds a little odd, because usually you think that the immune system *should* become activated. But in people infected with the AIDS virus, a more activated immune system is actually associated with a greater likelihood of developing AIDS. It's an indication of a weakness in the immune system.

MOYERS: So the prolonged grief of these men, edging into depression, had a negative impact on the immune system, inviting further deterioration?

KEMENY: Well, we also looked at their psychological reaction to those bereavement events. And to our surprise, we found some indications that depression may be related to these negative changes in the immune system, but that grief may not.

MOYERS: Why should this surprise us?

KEMENY: I think the surprise relates to how embedded we are in the notion that exposure to negative life events and our emotional reactions to these negative events always has a negative impact on our bodies. We've tended to forget that we have a whole host of different kinds of reactions we can experience. You and I can confront exactly the same experience, and you can feel one way, and I can feel a very different way. And those two reactions might have very different physiological accompaniments. So we need to focus on the specific nature of the psychological reactions we have to events. Studies in this area need to determine whether the immune system responds differently to a grief reaction as compared to a depressive reaction to the same kind of event.

MOYERS: Does research point to certain personalities who are prone to illness? Some scientists are looking at that and suggesting that some of us with the so-called "Type-A" personality are more prone to heart attack than others.

KEMENY: I think it's very important to know if there are certain characteristics, such as depression, that increase vulnerability to diseases, but this happens to be an area of science that's relatively weak at this moment. It's really unclear whether personality is related to diseases such as cancer. Probably the best area of research is the Type-A behavior pattern and heart disease. There is some evidence that individuals with the Type-A behavior pattern are more likely to develop heart attacks than individuals with the Type-B behavior pattern.

MOYERS: There are personalities who tend to keep too much in themselves. If in the fight-or-flight response there are hearts that will break, so to speak, if that tension is held too long, aren't there immune systems that are likely to buckle if an emotion is kept too long at attention inside?

KEMENY: It's interesting to think about it that way. You could speculate that the Type-A behavior pattern is characteristic of an individual who manifests the fight-or-flight response on an ongoing basis. They feel fight-or-flight responses when someone cuts them off on the freeway, for example, whereas Type-B persons can experience all kinds of negative events and not mobilize their physiology. If we stay in that fight-or-flight response all the time, it's possible that we produce stress hormones more frequently over the course of a day, and that those hormones then affect our immune system.

MOYERS: Dr. Spiegel's study on the effects of group support on cancer patients suggests that an environment of mutually sharing and giving and caring can have a positive effect on the chemistry of the body. That's the other side of it.

KEMENY: Yes, I think Dr. Spiegel's data suggest a couple of things. One is that mutual support and connection with other people may have a positive impact on health. Another is that the relaxation that comes with group support can counteract the fight-or-flight response. And that may be the reason he showed an impact on survival in those cancer patients. The third is that Dr. Spiegel's intervention was oriented toward people allowing themselves to experience negative feelings and to express them. And that may have been the critical dimension—that experiencing and expressing feelings led to the positive health benefits.

MOYERS: Do you think we'll be able to learn how to trigger our own immune system with our thoughts and our feelings, and that through meditation, hypnosis, and imagery, we could have a positive effect upon our system?

KEMENY: That's a very tricky question because two issues are involved here. One is the commonly held notion that if we have a particular thought, for example, if we imagine a natural killer cell killing a tumor cell, that thought could lead to the killing of the tumor cell. A lot of the imagery work is based on the notion that this kind of direct intervention is possible. But I'd have to say that nothing in the research data and nothing that we understand about physiology leads us to believe that kind of intervention could happen. We have no way even to speculate on how a particular thought about a particular physiological process, such as the activity of a killer cell, could get to the cell and alter it. However, that doesn't mean that it's not possible, just that we have no way of conceptualizing such a possibility at the moment.

MOYERS: Are we on the frontier of something?

KEMENY: Yes, I think we're on the frontier of a really fine-tuned understanding of how psychological changes relate to very specific changes in physiology. The state of science in this area is very global and very coarse in a way. We understand the major life change events and very chronic kinds of experience have physiological effects. But the territory we're entering into now allows us to distinguish between different kinds of emotional states, and how they are related to very specific physiological processes.

MOYERS: But you have no doubt in your own mind, as a researcher, that the mind and the body do the same dance?

KEMENY: From my own viewpoint, the mind and the body are two manifestations of the same process. Even to say they are "interconnected" is improper, because they are two parts of one whole.

MOYERS: Finding a language for this is part of the problem, isn't it?

KEMENY: I think the language is one factor that has prevented us from being able even to conceptualize mind/body processes. Just the fact that we use one kind of intangible language to describe the mind and another kind of material language to describe the body—languages that don't even have a way of connecting—prevents us from seeing that these two kinds of phenomena are actually two manifestations of the same process, neither one more important than the other, and neither causing the other. If we can figure out ways to talk that allow us to think about the mind and body as one and the same, we'd be better off.

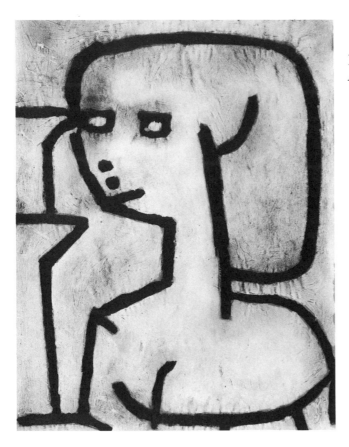

Paul Klee, *Girl in Mourning,* 1939

MOYERS: Are you convinced that there is a science beneath the mind/body connection?

KEMENY: There is certainly an ability now to scientifically investigate the neuropeptides and hormones and cells responsible for linking the mind and brain to the immune system, for example. The question is whether we can use those technologies to answer some of the questions about, for example, emotions and the immune system.

MOYERS: Can we see through a PET scan whether a subjective experience like feeling happy or sad has a physical impact on the brain?

KEMENY: We tend to think that feeling happy or feeling sad is intangible. We experience these emotions, but we don't imagine that they have physical correlates. But in fact, when we feel happy or sad or angry or afraid, very specific changes take place in particular regions of the brain. For example, with major severe psychological states like major depression, certain regions of the brain light up, indicating that there's activity in those regions. But we really don't know yet whether those same regions will light up if someone is experiencing a normally sad or happy state.

MOYERS: How is it that something as intangible as a feeling or a thought can change the chemistry of the body?

KEMENY: Although feelings and thoughts seem intangible, the brain is active anytime we feel or think anything. That activity can then lead to a cascade of changes in the body. The brain, as you know, regulates the heart, the gastrointestinal system, the lungs, and probably the immune system, and each change in the brain can lead to a sequence of changes throughout the body that can have an impact on health.

MOYERS: How is all of this connected to the health or the illness of the body?

KEMENY: Well, for example, it's possible that during certain psychological states like severe unhappiness, you have changes in the brain which then result in changes in hormone levels. Those hormones, circulating throughout the bloodstream over the course of the day, then have an impact on the immune system, because the hormones and the immune cells are all floating around in the bloodstream together. Potentially, that impact of the hormones on the immune cells may alter the ability of the individual to fight a flu infection or a cold. That's one potential sequence of events that might have an impact on health.

MOYERS: But it hasn't been up until recently, has it, that we thought emotions had an impact on the immune system?

KEMENY: Right. Earlier on we believed that we could feel even very severe states with no effect on the immune system. It was as if the brain and the immune system couldn't talk to each other. But now we're learning that in fact, the brain and the immune system do talk to each other and that they're in dialogue with each other all the time. It's a two-way conversation.

MOYERS: What does Athens have to say to Jerusalem? What does the immune system have to say to the brain?

KEMENY: Let's say you get exposed to a cold virus. The immune system would want to say to the brain that the body had just been infected with a particular type of virus so that the brain would set in motion a whole sequence of events that would allow the most effective response to that virus.

MOYERS: Is this area of research expanding? Are we going to learn a lot more in the next ten years?

KEMENY: I think the next ten years will be very explosive in terms of our understanding, not only of how psychological factors relate to changes in physiology, but of the mechanisms that allow that to happen. I think we'll begin to get a different understanding of how physiology works and how these cascades of processes linking the brain to the immune system really take place.

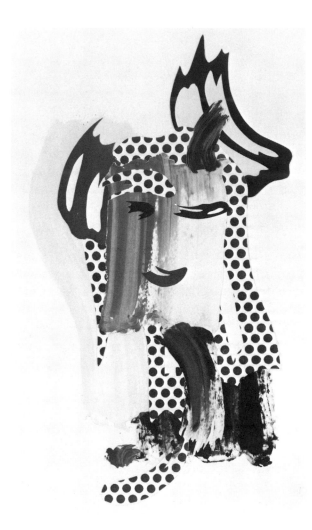

Roy Lichtenstein,
Head, 1986

MOYERS: Where is all this new understanding leading science?

KEMENY: Science is being led in a couple of new directions. One is to move away from the global concepts about the effects of stressful events on physiology and to move toward a really finely differentiated look at how different kinds of psychological reactions and emotions and cognitive states may have very different correlates in physiology. That's one important direction.

I think the other implication of this research is in education. It's no longer sufficient to train individuals in single disciplines, to train a neuroscientist to study only the brain, or to train an immunologist to study only immune cells, or to train a psychologist to study only the psyche. The very, very important questions in science, the ones that will be the cutting edge of the future, and that will lead to very important discoveries, cross the disciplines. We need to allow neuroscientists to talk to immunologists and to psychologists so that kind of communication can lead us to address the questions that span disciplines, and that link the brain to the immune system.

MOYERS: The whole person.

KEMENY: Yes, we need to look at how these linkages are taking place in the whole person and to conceptualize the whole person rather than parts of the person.

MOYERS: Could this also have a practical impact on doctors? So many patients complain that doctors just seem to treat them as if they were machines—you fix a part on this one, and then you turn to the next machine. But if you begin to understand that emotions have an effect on your health, might you not treat patients differently?

KEMENY: One of the most important implications of this work is that medical care needs to incorporate an understanding of how the psychological response of patients may have implications for their health. And health care delivery needs to include not only the very important aspects of medical science, chemotherapy, and surgery, but also psychological approaches that will aid patients in dealing more effectively with whatever disease they may have.

MOYERS: We're likely to learn that some of the old folk wisdom was fairly accurate. You know, I once heard it said of one of my neighbors in Marshall, Texas, that she grieved herself to death. Of course, from what you've said, that was probably depression rather than grief. Are we finding these folk wisdoms to be true?

KEMENY: Well, we may discover that some of the understandings that we have intuitively are also true scientifically—and some of them aren't. We have all kinds of biases through which we look at the world. There are things that we want to believe are true, that may very well not be true. But I do think that some of our intuitive understandings may be scientifically documented.

MOYERS: This is almost a cliché, but it was true in my culture that men were not supposed to express their grief. I remember seeing pain on my father's face after my brother died—he kept his grief bottled up, and it seemed to invite depression.

KEMENY: A lot of data suggest that men and women respond very differently to negative events, and that women feel much more comfortable expressing their feelings. Now, there are also differences between men and women in physiology and in health. It's possible, although certainly not proved, that those expressive differences may be correlated with physiological differences and have different health implications.

MOYERS: It's really an old wisdom—as a man thinketh in his heart, so is he.

KEMENY: Yes, it's an old wisdom, but it's a very important and essential wisdom that I think we need to relearn now and really begin to incorporate in medical care.

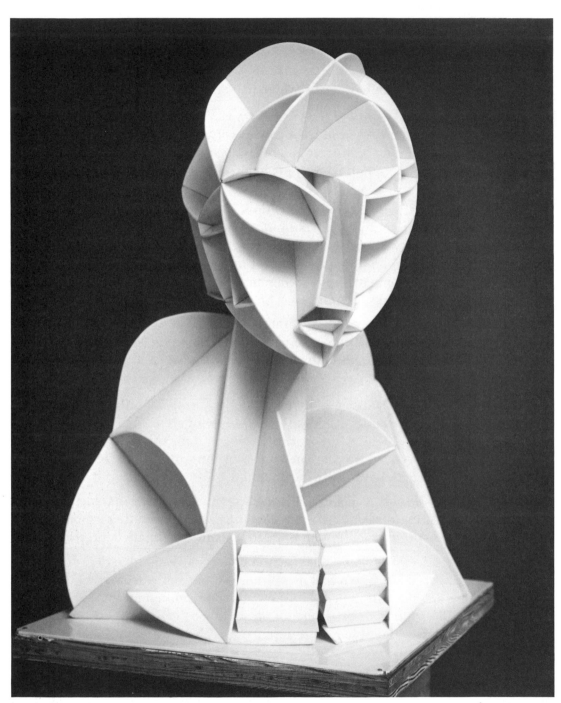

Naum Gabo, *Constructed Head No. 2,* 1916

THE BRAIN AND
THE IMMUNE SYSTEM

David Felten

DAVID FELTEN, M.D., Ph.D., is Professor of Neurobiology and Anatomy at the University of Rochester School of Medicine. He and his wife, Suzanne Felten, Ph.D., have discovered nerve fibers that physically link the nervous system and the immune system. Dr. Felten was the recipient of a MacArthur Foundation Prize Fellowship in 1983 and is Associate Editor of the journal *Brain, Behavior and Immunity*.

MOYERS: How did you get interested in psychoneuroimmunology?

FELTEN: Almost by accident. I came to it with an M.D. and a Ph.D. directed toward neurosciences. I had always been interested in the brain and had studied some of the chemical mediators—called "neurotransmitters"—that communicate from cell to cell in the brain.

One day I was looking through a microscope at tissue sections of liver in order to identify nerves that travel alongside blood vessels. I was having trouble seeing what the cells really looked like, so I said, "Let's go to the spleen. Everybody knows what the spleen looks like." So I started looking at blood vessels and some of the surrounding areas in the spleen. And there, sitting in the

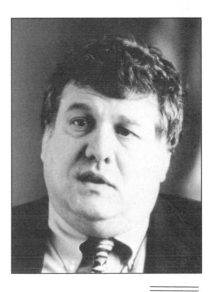

middle of these vast fields of cells of the immune system, was a bunch of nerve fibers. I looked at them and thought, what is this? Nerve fibers aren't supposed to talk to cells of the immune system. What are they doing here?

So we cut some more sections, and looked—and there they were again. We tried other blocks of tissue, and there they were again. They kept showing up again and again. We and others eventually discovered nerve fibers going into virtually every organ of the immune system and forming direct contacts with the immune system cells.

MOYERS: What was the significance of this?

FELTEN: Well, it suggested that the nerves might influence the immune system.

MOYERS: So when you were looking into that microscope, were you seeing something about the healing process for the first time?

FELTEN: I didn't realize it at the time, except that I was struck by the possibility that the nerves might be controlling some aspect of the immune response. A student of mine, John Williams, carried out some of the first studies demonstrating this. But in those days it was almost dogma that the immune system is autonomous and doesn't have any outside controls. We were almost afraid to tell anyone for fear people would say, "Oh, jeez, don't you know the work of Glutz and colleagues?" —or they'd come up with some reference that we had never found and make us look like a bunch of dufuses because we didn't know what we should have known. So we scoured the literature and searched high and low and tried to find every citation on the subject. And the more we looked, the more we realized that if you looked carefully at some of the photographs in other people's publications, you could see nerve fibers sitting out among the lymphocytes—but nobody ever commented on it.

When we went to the immunology literature, we found that the immunologists had discovered receptors for neurotransmitters sitting on the surface of cells of the immune system, but they couldn't quite make sense out of it. Why would a lymphocyte have a receptor for a neurotransmitter? The question just fell by the wayside. Nobody really put two and two together and tried to make a story about the brain having a direct influence on the immune system.

So we joined some of our colleagues, who are immunologists, and started studying immunologic changes that occur when you use drugs to affect the neurotransmitters or when you take the nerves away. Much to our surprise, we found that if you took the nerves away from the spleen or the lymph nodes, you virtually stopped immune responses in their tracks.

MOYERS: Meaning that the mind was carrying on a conversation with the immune system.

FELTEN: That was how we interpreted it. The practical implication was that the many stressors we face in life, which affect the autonomic nervous system, might have an impact on the immune system.

MOYERS: The mind controlling the body?

FELTEN: Yes, and this was the first hint we had. Since that time, Suzanne Felten and I have found a whole host of additional communication molecules. We have many players, many different neurotransmitters talking to many different cell types.

MOYERS: But I had always thought there was a lot of traffic between my brain and the rest of me. I just assumed that something was directing the movement of these arms, for example.

FELTEN: That was known for almost every system except the immune system. For a long time, immunology grew up believing that it was an autonomous field because a lot of experiments were done in the equivalent of test tubes. You can generate an immune response in a test tube. What researchers didn't realize at the time is that other signals come from the brain that may regulate what goes on. In fact, many immunology textbooks still talk about the immune system as an entirely autonomous, self-regulating system. Similarly, the brain scientists approached the neurosciences without taking immunology into account. So the two systems grew up ignoring each other.

MOYERS: And what you found suggested that they don't exist in isolation.

FELTEN: No, they clearly do not exist in isolation. Now there is overwhelming evidence that hormones and neurotransmitters can influence the activities of the immune system, and that products of the immune system can influence the brain.

MOYERS: Does this mean that the mind is talking to the immune system, saying "Hey, there's something dangerous down there. Be alert, be on your guard"?

FELTEN: I'm not sure it's saying it in that precise language, "Be alert, be on your guard." But certainly the brain is capable of signaling to the immune system in times of stress or loneliness, and perhaps under nonstressful, ordinary conditions. The higher centers of the brain can generate signals that very clearly influence hormonal outflow. In certain psychiatric disorders there are changes in some of the hormones. And when you're frightened, for example, there's a huge outpouring of adrenaline and noradrenaline from the sympathetic nervous system and the adrenal gland. What we hadn't contemplated before is that some of these signals that leave the brain when we feel certain emotions may well have an impact on the immune system.

Some of the researchers in this area are studying whether the stress that accompanies certain experiences, such as taking a medical exam, or divorcing, or going into a nursing home, are accompanied by changes in immune response. They've found that one factor contributing to a diminished immune response is whether or not an individual is in control of the situation; another factor is whether or not the individual feels lonely.

MOYERS: How does this affect the old notion that's been around the Western world for a long time—that the mind and the body are separate?

FELTEN: Well, I think that notion is down the drain. I can't imagine anybody thinking that the mind and the body could be separate in view of the multiplicity of connections from the brain to virtually all systems.

MOYERS: What does that mean for medicine?

FELTEN: It means that we have to pay very close attention to the feelings and perceptions of patients, and how they view their health, their disease, and the status of their illness.

MOYERS: And the further significance is that since the immune system defends us against disease—

FELTEN: Yes, our immune system defends us against invading bacteria, invading viruses, and inflammatory responses, for example. It also guards us against tumor cell formation. We depend on it to combat infectious agents that come in through the air, or through our gastrointestinal tract, or through our skin when we get a cut. The immune system has to kill off these invading infections or cells, or the body can be overwhelmed by the infection or the tumor. You can end up dying. We have a natural immunity, which is a generalized attacking mechanism, to try to get rid of some of these invaders, and then we have specific immunity, which generates an immune response against a very particular portion of molecules on the surface of some of the invading cells. The specific, acquired immunity allows you to recognize those same molecules again and again and to attack whenever they come in.

MOYERS: So the immune system is a kind of Maginot Line.

FELTEN: Yes, but it's not just a line. It has many fallback positions, so that if one thing doesn't work, then another mechanism comes into play, and another, and another. The immune system is wonderfully plastic. There are many different ways in which the immune system can try to attack or approach a problem. We have front-line defenses, and then we have backup defenses if the front-line defenses don't work.

So here we have this great defense system, which has a wonderful memory, and can generate responses to past insults that have come in again. And we also have the

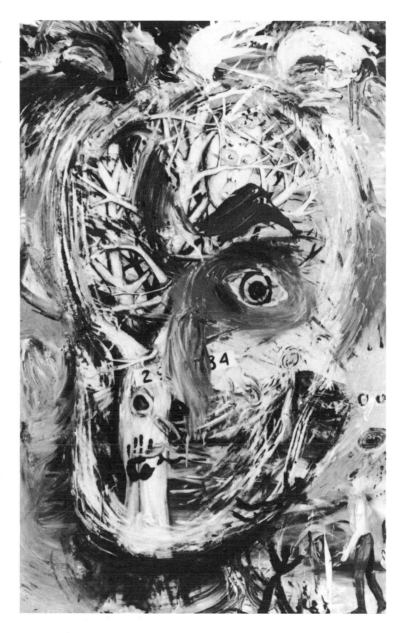

Jonathan Borofsky,
*Self-Portrait with
Head in Tree at
2,987,784,* 1986

brain with its wonderful memory of past experiences. We had thought these two great memory systems were independent. But now it turns out they're not—they talk to each other extensively.

MOYERS: In a football analogy it would mean that it's not just the offensive team that's getting its instructions from the coach, but the defensive team as well. And that's a revolutionary breakthrough?

FELTEN: It's a different way of looking at things, although, in a way, it isn't so revolutionary. It's common sense that what affects the mind or brain might have an impact on our health. You know, we hear people say all the time, "Don't get yourself so stressed out that you become sick." They probably don't realize there is an actual biological basis for that.

MOYERS: In the epilogue to a recent book on this subject, you ask, "Can we afford to ignore the role of emotions, hope, the will to live, the power of human warmth and contact just because they are difficult to investigate scientifically and our ignorance is so overwhelming?" What's the answer to that question?

FELTEN: Of course we can't afford to ignore these things, because if we do, we'll miss wonderful opportunities to help our patients. It turns out that these things do make a difference. Now I can't tell you the mechanism by which they make a difference because we have an abysmal lack of understanding here. There are big holes all over the place. We don't understand some of the brain chemistry of emotion. We don't even understand what measures of our immune response mean in relation to our ability to fight off an infection. We have some guesses, but we don't really understand that yet. Yet we observe individuals with this blazing determination to make it, to survive, to pull through an illness—and they somehow do. We can't afford to overlook that. But it seems as if medicine is going more and more in the direction of high-tech for evaluation and diagnosis at a time when people are crying out for someone who cares for them, someone who will sit down and actually listen to them, and hear how their condition affects them in their social environment and with their family and friends. That can't be accomplished by robots just cranking somebody through the medical system.

I'm not suggesting we abandon the high-tech diagnosis or pharmacology, but that we should add more of a humane and personal touch to medicine. The art is still important.

MOYERS: Because what the patient thinks and feels affects recovery?

FELTEN: It appears so. What we are trying to do now is find the factors that impact on the brain, which then sends signals that change the immune system. Of course, a change in the immune system makes a difference in the patient's disease. Now all of those links have not been made, or we'd understand all of medicine.

MOYERS: Are you suggesting that every time we have a thought or a feeling, hormones are released that somehow send a message to the immune system?

FELTEN: Yes, a constant traffic of information goes back and forth between the brain and the immune system. And certainly we know that hormones are continuously being produced and released, and neurotransmitters are continuously talking to target cells throughout the body. There can be subtle changes and shifts in activity in response to an individual's inner-generated thought process. One study at UCLA used actors and actresses who were told to think about a scenario, and generate in their own minds a feeling that comes with it. While they did this, their hormones in the blood were tested, and you could see changes in some hormones and indications of subtle changes in the immune system, depending on what they were feeling.

Now the big question is, does that make a difference in how the immune system responds to an invader? We don't yet know. We suspect it might, but we really can't say that if you think in a certain direction, and change your lymphocyte activity by X amount, that means you're susceptible to catching a certain type of disease. Where these subtle changes in the immune system may become particularly important is in individuals who are at the very edge of their capacity to respond—someone who's very elderly, for example, or someone who has viral diseases, or someone who has to take drugs that suppress the immune systems. In those circumstances the added impact of a stressor, or some psychosocial factor, or some feeling or mood could push them over the edge.

MOYERS: So if they began feeling more depressed, they might go over the edge into actually feeling worse physically?

FELTEN: Studies suggest that depression as a psychological state is not sufficient in itself to predict diminished immune response and increased susceptibility to illness. But depression does play a role in that the more severe the depression, the more likely you'll find a decreased measure of immune response. In the elderly, depression is more likely to be accompanied by decreased measures of immune response.

MOYERS: Are those studies showing that if I think I'm going to get worse, I'll get worse, and if I think I'm going to get better, I'll get better?

FELTEN: That's what we're trying to find out. I'm not sure that you can generalize that to everybody in every situation, but certainly those of us who have dealt with patients know that a patient's will to live makes a difference. I don't think there's any physician who would deny that. Yet we don't understand how that works. Perhaps some of it works through the cardiovascular system, perhaps some of it through peripheral vasculature, perhaps some of it through the immune system— there are many different systems that can go bad and cause trouble. But the immune system is one that we're particularly interested in with regard to viral infections, bacterial infections, pneumonia, and autoimmune diseases like rheumatoid arthritis—the immune system has an impact on a lot of diseases. So it is obviously of great interest to us to try to pursue the idea that hormones and transmitters flowing out of the brain may have an impact on how the immune system functions.

MOYERS: But hasn't the notion been around a long time that our state of mind affects our health?

FELTEN: Sure. Science is rediscovering what our grandmothers knew years ago. For example, they would tell you not to get yourself stressed because you'd catch a cold. Now studies of the cold virus show there may be something to this.

MOYERS: What's the most striking evidence you've seen that how we think influences how we feel?

FELTEN: Well, one of the most striking pieces of evidence is in the conditioning studies of Doctors Robert Ader and Nicholas Cohen that have been done in laboratory animals and now are being applied to humans. The fact that one can classically condition an immune response is phenomenal. Studies show that you can take a genetically autoimmune animal which will die if it's not immunosuppressed, and you can condition that animal to live on a relatively low level of drug that would not even come close to keeping an unconditioned animal alive. This suggests that the brain knows how to manipulate the immune system. We just haven't figured out how to convince the brain to do that under all circumstances.

MOYERS: So the brain can teach the immune system how to respond?

FELTEN: It can help to regulate the immune system, yes. Your brain can learn how to change immune response.

MOYERS: And what does that mean to me?

FELTEN: What it ultimately means is that we can have any variety of signals into the brain that we might be able to use to therapeutically benefit a patient. We can certainly intervene with drugs, which is one of the common ways that medicine intervenes—but how about intervening by giving somebody social support? How about having some of the social care-givers provide enough counseling and warmth and support to those who are at risk so that they don't feel lonely? Some studies indicate that even very small interventions can make a difference. For example, having college students visit someone in a nursing home on a weekly basis really makes a difference. Now most family members and social workers probably don't think of themselves as actually affecting the chemistry and pharmacology of a patient's nervous system and immune system, but that's probably what they're doing.

MOYERS: You keep returning to this issue of loneliness. I don't quite understand the role it plays.

FELTEN: Loneliness keeps showing up in the studies as a predictor of diminished measures of immune response.

MOYERS: If I'm lonely, what happens?

FELTEN: In one study, of medical student immune responses and examination stress, those students with chronically diminished immune measures were not those at risk of flunking out of school, as you might have guessed, but were those who said that they were lonely and had poor social support. Loneliness shows up again as a factor in lowered immune responses when people in nursing homes have been studied.

MOYERS: Are you saying that patients who feel lonely may in fact be affecting their own immune system, so that if they really feel bad about feeling lonely, their

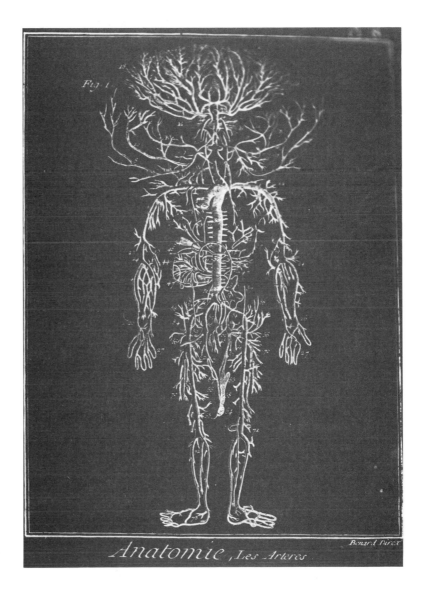

Anatomie, Les Artères, French, 18th c.

immune system doesn't fight the disease, or doesn't fight the illness as vigorously as it might otherwise?

FELTEN: That is certainly a possibility. We don't have absolutely iron-clad demonstrations of that yet, but the trends are pointing to the likelihood that loneliness may leave the immune system somewhat low in its responsiveness. Now one of the difficulties we confront is trying to interpret what measures of the immune response mean. We take peripheral blood, we count lymphocytes, and we look at some of their activities, and their ability to produce more lymphocytes—but we have to ask, what does that mean to a patient with hepatitis? What does that mean to a patient with bronchial pneumonia? Those answers haven't come forward very well. There are still gaps in our understanding of what immune measures mean to a patient's susceptibility to disease. So that's one point where I hesitate a bit, because these studies of loneliness have been done on measures of the immune system taken from peripheral blood. What that ultimately means to a patient's susceptibility to illness, or to their continued downhill course if they are already ill, remains to be worked out.

This is a new field, and there are still lots of holes in the system, because we have to go from a patient's perceptions to a common pattern of hormone and transmitter outflow that we can understand. We're just now struggling with how the measurable impact on the immune system actually makes a difference in whether a patient becomes ill or not.

MOYERS: Your caution suggests that even if we know, for example, that the nervous system and the immune system are connected, those connections may not be clinically significant.

FELTEN: They may not be clinically significant in a number of individuals, but we think they are clinically significant in some people. For example, Dr. David Spiegel did a rather well-known study on women with breast cancer, who were given counseling and peer-group support, along with appropriate medical care, versus appropriate medical care alone. He found that not only did the women report that they were better adjusted and had a better quality of life, but that they lived longer. Now if someone had discovered a drug that did that, they would have had their face on every major newsmagazine in the world as the next Jonas Salk in medicine. But because the difference was correlated not with a drug but with something psychological, his study was met with a certain degree of "Well, let's wait and see"—which perhaps is appropriate.

Now whether or not those hormonal and transmitter influences that were generated by the counseling and peer support acted on the immune system and assisted it to combat some of the metastases from breast cancer remains to be demonstrated, because they did not measure the immune system in that study. But certainly when something is immune-mediated as a disease and responds to psychological inputs coming into the brain, we have to suspect that the brain is having an impact on the immune system. And whether it's a direct impact on cells of the immune system, or an indirect impact through blood flow or whatever, what's the difference, if it works? Of course there's a big difference to us researchers, because we want to find out what the mechanisms are. The better we understand the mechanisms, the more likely we can intervene to make a difference and to change the system.

But an interesting question arises if we see that we can replicate Spiegel's results again and again, and show that counseling does make a difference. Should not counseling then become a standard therapeutic approach to women with breast cancer? Some of my colleagues think not—that if we don't know the mechanism by which it acts, perhaps we'd better be cautious and wait. But I think that if it continues to work, we are honor-bound to use it for the benefit of the patients, and then work vigorously to understand the mechanisms behind it.

MOYERS: But science rests upon knowing or discovering the mechanisms by which cause produces effect.

FELTEN: That's right, but part of medicine is beyond the immediate science at hand. We may not know how counseling, for example, might benefit someone who's depressed, but we also don't know how some of the drugs that we give for depression affect the brain. In some cases we don't have a clue. We can say, "Yes, it affects such-and-such a transmitter"—but what does that mean? We haven't worked it out yet, even though we still use the drugs.

MOYERS: Some critics have said that patients in this kind of research get better because they want to believe they will—you know, the placebo effect, based on the power of suggestion and the response of belief.

FELTEN: A simple effect is a very powerful effect, not to be demeaned. To appreciate the power of such an effect, look at terminal cancer patients who are allowed to give themselves their own morphine injections versus those who receive it from a nurse or doctor. They generally end up with better pain control even though they give themselves less of the narcotic. Their control makes the difference. Now we don't understand the mechanism of that. Does the feeling of being in control result in an increased production of our own endorphins? Maybe. We just don't understand the mechanism yet—but we use it, and we benefit patients. I think that to deny that there are interactions between the brain and the immune system is to play ostrich, to stick your head in the sand. We have unequivocal evidence that these two systems communicate. What we don't yet understand is how much difference that makes in certain illnesses.

MOYERS: Do you think we'll know ten years from now?

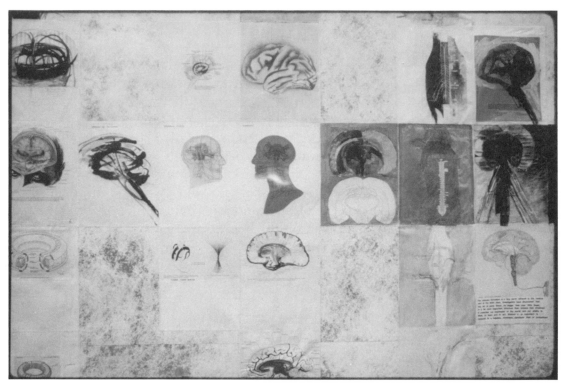

Todd Siler, *Progression and Development of an Intuition* (detail), 1981–82

FELTEN: Oh, yes, absolutely.

MOYERS: But aren't you simply groping toward the obvious? If I'm in the hospital, and I'm feeling bad, I feel better if a doctor comes and sits by the bed and talks to me and shares information with me. If I'm lonely and feeling depressed, I perk up when someone who loves me comes and spends time with me, and we confide in each other. Isn't all this "the world is round after all"?

FELTEN: Yes, it's reinventing the wheel, but it's reinventing the wheel from a much more mechanistic point of view. We're now at least in a position to know that there are mediators, molecules that communicate between the brain and the immune system that might play a role in this. And we are able to look at experimental animals and identify which stress hormones and which neurotransmitters are actually necessary for the animal to respond to that stressor and produce a decrease in immune response. The classic way to study control and stress is to produce a very mild shock that the animal can then shut off. The animal that shuts the shock off does better than the animal that gets exactly the same shock but can't shut it off.

We're not talking about horribly painful shocks, we're just talking about a minor annoyance that the animal can shut off or not shut off. The controllability of that stress makes a difference.

We face many varieties of stress in the hospital. Patients coming into a hospital have the stress of wondering if they're going to have to change their housing conditions, or they may have the stress of a life-threatening illness, or they may have what we would view as perhaps a milder form of stress, which is just an annoyance, with all of the beeps and other noises that we have. Or for some very vigorous people, simply being put into bed may be a terrible restraint and cause stress. Interestingly enough, that has ramifications not only on the immune system side, but on the amount of brain damage that could occur during reduced blood flow. Our working hypothesis is that with stress hormones on board, a decreased blood flow to the brain produces far worse brain damage than what would occur in the absence of those stress hormones. So it may be that both systems are getting damaged in the presence of some of these stress hormones, especially in the elderly, who have susceptibility in both the immune system and the nervous system.

MOYERS: Is this research leading us toward a different way of looking at health and disease?

FELTEN: Well, I think it has to, because if a patient's attitudes and perceptions and emotions make a difference in how the immune system functions, or in how the brain reacts to a given condition of decreased blood flow, for example, then the patient is at the center of medical treatment and care, and we have to talk about the patient as an active, vital participant in healing. It doesn't come from the physician. It comes from the patient. The physician is just one other participant in the process of healing.

It's interesting that, as Norman Cousins pointed out, you rarely hear the word "healing" in medicine anymore. That's a shame. The patient has to be at the heart of healing. And the physician and nursing care-givers and social workers and even family members all have a role to play in the overall healing of a patient.

MOYERS: The very word "patient" has a passive connotation, whereas the word "person" suggests someone who is an active agent in his or her own life.

FELTEN: Yes. I guess the medical profession has become very used to thinking in terms of doing something to a passive recipient. But patients have to be very active participants in their own health. A message has gotten across with regard to diet, exercise, smoking, drug abuse, and so forth—but the message can be extended beyond just those immediate issues at hand. Patients have a vital role to play in their own healing and in many other circumstances, such as autoimmune diseases, or infections, or things of that nature.

MOYERS: What are some of the diseases this information might help us to deal with?

FELTEN: I've been thinking for a long time about what diseases we might target first. The autoimmune diseases, like rheumatoid arthritis or multiple sclerosis, involve a disregulation of the immune system so that it attacks some tissue in the person's own body. In autoimmune diseases you're generating responses against "self." The purpose of the immune system is to protect "self" by generating responses against foreign invaders. But when autoimmune disregulation occurs, right now, you have only one real option—to suppress the immune system so that it can't attack anything, including "self." What we are working on right now is a model of rheumatoid arthritis in rats. We're finding that just by giving drugs that affect nerves in organs of the immune system, like the lymph nodes, we can make the disease either much worse or much better. In other words, we may have a whole new group of drugs that are directed at the nervous system rather than the immune system so that patients with these autoimmune diseases won't have to take drugs that have such a terrible, devastating effect on the entire immune system.

MOYERS: In doing the reporting and research for this series, it has occurred to me that bogus remedies are the most prevalent for those problems that orthodox medicine has been unable to do much for—for example, cancer, arthritis, aging. But you're talking about possible hope for coping with these.

FELTEN: Yes, there's hope if we pursue this research responsibly and carefully, scientifically. Certainly, there's the opportunity for a lot of bogus approaches, and that worries us. A lot of us in this field tend to be exceedingly conservative because of the charlatans and the snake oil salesmen, who figure, what have they got to lose? They prey on the desperate, and the elderly, and the dying, promising them all kinds of cures if only they follow their remedy, for the low, low price of whatever it turns out to be—all without any substantiation whatsoever. That's why I try to stick to those factors that can be identified from careful studies of humans, or from some of the animal studies that really point in a responsible direction. I don't know what can be done about some of the charlatans who'll tell somebody that they're going to give them guided imagery that will cure their cancer, or whatever there is. I want to see the studies showing that what they do actually produces a difference in the patient's sense of well-being, or in longevity, before I start recommending anything to patients. I would particularly caution individuals not to abandon appropriate medical therapy in order to go chasing after something someone promises them. Anyone can find testimonials for anything. Let's see the controlled scientific studies first.

That's the plea all of us make in this field, because all kinds of folks have started hanging out their shingles, claiming that they are now practicing psychoneuroimmunology because they have some program they've developed, even though they don't have one shred of evidence that their program is effective. I don't like that. That is essentially fleecing people and taking advantage of them.

MOYERS: You've written about the "dark side" of mind/body medicine. What do you mean by the "dark side"?

FELTEN: I mean by that people who promise patients things they can't deliver. For example, promising cancer patients that although traditional medicine can't help them, their regiment of diet plus imagery plus whatever else they add will help cure them of their cancer. That is totally unsubstantiated. It's a cruel hoax to try to pull people away from traditional medicine into totally unfounded and unsubstantiated approaches to cancer. Usually, what you find is that the people who are practicing this kind of approach are lashing out at medicine, claiming that medicine has totally failed in the treatment of cancer, which, of course, is ridiculous. Tremendous progress has been made in treating several kinds of cancer, even though in other kinds of cancer we really have made precious little progress. In those diseases where even the strongest of drugs and chemotherapy and radiation therapy don't work, why would we suspect that hormones and neurotransmitters would do any better? The dark side involves an exploitation of this to make money.

MOYERS: Isn't there also the issue of blaming the victim for the victim's illness? If you don't get better, it's something to do with your attitude.

FELTEN: Oh, absolutely. An article in *The New England Journal of Medicine* argued that we should not make patients feel guilty if they can't help themselves recover from an illness. I appreciate that warning—but I also think that we can't let a patient totally reject all responsibility for getting in there and fighting. Patients are responsible for bringing their best to medicine so that medicine can do its best for them.

   Of course we don't want patients to feel guilty if they have a disease that overwhelms them. And eventually we all have to face death, so someday each of us will have our physiology totally overwhelmed by some disease process that we can't stop. The fact that a patient can't recover from a serious cancer, for example, is not a failure on the part of the patient, or a failure in the field of psychoneuroimmunology; it's just a demonstration that in some situations, no intervention of any magnitude will do any good.

MOYERS: What about the possibility that we're better off with an immune system that ignores our conscious thoughts? Some people, hearing bad things, might react as if those bad things are going to happen to them. They might get depressed, close down the immune system, and just quit. Are you worried about that?

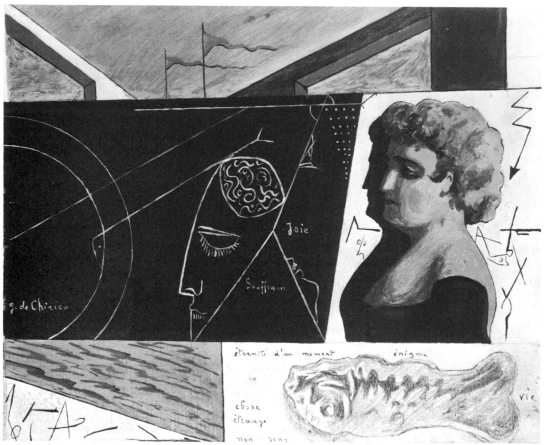

Giorgio de Chirico, *The Fatal Temple,* 1913

FELTEN: No, I'm not worried about that because I'd rather have some degree of control than just leave it to the whim of my immune system to do whatever it wishes to do. I'd like to think that I could boost it a little bit now and then.

MOYERS: How am I going to get control of my immune system?

FELTEN: That's what we're trying to learn. We know that the brain can be conditioned to respond as if a certain drug has been given, even when it hasn't. That suggests that the brain can be trained to regulate its own immune response.

MOYERS: The mind telling the immune system what to do.

FELTEN: Yes. Emotion, of course, is a very powerful stimulus over the peripheral parts of the body. We are reminded of that every time we see something really frightening. The reason emotion may play such a role is that the autonomic nervous system—that automated, unconscious part of our nervous system that controls our viscera—has direct physical connections to cells of the immune system. If you take those nerves away, the organs of the immune system don't respond to a challenge in the same way.

MOYERS: You're looking at complex operations of the body for evidence of the relation of the mind to the body—but aren't there suggestions from common life that the body is responding to the emotions all the time?

FELTEN: We certainly know from some very simple examples that our past perceptions make a difference in how we react to a given stimulus. For example, if you see a dog walking down the street, and if you happen to own a dog, and like dogs, and you particularly like that breed, you'll have a very warm feeling, and you'll want to go over and talk to the dog. If you don't care one way or another, you may have no response, or a neutral response. If, on the other hand, you were just bitten by a dog of that breed, you may experience a full-blown arousal response so that the adrenaline starts flowing, and your sympathetic nervous system activates at a sky-high level, and the pituitary releases stress hormones that affect the immune system. The heart rate goes up, the pupils dilate, the bronchials dilate to let more air in, the blood gets shunted to the muscles so that you're ready for a fight-or-flight response, and neurotransmitters are dumped into the circulation. Clearly, the difference is not in the stimulus, because the dog evokes different responses in different people, depending on their past experiences. That's why I think a patient's perceptions of what is going on are important, because patients react in very novel, individualistic ways that are affected by their past experience, their attitude toward doctors, and their feelings about such things as illness, hospitals, and their current situation in life. Given all that, there is room for incredibly different impacts of these stress mediators on the immune system. What is a stressor to you may not be a stressor to me.

MOYERS: If, as a child, you'd had a pet like that dog, you'd want now to go over and pet it, but if I had been bitten by a dog like that, I'd want to run: my mind has stored the memory and is calculating what to do at lightning speed.

FELTEN: Yes, the memory of being bitten is stored somewhere in your cortical banks, so that seeing the dog on the street triggers an emotional response through your limbic system, and your limbic system tells other parts of your brain, "Turn on the hormones, turn on the autonomic nervous system, get ready for a fight-or-flight response, because this is not good." The limbic system, or the emotional part of the brain, is what gives you the opportunity to react to a specific stimulus, like seeing a dog, in an individualized fashion that is yours and yours alone. That part of the brain gives you the first real individualized reactivity to the outside world.

MOYERS: When does this mind/body connection begin?

FELTEN: It can occur as soon as we're capable of perceiving sensory stimuli. Apparently, babies are quite capable of reacting to signals coming from the mother, so the mother's input to the baby makes a difference as to how the baby reacts.

MOYERS: This is why people talk about the importance of bonding with a baby, and communicating with the baby physically as well as emotionally.

FELTEN: Yes, and that touching makes a difference. Studies have shown that even in rodents, physical touching during early development, before weaning, greatly increases the number of small neurons in certain parts of the brain. Now that's a very powerful impact. Once again we rediscover that Grandmother knew what she was talking about, that you need to touch and love and nurture a baby. I'm sure that Grandmother didn't know that involved postnatal proliferation and migration of small neurons into the brain, but nonetheless, she knew the effects were real.

MOYERS: Well, if Grandmother knew it, why do you need to study it?

FELTEN: Because we need to understand how it happens, and whether nutritional factors could play a role, and whether we can help kids who are at risk. And we need to know whether we can intervene later on to stimulate the growth of more of those cells.

    All this speaks to the fundamental issue of the plasticity of systems. Our brain is amazingly plastic. We can afford to lose a fairly sizable amount of some of the major systems of our brain, and the remaining portion can still work. For example, the dopamine systems of the brain have to be knocked down by approximately eighty percent before the symptoms of Parkinson's disease come out.

    The immune system also has that kind of incredible plasticity, so it may well be that a stressor may make no difference in somebody who's young and vigorous, because they just adjust their immune system and go on their way. But to someone who is right at the edge, and who simply cannot take another hit, this stressor may be the final insult, and the whole system may fail. For example, AIDS patients are already right at the edge, so we're always worried that they'll get opportunistic infections. Does the stress of AIDS, and the stress of the social rejection and stigma, and some of the difficulties that AIDS patients face add the final straw that makes their demise more rapid? That's an issue of great importance. What we have discovered, once again, is that those patients who have a tough, fighting, blazing determination seem to do pretty well compared to those who don't.

MOYERS: When you talk about this, you get very excited.

FELTEN: Because I like science. It's an act of discovery. Three or four hundred years ago, we could go off and explore new land. Now we have an even more interesting new land to explore—the land of the brain and the land of the immune system. I have become passionately interested in how the brain and the immune system interact, and I'm also very interested in how age-related changes fit in with both systems. The immune system and certain parts of the brain run downhill with age. Two of my colleagues, Doctors Denise Bellinger and Suzanne Felten, have found that the nerve fibers that talk to cells of the immune system disappear with age. And we wonder, does that contribute to the diminished function of the immune system? So now we're trying to get the nerves to grow back to see if we can get the immune system to function better.

MOYERS: Is medicine really open to this new frontier?

FELTEN: Yes, I think many doctors are very interested in this, even though they were cautious originally—they'd say, "Interactions between the brain and immune system? No way. Show me." But now we have an overwhelming body of work with conditioning, we have stress-related studies in animals and in humans, we have work showing direct hormone influences on the immune system—all have come together in a new merging of immunology, endocrinology, and neurosciences. We can no longer each go back and sit in our laboratories and say, "I'm a neuroscientist, I'm interested only in neurotransmitters" or "I'm an endocrinologist, I'm interested only in hormones" or "I'm an immunologist, and I know that the immune system is autonomous, so I'm going to study only cytokines as the messengers." You can't get away with that anymore because we've seen that these systems talk to each other abundantly.

Now that's good news and bad news. The good news is that it opens up a wonderful discipline with incredible opportunities for discovery and for using new combinations of treatments to get at diseases of the system. The bad news is that now we have to start talking each other's language. And in the past, heaven forbid that immunologists and neuroscientists would ever use each other's language. They'd rather use each other's toothbrushes. But that's no longer a viable approach. We have to learn how to talk to each other and to educate each other.

MOYERS: I see a lot of young people in your lab. What does that say about the future of this research?

FELTEN: One of the most heartening aspects of doing this research is that our very finest graduate students and our brightest M.D. students are drawn to this field as if by a magnet. They're interested in studying everything from physiological and psychological correlates all the way down to the intracellular molecular biology. And they don't have the old biases that some of us grew up with about the immune system being autonomous or the brain not being able to communicate with lymphocytes and macrophages. They say, "Why not?" They're always ready to challenge us. That gives me hope, because I don't know if what we do will ever make a difference—but

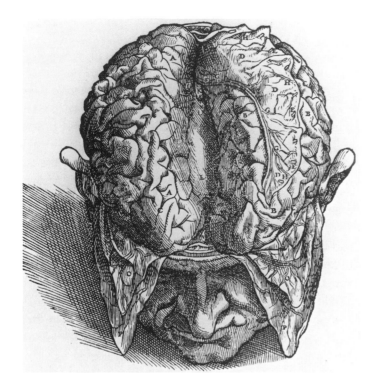

Andreas Vesalius,
*Two Cerebral
Hemispheres,* 1543

I do know that if we can train bright students to start doing really great things, that is an accomplishment.

At the same time that we have these wonderful students, we're observing colleagues who had initially told us, "It's too bad you've left mainstream research for this psychoneuro—whatever-it-is." Now they're beginning to come back to us and say, "Well, it's actually quite interesting that there are direct contacts between the nervous system and the immune system." They're starting to show up at seminars and to ask questions here and there. A few of them have actually come over and expressed an interest in doing some experiments. So people are getting intrigued. Many skeptical scientists are still open-minded enough that when you can show that cells have receptors, and that neurotransmitters are released, and that taking nerves away changes an immune response, they can believe it because they know they're seeing hard-core data.

MOYERS: When you're chasing a hypothesis, how do you know that you've come upon something?

FELTEN: When I first stumble onto something, it's just a gut feeling. It's sheer excitement. For example, we began looking at some published studies by Dr. Robert Sapolsky, showing that stress hormones from the adrenal gland can kill off cells in a part of the brain that is extremely important for short-term memory. We have tried to expand this concept to include some important brain neurotransmitters that may exacerbate this response.

MOYERS: You mean if I react too strongly to something, I can actually kill my brain cells?

FELTEN: Well, a long-term presence of this stress hormone can lead to the gradual death of some of the brain cells. We began to wonder what happens in the elderly who have the beginnings of what we commonly call "hardening of the arteries." They're not at the point where they have brain damage from decreased blood flow, but they're getting close. And we know that decreased blood flow to the brain first affects those very cells that the stress hormones affect. The combination of decreased blood flow plus stress hormones and increased brain neurotransmitters is big trouble compared to either alone. So what happens to some of the elderly, who come into the hospital at risk and are exposed to all kinds of stress phenomena? The general anxiety may produce terrible levels of stress hormones. And at the same time, whenever you go into a hospital, you always meet all of the organisms that hang out there, like staph and strep. Interestingly, an immune response also increases the level of these stress hormones, and increases the turnover of certain transmitters in the brain that actually synergize the damage that's done during decreased blood flow. So the last thing you want to do to somebody who is at risk for decreased blood flow is to increase their stress hormones, arouse their immune responses, and exacerbate the turnover of some of these vital transmitters, thus increasing the damage caused by the condition. But that's exactly what happens when they go into a hospital.

MOYERS: So when you bring people to the hospital, think hard and carefully about how you treat them.

FELTEN: Yes. For example, studies suggest that a patient who can look out the window during recovery from some specific types of surgery stays there a shorter time than the patient who can't look out a window. The environmental circumstances of the hospital make a difference in how well a patient recovers. There's a lot of literature on that, although basically it's been ignored, because for many decades we've practiced medicine more for the benefit of the staff and the hospital than for the benefit of the patients. And that is something that has to be changed. We have to start looking at the impact of the environment on how a patient recovers.

MOYERS: If you really believe that there's something to this mind/body thing, what difference does it make to you in how you practice your profession, or your calling?

FELTEN: I think it means that we have to pay attention to the patient directly. We have to care about how that patient perceives what is going on. It also means that we have to ask whether there are adverse circumstances, like lousy housing conditions, or poor nutrition, that may be stressing them. If we really believe the patient is the center of the healing process, then we have to go after whatever circumstances contribute to a bad outcome. And if that means taking social action, fine, then let's take social action to change some of those factors that have an adverse impact on a patient's ability to recover from disease.

MOYERS: What do you mean?

FELTEN: Well, think about the early days of industrialization, when ten-year-old children were developing pneumonia from working in dark, dank factories eighteen hours a day. The solution is not to come up with better antibiotics for treating pulmonary diseases in children, but to pass child labor laws so that children are not exploited. We may have more subtle aspects of that, where poor living conditions may contribute to a patient's poor health. Isn't it the job of society to try to go after those factors and eliminate them so that the general population can have the best health status possible?

MOYERS: That's politics, not medicine.

FELTEN: Sure, it's politics—but politics inevitably get involved in the practice of medicine. Are we treating geriatric patients, or aren't we? Are we going to use fetal tissue, or aren't we? Politics is so heavily imbedded in all of medicine and research that it can't be extracted.

MOYERS: So you're talking about changes that go beyond meditation and other techniques for altering our inner perceptions. You're talking about the environment in which we live.

FELTEN: Yes. Maybe changing the living environment helps people recover from autoimmune disease, for example, or helps people have a better immune response in old age.

MOYERS: What does science really tell us about healing?

FELTEN: We understand how an immune system will respond to a foreign invader, and we understand a little bit about how the brain responds under certain adverse circumstances. But beyond that to the elusive aspects of the mind that contribute to healing, we know very little. And we know very little about what gives some people the determination and perhaps the will to recover from a disease.

MOYERS: But you already know enough to say that healing is not just something that a doctor does to you or for you. I'm intrigued by the epilogue you wrote in a recent book. Would you mind reading this section?

FELTEN: "Just as the physical world of rainbows, lightning, and stars was not understood in the centuries before modern physics and astronomy, so also the more elusive and complex aspects of the human mind are not understood at present, even with the impressive technology we have at our command. Can we afford to ignore the role of emotions, hope, the will to live, the power of human warmth and contact just because they are so difficult to investigate scientifically and our ignorance is so overwhelming?"—I'm not sure I can do this. . . .

MOYERS: Well, let me. "I am one such basic scientist who has been touched personally by the example of my mother, Jane Felten, a courageous woman who faced life crippled with polio and beset with medical problems, but whose determination and irrepressible spirit seemed to carry her through almost unbelievable medical adversity. Paralyzed at eight years of age, she faced more than ten orthopedic procedures to fuse bones of the lower extremities to allow her to stand with crutches. She never thought anyone would want to marry her till she found a kind, gracious, and loving man, Harold Felten, whose example has been an inspiration to all who know him. She was told . . ." and you go on with a beautiful description of your mother's life, lived despite enormous and painful adversities. What did your mother's life teach you about this field?

FELTEN: I don't know that we can explain any of what I watched my mother go through by what we now know. She had her bones fused so she could bear weight on her lower extremities. And she then learned how to walk on her crutches and developed fantastically powerful arms doing that. Later, as part of the process of raising children, she had to learn how to hold her weight on the crutches, which of course induced problems in the brachial plexus that affected her arms. Then she had congestive heart failure. Finally, she ended with poor profusion of her brain, which caused her to have dementia. She died brain cell by brain cell. And in the meantime, as she was going downhill, she would get bout after bout of pulmonary edema, and intermittently have such incredible bouts with pneumonia that you would swear someone as ill and debilitated as she was just couldn't possibly recover. But she'd stick her jaw out with this incredible determination. She was not going to give up. And she'd recover again and again and again, until the very end, when, obviously, one reaches a point where adverse physiology overwhelms everything.

Maybe she's an example of psychoneuroimmunology in action. We don't know that. But we do know that she struggled back under conditions that ordinarily would overwhelm anyone. And she's one person among many people who have the same kind of tough determination, who fight back, who really seem to help themselves through circumstances that are almost unbelievable. Then there are other people who just give up and decide it's time to die. They run rapidly downhill, and they do die.

MOYERS: Do you think you can find out the difference through the microscope in the lab?

FELTEN: I think we can discover correlates. But I don't think we'll ever causally understand what goes on, because when we're doing work with humans, so much depends on inner thoughts and emotions and attitudes—and we can't really study the brain chemistry involved with that, at least not with the technology we now have. Things that can't be brought down to the level of an animal model are very difficult to study mechanistically, which is why diseases like AIDS are so incredibly difficult to approach. Perhaps someday we will understand what the will to live correlates with in relation to our hormones. But I'm not sure that we'll ever understand the brain circuitry involved and what all the individual signaling is. Maybe the people in artificial intelligence will help us understand that someday. But right now it's beyond what we can strive for.

MOYERS: Have you come to any tentative conclusions about the mind in relation to the body and healing, other than that there's something there?

FELTEN: I haven't come to any conclusions about the exact sequence of events because we're just in the infancy of our explorations in this field. But all of us have seen mind/body interactions. And that is enough of a stimulus to keep searching, even though we can't explain it right now.

MOYERS: You say "mind/body." A lot of people say "mind *and* body." It seems to me that we need to eliminate the "and," because we know the mind is of the body and the body is of the mind.

FELTEN: Yes, it's all an interactive process. The brain just happens to be the real person, as we define an individual. I always think of the rest of it as peripheral. You know, there's a pump, there's a filter, there's a community of cells that act as guards. You can picture all the rest of the body as there to protect the brain, which is your personality—what makes you human.

Now that's obviously coming from the bias of a neuroscientist. Our immunologists would say it's really the immune system, and the brain is there just to protect the organisms so that the immune system can continue to function. You know, we all have our ways of looking at this. But certainly we have been impressed with the fact that the brain controls a lot more than we thought it did. Fifteen years ago we didn't even realize that the brain might be able to regulate metabolic cells like liver cells and fat cells. Now we know it does. So we're learning piece by piece.

MOYERS: In China the other day I witnessed the removal of a tumor from deep within the brain of a thirty-seven-year-old schoolteacher. After the surgeon had opened the forehead and removed the bone, he let me look into the brain. There in that mass of white tissue I saw the ugly intruder—the cancer. I was looking at the brain. But I couldn't see the mind. Somewhere in there, I said to myself, there's a mind at work. Where is it? I wondered.

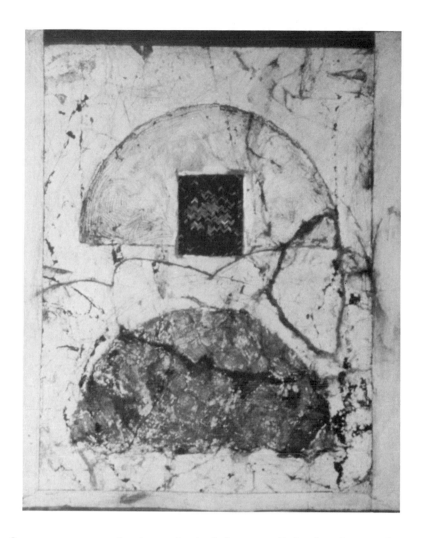

Terence La Noue,
Kashmir, 1979

FELTEN: Well, I tend not to separate brain and mind, because I think, ultimately, they're one and the same.

MOYERS: And you don't separate mind and body the way we used to.

FELTEN: No, we don't separate them neatly.

MOYERS: When you described your mother with her jaw jutting out with determination, you were describing what once upon a time we thought was primarily, if not purely, a physical reaction. But something more was going on back there—intelligence and emotion and body, acting in concert. A will at work.

FELTEN: Yes. We don't know all of the peripheral accompaniments that go along with that determination—for example, what hormones and neurotransmitters are at work. I wish I knew. I'm insatiably curious to know. But we just don't know that yet. We're working at it, though, and piece by piece it's falling into place.

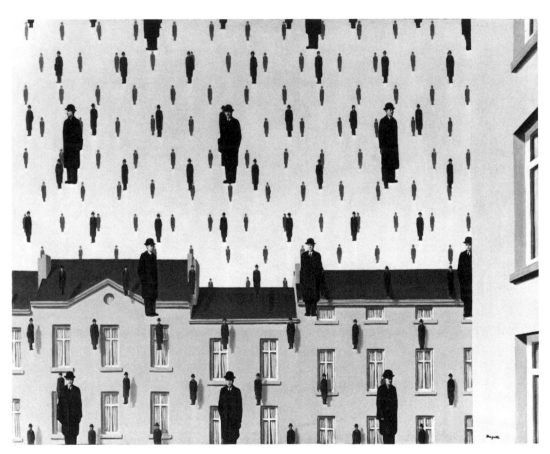

René Magritte, *Golconde*, 1953

CONDITIONED RESPONSES

Robert Ader

ROBERT ADER, Ph.D., is Director of the Division of Behavioral and Psychosocial Medicine at the University of Rochester School of Medicine. He conducted a landmark experiment showing that mice could be given a drug to suppress their immune system and then be conditioned to continue suppressing their immune system after the drug was taken away. The experiment expanded understanding of what humans might be able to control in their own bodies.

MOYERS: You were originally trained in psychology. How did you get interested in immunology, especially since it is such a different specialty from psychology?

ADER: Well, I got into it by accident, really. I was doing some studies on learning that involved giving an animal a distinctive flavor—saccharine, in this case—and then injecting the animal with a drug that induced a stomachache. Very quickly the animal learns not to drink anything that tastes like saccharine. It's a powerful learning procedure that occurs in every animal species in which it has been tested. If you think about it, an animal in the real world that cannot learn very quickly what is safe or unsafe to eat and drink simply will not survive.

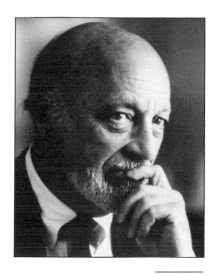

MOYERS: I learned a similar lesson as a child when I touched a hot iron—after being burned, I never touched the iron again.

ADER: Yes, and what you learned was not simply to avoid touching that particular iron, but to avoid touching any iron. You learned in one trial that there is a negative effect if you engage in certain behaviors.

Of course in this instance the stomachache was induced not by the saccharine, but by the drug. But because the saccharine was administered in association with the drug, the animals responded to it as if it were the drug. In this particular study we were trying to discover if the amount of saccharine the rats drank in conjunction with the drug affected their learning. As we expected, the more saccharine they drank before being injected with the drug, the stronger was the subsequent aversion to saccharine.

But something else happened during the course of this experiment. We knew that the drug we were using to induce the stomachache in the rats also suppressed the immune system, so we gave it in small enough doses not to affect the mortality of the animals. Yet, in this experiment, some of the animals died after being re-exposed to saccharine. This was troublesome because it meant that there was something going on in the experiment over which we had no control. Soon it became apparent that the mortality of the animals varied directly with how much saccharine they had drunk. Those who had drunk the greatest volume of saccharine died the soonest.

Now that was an orderly relationship, so presumably it had some explanation. You have to understand that as a psychologist, I was not aware of the general position of immunology that there are no connections between the brain and the immune system. So I hypothesized that at the same time that we were conditioning the aversion to saccharine, we were also conditioning the immunosuppressive effects of the drug we had given them. That meant that every time the animal was re-exposed to saccharine, there would be a conditioned immunosuppressive response, and the animal would not be able to mount a strong reaction to pathogens, or foreign proteins, in the environment. The stronger the conditioned response to saccharine, the greater the immunosuppression, and the greater the mortality.

At that point I found Nicholas Cohen, an immunologist with whom I've been working for the past seventeen years. Dr. Cohen thought my hypothesis was worth exploring, so the two of us set out to do an experiment to determine if in fact we could condition a suppression of the immune system.

We took a group of animals and gave them a drug that suppresses the production of antibodies—an immunosuppressant. At the same time, we gave them saccharine. In other words, in this group of animals the saccharine and the immunosuppressant were paired.

We then injected these animals as well as a control group of animals with an antigen to induce them to produce antibodies. Next we gave the control group the immunosuppressant drug, while we gave the experimental group only the saccharine that had previously been paired with the drug. The control group reacted by suppressing antibody production—but so did the experimental group, which had been given only the saccharine. In effect, we had demonstrated that learning processes could influence immune responses. The experiment was a direct and rather dramatic demonstration of a relationship between nervous system function and immune function.

MOYERS: Once you realized that the rats could shut down their immune system, what were the implications for us human beings?

ADER: One of the immediate clinical implications had to do with placebos. Here we had a conditioning effect that had a major biologic impact on the survival of the animal. That suggests that the placebo effect is a learned response available to anybody under the appropriate circumstances.

MOYERS: So, for example, if we are taking certain drugs for an illness, we might also condition ourselves to respond to a smaller dose as if we were taking a larger one. We could get the same therapeutic benefit without as many side effects. Is this kind of conditioned learning similar to the experiment with Pavlov's dog?

ADER: In principle, it's identical. Pavlov put food powder in a dog's mouth. That's an unconditioned stimulus because it unconditionally elicits salivation. And then he rang a bell before he gave them the food powder. Now a bell normally does not produce salivation. But by repeatedly pairing the bell and the food, eventually the bell began to elicit salivation.

Our experiment was an example of classical Pavlovian conditioning applied to the modification of a physiologic response that people thought was not regulated by the brain. And I say "physiologic response," because for integrationists such as myself, immune responses are not something apart, although for years they were treated as if they were. A few years ago you couldn't find a textbook in immunology that mentioned the brain. Not only was there no chapter on the brain, you couldn't even find "brain" in the index. Recent textbooks are now coming out with statements like "The current data coming from psychoneuroimmunology indicate that, as we have long suspected, the immune system may not be completely autonomous." Even though it may sound a little begrudging, there is increasing acknowledgment of the role of these other influences on immune system behavior. And that has phenomenal implications for the way the immune system is studied.

What we did was described as "dramatic"—but I don't think it was. What's more surprising is that the immune system should have been thought of as autonomous in the first place. All we're suggesting, consistent with everything else we know about every other system in the body, is that this is just another physiologic response

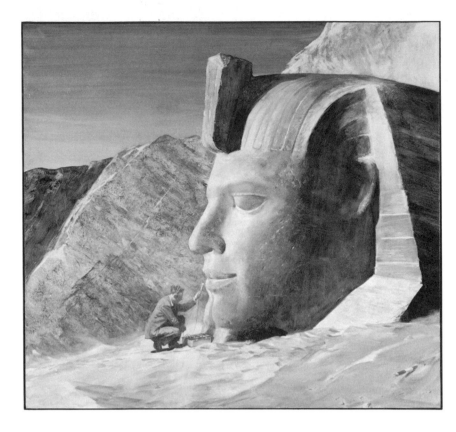

Mark Tansey,
*Secret of the
Sphinx*, 1984

integrated with all other physiologic responses. I don't find that dramatic at all. I find it intuitively self-evident.

A number of demonstrations provide overwhelming evidence that there are interactions among the nervous system, the endocrine system, and the immune system. Some of that evidence is at the anatomical level, for example, the kind of research that David Felten does in documenting "hardwired" and neurochemical connections between the nervous system and the immune system. Some of the evidence is at the other extreme, on the level of the whole organism—for example, studies of the influence of psychosocial factors on diseases that we think are mediated by the immune system. Now, although we have this information about anatomical connections and neurochemical signaling between the nervous system and the immune system, we don't know the functional significance of these connections. And although our experiments demonstrated a functional relationship between the brain and the immune system, we don't know what the mechanism is.

At the level of the whole organism, this work demonstrates the possibility that the immune system could mediate between psychosocial factors, like stress in the workplace and altered susceptibility to disease. That mediation is basically unknown, even though we do know that events in the real world, as they are perceived by the individual, will influence both the susceptibility to disease and the recovery from disease. We've now demonstrated that the brain is capable of exerting some regulation, modulation, or control over the immune system.

MOYERS: We've long known that the state of mind can affect the state of health. But here we see that the immune system itself is directly receiving messages.

ADER: Yes. We know from the neuroanatomical data that substances released by nerve endings are capable of modifying lymphocytes. And we know that lymphocytes can receive these signals, because they have receptors on their surfaces that are capable of doing that. And we certainly know that an activated immune system produces chemicals that can be perceived by the nervous system. So there is a communication among these systems. They are interacting, and that can be demonstrated. But, as I say, the functional significance is not fully understood.

MOYERS: Are you saying that we can consciously turn something like a sugar pill into a powerful drug?

ADER: No, I don't mean to imply that humans can voluntarily or willfully modify their immune system. That may be a reasonable hypothesis, but it would be very difficult to demonstrate at this point. What we do know is that neutral events, like drinking saccharine, can be associated in such a way with events that do influence the immune system that the neutral events can modify the immune system. That has to be a central nervous system process.

MOYERS: What are you finding that has a practical relevance to us now?

ADER: That depends upon the bias or the orientation with which one starts. The word "psychoneuroimmunology" is sometimes used now as a substitute for psychosomatic medicine. I've been called a "psychosomaticist," but I don't believe there is any such thing as a psychosomatic disease. I don't accept the notion that psychological factors alone cause disease. You see, if I allow you to label certain diseases as psychosomatic, then, implicitly, I'm allowing you to say that certain diseases are immune—pardon the expression—immune to the influence of psychological factors. But if psychological factors can be shown to influence the susceptibility to or progression of any single disease, one must at least entertain the logical possibility that psychological factors could play some role in all disease. All disease is multidetermined, and one of the determining influences is the psychological state of the individual.

MOYERS: So if psychoneuroimmunology is not psychosomatic medicine, what is it?

ADER: In general, it is a new direction in the study of the relationship between mind and body. Of course, the relation between mind and body has been studied for a thousand years. Nevertheless, what we don't know is how the relationship works.

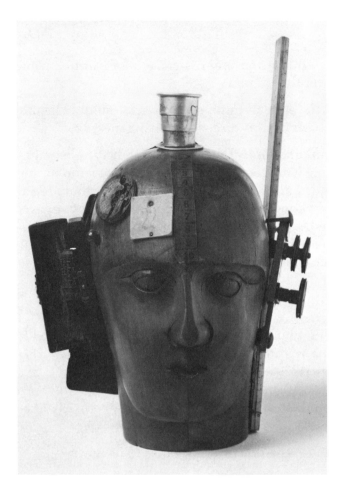

Raoul Hausmann,
*L'Esprit de Notre
Temps. Tête
Méchanique,* 1919

As a component of psychosomatic medicine, if you will, psychoneuroimmunology is the study of the interactions among behavioral, neural and endocrine, and immune processes of adaptation.

Another significant result of research in psychoneuroimmunology is that it is altering the way we study the workings of the immune system. It's one thing to study a phenomenon in a test tube, but the real question is, how does it work in vivo, in the body? How it works in vivo is modified by nervous system activity, and you don't see nervous system activity in a test tube. You work in vitro—with the test tube method, so to speak—in an attempt to eliminate all the variables except the one you want to study. That has been an effective strategy for the study of many diseases. But it has not been effective for today's killers, like cardiovascular disease and cancer. The immune responses that we should really be concerned with take place within the living organism—within a neuroendocrine environment—that is exquisitely sensitive to the demands of the environment as these are perceived by the individual.

I can set up experiments to produce disease in the laboratory. I can inject you with enough pathogen to make you ill, no matter whether you are happy or sad, under stress or not under stress. You will develop that disease because I guaranteed it when I injected you with that quantity of pathogen cells.

But that's not the way disease occurs in the real world. Germs are a necessary condition for disease, but apparently they're not a sufficient condition for disease. If they were, most of us would be sick most of the time. Why is it that when an entire population is exposed to the same set of pathogens, some people become ill and some people do not become ill? What are the other contributing factors? If you set up your research strategy in such a way as to unconditionally produce disease, that's okay for studying some of the mechanisms of disease, but it won't tell you about how the disease develops in human beings in the real world.

The biological sciences have become compartmentalized and bureaucratized— and that simply reflects our own ignorance. I'm a psychologist, you're a biochemist, somebody else is a pharmacologist, someone else is an immunologist. We've divided up the pie into manageable pieces. But this division has no bearing on the biology. The biology doesn't recognize these disciplines. There is only one organism, and the nature of the relationships among systems is every bit as important, functionally, as the relationships within a system.

MOYERS: That's the body?

ADER: The mind and the body—that's the same thing. They're inseparable.

MOYERS: It was interesting that when I said "body," you referred to the mind/body. The mind and the body are one and the same.

ADER: Yes, they are inseparable components of the whole. And the same is true for adaptive processes. They are integrated. For example, if you start with the assumption that the immune system is autonomous, there are certain questions you don't ask. But if you think of the immune system as an integrated part of our adaptive processes, then there are all kinds of new questions you can ask. And these questions are being asked now. Every time we turn over a new rock, there's something there. It's amazing to see the amount of new information coming out of integrated research in this field now.

MOYERS: What's your response to the growing conviction that we can think ourselves well?

ADER: That is an extreme statement that reflects a total confidence in the ability of the mind to influence the body. I can differ with it only at a quantitative level, because, in fact, the evidence does suggest that mind influences body, just as the body influences mind. You see, we have a funny language. To talk about mind and body is to set up a dichotomy. It implies a separateness that we don't mean when we discuss this subject. We have a one-dimensional language for a three-dimensional concept.

If you ask, "Can a person exert will to influence body and therefore disease?" I have to say that I think it may be possible in some individuals, and, if it's possible in some, it's potentially possible in all. But I think such claims are exaggerated. Like many other odd coincidences, only the positive instances are reported. How many times does a person exert will and *nothing happens?* These cases are not reported.

On the other hand, we used to think that we could not control certain autonomic responses like heart rate, blood pressure, temperature in the extremities—things like that. But we now know that these responses are subject to a certain amount of voluntary control.

MOYERS: Biofeedback has shown that.

ADER: That's right. Biofeedback is predicated on a learning process, so why can we not extend the same principle to the immune system? Well, I would argue that in principle, it would apply to the immune system. Autonomic nervous system responses are very rapid. All you have to do is to place electrodes on appropriate parts of the body, and you can measure changes in muscle tension, or heart rate, or what have you. It's a very rapid response to external stimulation. Hormonal responses, however, are

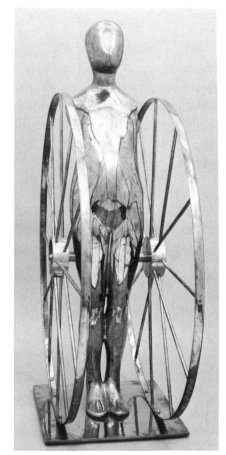

Ernest Trova, *Study: Falling Man (Wheelman), 1965*

much slower, and immune responses are much, much slower than that. The production of antibodies, for example, takes days. Feedback to the individual could not occur in proximity to any response that the individual made in an attempt to alter immune activity.

MOYERS: But let's assume, for the sake of the discussion, that we could do with the immune system what biofeedback does for heart rate and blood pressure. What would that mean for healing, potentially?

ADER: Potentially, it would mean that you could exert some control over how fast you produced antibody-specific responses to pathogens in your environment. At the moment this possibility remains at the level of science fiction.

MOYERS: I'm asking these practical questions because it seems to me the public may be a little overenthusiastic about the medical implications of the new mind/body research.

ADER: Well, yes, that's exactly what's happening. The clinical implications will depend on the basic research. But the potential to regulate the immune system by the brain is so dramatic that the public has embraced the possibilities far beyond what the data so far can support. For example, there are all kinds of advertisements for interventions to enhance your immune function and protect you against disease. These interventions may be based on reasonable hypotheses, but there are no data whatsoever to support those claims.

MOYERS: I understand that, and yet there's something beckoning you on, or otherwise an intelligent, committed, and credentialed man would not keep spending so much of his life on what is mere potential.

ADER: Well, potential is a lot, but there is also the desire to understand the nature of what is not yet known.

MOYERS: But you're not prepared to say now that we can learn to direct our minds to help in the healing of our bodies. On the other hand, you also wouldn't rule out the possibility that someday we might be able to learn to do that.

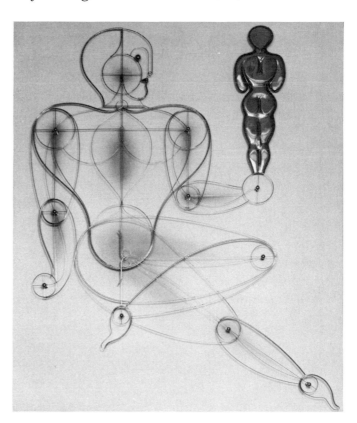

Oskar Schlemmer,
"Homo," 1931

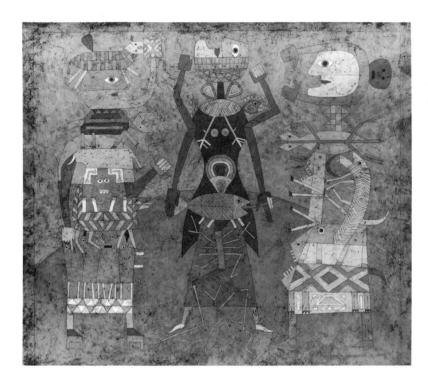

Victor Brauner,
*Mémoire des
Réflexes*, 1954

ADER: I would put it this way: it is possible that we can learn to influence the balance that maintains health in relation to the outside world. I find it a little bit unbalanced that we talk more about how the mind can be taught to influence the body than about how the body can influence the mind. The statement that we can learn to use the mind to influence the body implies a dualism that does not exist.

MOYERS: Isn't there a danger in assuming that what you see in rats and mice is also true for human beings?

ADER: You invariably see objections to extrapolations from animal research to human research, although in the specific case of the immune system, the similarity between mouse and man is quite striking. But you also have to remember that the extrapolations we've made from animal research are based not necessarily on the specifics of the intervention or the outcome measure, but on the principle of the interaction among systems that influence disease, or recovery from disease, or the response to drugs. Those principles, rather than any particular results, can indeed be extrapolated to humans.

MOYERS: So what are the questions we want to keep on asking?

ADER: The most basic of those questions is: what is the extent and nature of the relationships among these systems? It's now time to study the immune system as an integrated component of adaptive responses. We need basic research to understand the nature of these relationships before we proceed to clinical applications.

IV

THE MYSTERY
OF CHI

"Mind moves matter."
—VIRGIL

An operating room in Beijing: in a surgical gown, complete with mask and slippers, I watch as a scalpel cuts slowly across the hairline of a young woman, a schoolteacher. She is barely visible beneath the swaddling around her face. A large tumor has invaded her brain, and shows up plainly when the doctors check the CAT scans on a nearby light box. The surgeons are well acquainted with Western technology and probe faultlessly toward the tumor.

I look at the woman and see six tiny needles protruding from her forehead, calves, and ankles—needles to ease the pain of metal cutting into human tissue. For anesthesia, she has been given a mild sedative and a small amount of narcotic—less than half the standard amount she would have received in a Western hospital—and the acupuncture needles, administered by doctors trained in traditional Chinese medicine. The young woman is awake but doesn't flinch under the surgeon's knife. The doctors talk to her as they guide their instruments toward their prey. The chief surgeon motions to me to peer through a magnifying lens directly at the ugly black growth, which is visible through the cavity his assistants have opened in the woman's forehead.

I walk around the operating table and lean under the large green sheets that cover her like a tent. "How are you doing?" I ask through an interpreter. She answers, "Okay." By noon the tumor has been successfully removed. Because a portion of the anesthesia has been provided by the stimulation of the needles, the woman has been able to cooperate with the doctors throughout the surgery; there will be fewer side effects from drugs, and she will bounce back more quickly, although the operation has taken more than three hours.

As I have just witnessed, there are other geographies of the body, other maps, that guide healers in other cultures. I will meet here traditional Chinese doctors who do not sample blood, look at X rays, or make distinctions between physical and mental disorders. Instead they talk about a mysterious force called chi (pronounced "chee"). To them, the body is an energy system, its architecture so foreign to our Western way of thinking that we would pay no attention at all except that traditional Chinese medicine, based on chi, seems to work for millions of people, and to have worked for centuries.

As we are filming in China, the International Traditional Medicine Congress, attended by 700 doctors and scholars from 40 nations, is meeting in Beijing. It will proclaim October 22 as World Traditional Medicine Day and affirm that traditional Chinese medicine (officially called TCM) "is by no means inferior to synthetic drugs and antibiotics." Rooted deeply in China's past, traditional medicine was outlawed in the 1920s by the Nationalist government on the grounds that such practices were "backwards and superstitious." In the 1950s Mao Zedong, then governing a country with 500 million people and only 38,000 Western-style medical doctors, restored traditional medicine to official status and called for a "solid front" between Western-trained and traditional physicians. Western medicine became the preference of the elite, but TCM never lost its popularity with the masses and is today enjoying renewed vitality. The government says there are approximately 2,100 traditional medicine hospitals and an estimated one million traditionally trained doctors and pharmacists throughout China. They constitute a network that is an integral part of the health care system, coexisting with hospitals using Western medical theory and techniques. The state administration for TCM has been given funds that have spurred a boom in research. Reports presented to the international congress tell of hundreds of new drugs produced from herbs and animals such as musk deer, scorpions, and geckos; of new acupuncture techniques for the foot, face, scalp, nose, and ankle; of treatments for senile dementia and Parkinson's disease.

Acupuncture has fascinated the American public since James Reston of the *New York Times* had to undergo an appendectomy during President Nixon's trip to China in the early 1970s and wrote about its use as an anesthetic. I suspect that acupuncture is what we think of first when we conjure up a picture of Chinese medicine. But herbal medicine, massage, exercise, meditation, and an appreciation for "balance" in life-style are also part of this complex medical system, which I have come to explore precisely because it refuses to make distinctions between mind and body.

This is not a journey I could undertake on my own. Luckily, I have an experienced guide, Dr. David Eisenberg, instructor in medicine at the Harvard Medical School and a staff internist at Boston's Beth Israel Hospital. Shortly after relations were normalized in 1979, David became the first American medical exchange student sent to China. Working beside his teachers in traditional Chinese clinics, he studied acupuncture, massage, and herbal techniques, and he returns to China often to continue his research. In his book, *Encounters with Qi*, he asks some large questions that will guide our travels together:

- What can we in the West learn from the medical practices of the Chinese people that might improve our understanding of health, illness, and the healing process?
- Can Chinese medicine be integrated into Western medical practices as our practices have been integrated into Chinese medicine?
- Can Chinese medicine prove its assertion that life-style and attitude can significantly alter the natural course of human illness?

The park in Shanghai is empty and still. We are waiting for dawn. The last long shadows vanish quickly like rivulets of water in sand. From behind distant rooftops the light advances. But the sun has not yet made its debut when I see them.

I blink at the sight. The gates of the park have been flung open, and all of China appears to be heading toward us. Throngs of elderly people—I reckon many to be in their nineties—spread out in every direction. The scuffling of thousands of soft-shoed feet swells like the hum of cicadas on a summer morning in Texas.

The people ignore us. They have come, as they come every morning, every season, rain or shine, to practice an ancient art, t'ai chi ch'uan. Some form groups, like ballet dancers, and soon are gently and effortlessly swaying, gliding, weaving their arms, legs, and torsos, their feet, hands, and heads into a noiseless concert of bodies. Hundreds of others go solo, and the park is alive with motion, reminding me of waves lapping the shore, of clouds enfolding a mountain. Now the sun rises on a fantastic ritual dance of human harmony.

"Harmony, yes," says David Eisenberg. "But if you were to ask them, it is not a dance, or their muscles, or their limbs they would tell you about. And they wouldn't call it an exercise. They would tell you it's about that force called chi."

To these people, as to their physicians, the body is a series of energy conduits. Chi, the Chinese name for this energy, flows along systematic meridians, which do not coincide with any known physiologic structures. When a patient is ill, our Western doctors look for physical or chemical abnormalities. Chinese doctors search for hidden forces that are out of balance. Their task, as they describe it, is to restore unseen harmonies. Sticking needles into the body is obviously a physical intervention to Westerners, but not to the Chinese. They see it as intervening in an energy system. The same is true of herbs. For the Chinese, herbs are not a concoction of chemicals that influence other chemicals in the body; herbs help to "unstick chi"—to get the energy flowing again. Through pressing needles into specific points in the body, through using herbs, and through massaging pressure points, Chinese doctors, it is said, control the flow of chi.

As we see in the park, they also teach their patients to master the flow of energy in their own bodies through combined mental and physical practice. Chinese sages taught that treating someone who is already ill is like beginning to dig a well after you have become thirsty. The classical Chinese physician received a fee only as long as the patient remained in good health. Payments stopped when sickness began. The task was to teach patients to stay healthy by living correctly; temperament, diet, thoughts, emotions, and exercise were all important in a system in which the patient took primary responsibility for sickness or health. The physician was a role model. Patients went to him to learn about "energy medicine."

Eisenberg hadn't been prepared for anything quite like this. Everywhere he went after his arrival, he encountered chi. "Walk through a hospital in any city or countryside and you see an herbal unit, an acupuncture unit, and a chi gong unit. You go to the physiology laboratory of the best college of traditional medicine in

China, and you see a computer built by top Chinese biophysicists stimulating twenty different human pulses as a teaching tool for medical students learning pulse diagnosis. In another room there is a wall of IBM computers with colorimeters that measure the color of the tongue; they are a teaching aid for students learning to differentiate between hundreds of tongue-based diagnoses. A helium neon laser is used to stimulate selected acupuncture points, and precise physiologic responses are compared with stimulation from a needle or an electrical current. Go into the huge lecture hall and you find a twelve-foot-high human statue with hundreds of clearly marked acupuncture points, surrounded by students learning where to place acupuncture needles to intervene in a variety of medical, surgical, or psychiatric conditions." He still marvels. "What kind of vision of the body is this? None of this has any overlap with anything I learned in medical school."

To American doctors, of course, the existence of chi is unproven; as a physical reality, chi makes no sense at all. Out of respect for Western skepticism, and for their own intellectual satisfaction, researchers at the Shanghai Institute of Traditional Chinese Medicine, the Beijing Institute of Traditional Chinese Medicine, and the State Administration of Traditional Chinese Medicine are looking into the mechanisms of the ancient medicine. "Chi gong is an old practice," one Chinese physician tells Eisenberg, "part of the national treasure house of traditional Chinese medicine. We have tried these past few years to understand it by means of modern scientific principles and techniques. We do not yet understand it and would like your help in defining the nature of chi."

No small task.

Chi gong, the most perplexing of all the Chinese healing techniques, literally means "manipulation of vital energy." Chinese physicians use it to treat a variety of illnesses, typically chronic neurological and muscular disease, including multiple sclerosis. People learn to direct the "vital energy" in their body through special breathing and physical exercises. Chi gong is in effect a discipline whose practitioners are instructed in the art of "centering," of achieving a particular state of physical balance, and simultaneously of meditating, as Jon Kabat-Zinn's patients were doing when eating raisins.

Estimates of the number of people who daily perform chi gong and t'ai chi exercises like those we have seen in the park range to the tens of millions. But no well-designed, controlled studies have shown whether these millions of practitioners have changed their health status through daily chi gong exercises. As Eisenberg says, "The mere fact that ten million people get up at dawn to practice an ancient art does not prove that the practice can alter susceptibility to disease or its natural course. The fact that the exercise is thousands of years old, and a hallmark of Taoist, Buddhist, and imperial Chinese scholarship, does not necessarily mean that human beings hold within them rivers, streams, and pools of vital energy." Nonetheless, the mystery challenges him, calling him back to further study.

Traveling with him, I see remarkable and puzzling things and often wonder whether what I am witnessing really causes healing or is simply the result of the placebo effect—what happens when a person thinks that a fake pill is a powerful drug and experiences a real cure. It is astonishing to think that an entire medical system could be built on the placebo effect. But even if scientific studies of chi showed it to be only a mental construct, the power of that construct as it has been applied to hundreds of millions of human beings for centuries would point to the role of the mind in healing. So Eisenberg is now working with Chinese authorities to develop research on the principles of Chinese medicine using Western scientific methodologies. If it is truly effective, Chinese medicine will stand up to the most rigorous scrutiny. After all, as Eisenberg keeps reminding me, there is an ancient Chinese proverb: "Real gold does not fear the heat of even the hottest fire."

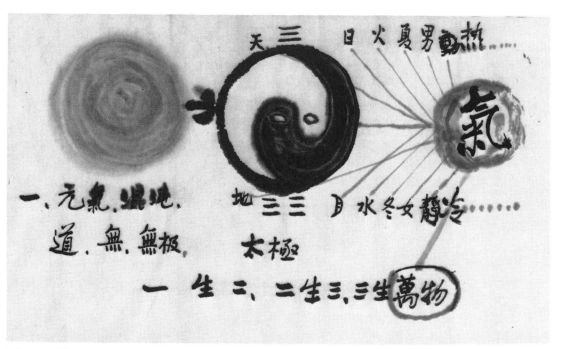

Master Wang,
*Creation of the
Universe; Yin and
Yang*, 1991

MEDICINE IN A MIND/BODY CULTURE

David Eisenberg

In Beijing, we visit the Dongzhimen Hospital, where David trained eleven years before. Dongzhimen is one of the three traditional Chinese medicine teaching hospitals in the city, where Western and Chinese medicine exist side by side. At eight in the morning, the waiting areas are already crowded. A long line of people stand in front of smoked glass windows with big Chinese characters posted above them: "Traditional Chinese Herbs." On the other side of the room, patients stand before another series of windows below another sign: "Western Medicine."

After talking with a few of the patients, David and I go behind the scenes into the herbal pharmacy where the medicines are being prepared. The floor is littered with baskets filled with a variety of herbs, and the walls are lined with dozens of herb drawers left half open. Five or six people in white gowns and baker-type hats are filling out prescriptions, typically scooping out as many as twelve different herbs to carefully mix together a single herbal remedy. We watch as they scoop, weigh, measure, and put the remedies into bags.

EISENBERG: This is the herbal pharmacy, the nerve center of the whole hospital, where the bulk of all the Chinese medical therapy is. Many of these herbs have been administered for thousands of years, and the effects have been documented and well studied.

MOYERS: What's in these remedies?

EISENBERG: Most remedies use plants, but some also contain deer antlers, snake gallbladders, shark fins, and other exotic substances.

MOYERS: What are these? They look like scorpions.

EISENBERG: That's exactly right—they're dried, whole scorpions.

MOYERS: And this? Look!

EISENBERG: It's a gecko.

MOYERS: That's a medicine? What is it good for?

PHARMACIST: It halts a cough and reduces phlegm.

MOYERS: And this?

PHARMACIST: The roots of a large-flowering skullcap.

EISENBERG: This one is called "milk vetch" in English. It's good for relieving fever. In Chinese, it would be said to diminish the "excessive heat" in the body and to take away the toxins.

Now, here's an important plant—ginseng root, used for increasing "chi," or vital energy, the life-force of the body.

MOYERS: Will it grow hair?

PHARMACIST: Maybe. But losing hair is not a sickness.

MOYERS: But how do you know the proper mix? Does it take a long time to study?

EISENBERG: Yes, and this is absolutely the hardest part of Chinese medicine. The doctors have to understand a complex set of rules which govern balance in the human body. The Chinese would say that if a certain internal organ doesn't have enough energy, then you need certain herbs to increase it.

MOYERS: Do any of these concoctions have a chemical base similar to Western drugs?

EISENBERG: They are not thought of in the same way. They're not prescribed because of their active chemical ingredients, but because one of them increases heat, and one of them decreases the stagnation of vital energy. That's the language the Chinese use. It has nothing to do with chemistry. It developed 2,500 years ago, before chemistry as we know it was described.

MOYERS: As a pharmacist, did you also study Western medicine?

PHARMACIST: Yes, first I studied Western medicine and then traditional Chinese medicine because some patients like to take this medicine. Western medicine is not very useful for some things, especially chronic diseases like certain forms of hepatitis, stomach trouble, and ulcers.

MOYERS: And what do they do with these ingredients?

Shen-nung,
legendary Chinese
god-emperor and
father of
pharmaceutics, in
drawing dated
1920

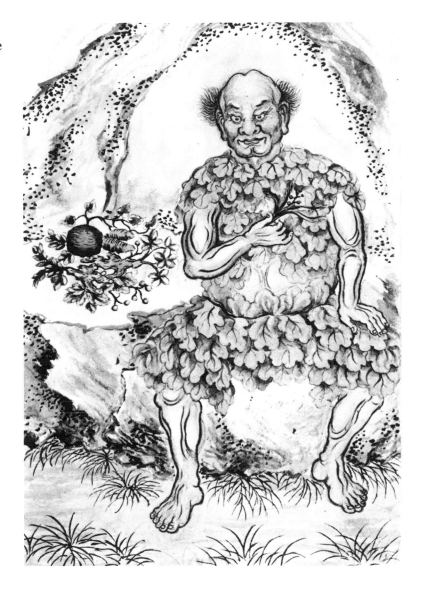

PHARMACIST: They boil them in water for about half an hour and drink the liquid like a kind of tea every day.

MOYERS: I count sixteen ingredients here.

EISENBERG: That's the herbal medicine for one patient for one day. Look at the shelves. How many different kinds of ingredients are here?

PHARMACIST: Maybe eight hundred or more.

MOYERS: How many are there in Chinese medicine?

PHARMACIST: Over two thousand.

MOYERS: Will some of the people taking this also take Western medicine?

PHARMACIST: Some patients do, but a lot of them take only this.

MOYERS: Is that the doctor's choice or the patient's choice?

PHARMACIST: The doctor's choice, just as in Western medicine.

MOYERS: Have these prescriptions been analyzed? We know the names of the ingredients and where they come from, but do we know what's really in them?

EISENBERG: The only one that has been analyzed to any extent is ginseng. That's not surprising, because when you think about it, a single herb, like ginseng, may have fifty or a hundred different chemicals in it. Sorting out which ingredient is doing what is not so simple.

MOYERS: So we know what herbs are in these prescriptions, but we don't know the active ingredients that make them work.

EISENBERG: We don't even know all the ingredients in each herb or how they interact when you boil twelve of them together in water.

MOYERS: We know that some plants in their natural condition contain digitalis — which we use for heart conditions. So there is a chemistry involved in herbal therapy.

EISENBERG: Right, but the Chinese weren't interested in "chemistry" as we know it. They didn't have organic chemists to analyze the active ingredients. They had people who observed whether whole herbs helped with certain problems. These herbs are prescribed based on a notion that the body is basically a system filled with energy—"chi." When a traditional Chinese doctor prescribes a specific herb, he's not attempting to correct a chemical abnormality, he's trying to restore the harmonious flow of chi. Each herb is given to increase chi when there's not enough, or to decrease it when there's too much.

> *From the pharmacy, David and I walk to the "kitchen," where herbal teas are steeped for each patient in the hospital. Treating a patient with Western medication in a hospital is a simple matter of prescribing premanufactured pills or hooking up a drip bottle. But herbal medications must be prepared fresh twice a day. In the kitchen there are four long rows of twenty-five burners, all the burners going at once, each one brewing a specific combination of herbs according to the recipe written on a slip of paper and tacked next to the brew.*

MOYERS: Some scientifically grounded person walking here would be reminded of the witches in *Macbeth:* "Boil, boil."

EISENBERG: And until these remedies are tested scientifically, that would be a fair sentiment.

MOYERS: Looks like a cure for every ailment.

EISENBERG: This is what they call the "boil the medicine room." Each of these pots contains herbs for one patient in the hospital. And in each pot are ten to fifteen different herbs.

MOYERS: And a different mixture of herbs—each patient has an individual prescription.

EISENBERG: Yes. The doctors will make their rounds in the morning, look at the pulse, look at the tongue, write the prescription, and send it here. And then each of these "cooks" has to mind twelve pots at a time, boiling each pot for about twenty minutes. The pots have to be copper, or, they say, you lose some of the effectiveness of the herbs. This hospital has five hundred patients, and each patient has one pot of herbs cooked here every day. Then the broth is put into thermoses and brought to the wards. That's the treatment.

MOYERS: I just can't begin to describe the smell of these boiling broths. It's every root I've ever smelled, every tea, gum, raisin, root. And each of these brews looks different. That looks like cabbage and collard greens, and this looks more like beans. That looks like acorns.

EISENBERG: I know. I think it's awful. I don't know how they drink any of this stuff.

MOYERS: Under what circumstances would you drink it?

EISENBERG: I think if I believed that this was the best medicine for me, I would drink it. But it really smells and tastes horrible.

MOYERS: I feel as if I've walked into a medieval alchemist's shop—boiling roots, boiling gecko, boiling scorpion.

EISENBERG: Well, the style of making these herbs is hundreds, if not a thousand years old. A lot of the general prescriptions are five hundred years old.

MOYERS: How much of the effect of these herbs is merely psychological?

EISENBERG: I don't think anyone could answer your question unless we test these remedies against something. But these people take the herbs because they've been helped by them. Chinese patients are basically very practical. If a remedy worked for them, or their brother, or their mother, or their grandmother, they're going to take it.

MOYERS: So that's the tradition.

EISENBERG: And it's worked a long time.

After visiting the herbal pharmacy, we scrub and dress for an operation on a young woman. The only anesthesia used is acupuncture and a small amount of narcotic and sedative—about half the amount used in the West. Later, we visit the acupuncture ward of the hospital.

EISENBERG: Most Americans think acupuncture is used only as an anesthetic, but Chinese medicine uses it to cure hundreds of different diseases. We also tend to think of acupuncture as using needles, but that's not always so. Here you see a variation of acupuncture using what are called "pulling cups." The doctor is putting glass suction cups on the acupuncture points along the patient's lower back. My grandparents in Russia had this same kind of treatment. I think suction cups have been used for a long time, all over the world, to treat disease.

MOYERS: The suction cups are pulling the patient's skin up into a mound like an ice cream cone.

EISENBERG: Yes, and it causes quite a bruise. But this patient says it doesn't hurt and that after the treatment, he could lift his arm higher.
    Now, the woman over there has paralysis of the face. The doctor is putting needles into her arm and face, into what is called the "large-intestine meridian."

MOYERS: I don't understand that.

EISENBERG: Well, the body in Chinese medicine is made up of circuits of energy. Each applies to one organ. In this case, the doctor is attempting to increase blood circulation along the energy channel of her large intestine.

MOYERS: What, exactly, does this do for her?

DOCTOR: It's difficult to explain this in light of Western medicine. But according to traditional Chinese medical theory, this woman's disease is caused by "wind" and "heat." It has to be discharged in order for her face to get better.

MOYERS: What does this do for her intestine?

DOCTOR: The acupuncture treatment clears energy imbalances which, in her case, primarily involve her large intestine. When her "wind" and "heat" are discharged, the passages will be cleared, and when the passages are clear, the energy will flow and her face will recover. This is the theory.

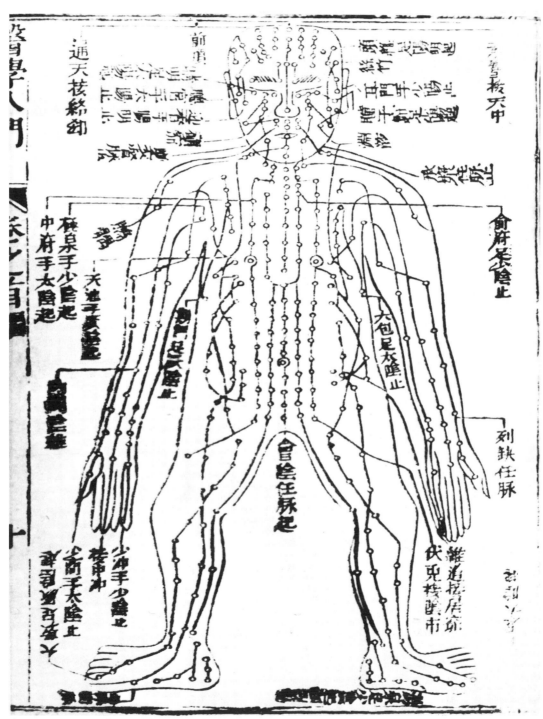

Acupuncture chart, Ming dynasty

MOYERS: What is the patient feeling now?

PATIENT: I feel a swelling during treatment. Then I feel better. When I came in, I was dizzy, and my arms had no strength.

MOYERS: Did you try Western medicine when you first got the disease?

PATIENT: I went to the hospital, very sick. I took some Western medicine and returned home, but the next day I returned to the emergency room of the same hospital. They said I had Ménière's disease.

EISENBERG: That's a disease of the inner ear. Did the Western medicine work?

PATIENT: No, I had to have intravenous feeding. After that, I came here.

MOYERS: So they've stuck needles into certain energy channels in her body.

EISENBERG: Yes. The channels are called "meridians."

MOYERS: We have nerve charts. Do they correspond to the pathways of chi in the Chinese system?

EISENBERG: No, the meridian system does not correspond to any anatomic map we have in the West. Some of the meridians are close to nerves or arteries, but no one in the West has been able to make a direct correspondence. Their diagnostic and therapeutic roadmap—the way they describe the workings of the human body— is totally different from ours.

MOYERS: How does the doctor know he's hitting the right point?

EISENBERG: It's an incredibly difficult thing to do. He asks her whether she feels the chi, and if she has a sensation, that's how he knows. He also has to feel it. My acupuncture teacher said it's like fishing. You must know the difference between a nibble and a bite. You put the needle in, and if it gets a little stuck, if there is a tension pulling back, then you know, even without asking the patient. But it's an art. A lot of the knowledge is really in the fingers.

MOYERS: What does the patient feel when she feels the chi?

EISENBERG: The patient usually has some sensation like fullness or numbness or tingling. It looks as if this might hurt, but if you put the needles in right, the patient doesn't experience pain, just a kind of swelling sensation.

MOYERS: But when she talks to the doctor, she reports feeling fullness all the way up her body, and not just where the needle went in.

EISENBERG: This is a part of acupuncture that I don't understand. You can put a needle in somebody's foot, and they'll feel numbness all the way up the side of their neck. Some people think that's how the acupuncture channels were first discovered: they put in needles at different sites, and the patients felt sensations in distant parts of the body.

MOYERS: Wouldn't we simply say that the doctor struck a nerve?

EISENBERG: Yes, that's the way you'd think of explaining it—but that doesn't work, because the nerves don't go all the way from the toe to the hip to the shoulder to the head. They have to go along different tracks. It doesn't make sense from the Western standpoint.

MOYERS: When the doctor does acupuncture, does he use his own chi?

DOCTOR: Yes, I have to use my chi in order to stick the needle in. I also spin the needle, which requires a lot of skill. If I do it with the emission of my chi, the patient will have an intense feeling.

When you first start learning, you can't use your chi very well. The patient will be afraid until you have mastered it. If you can get the chi centered in the fingers, the patient will feel comfortable.

EISENBERG: My acupuncture teacher says that a good acupuncturist has to use chi to make acupuncture work. If you put the needle in without using chi, it's like "putting a needle into a piece of steak." Nothing happens. You need to put your own chi through the needle, and you need to feel the chi through the needle from the patient's body.

Let me tell you that just putting the needle in perpendicular to the skin so that it doesn't hurt is unbelievably difficult. For me, as a foreigner, the practice exercise was putting the needle through ten pieces of paper without bending the needle. Until I could do that, they wouldn't let me near a patient. It took me weeks, just practicing with these needles. I think these needles are thinner than a hair, so to put them through anything like paper, let alone skin, without bending them is just incredibly difficult.

MOYERS: Did you finally learn?

EISENBERG: No. I got to the point where they let me put needles into people, but I never felt the chi. The whole thing is just incredibly difficult. These doctors first have to be trained in all the theory, and then they have to know the 365 meridians. For each patient, they have to make a precise diagnosis to know where the energy problem is. Then they have to get the needle in exactly the right spot, and if it's not right, they have to move it a millimeter or two until they do find the right spot, and then they have to use their own energy.

MOYERS: Did you learn the meridians when you were studying here?

EISENBERG: Yes, they painted me with iodine dots, and I had to recognize all the points on my own body, and then on my teacher's body. I got that far, and then I worked on a few hundred patients—but I never felt the chi. That level of skill takes years of apprenticing.

MOYERS: How many people in China have experienced acupuncture?

DOCTOR: About a third of the people in China have probably been treated with acupuncture at some point in their lives. That's a third of 1.1 billion people—so probably hundreds of millions of people.

MOYERS: So what's happening with this patient is as common to her as taking aspirin is to us.

EISENBERG: Yes, and you have to remember that acupuncture is found not only in China, but also in Japan, Korea, Singapore, Vietnam, Malaysia—all these places use acupuncture needles and this theory. So for hundreds of millions of people, this is not so strange.

> *Next is the massage unit, where we speak with Dr. Zang, once David's massage instructor. In the West, massage is, at best, a complement to standard medical treatment. Masseurs are not doctors. But in China, massage is a specialty, like radiology. The massage doctor first attends a traditional Chinese medical school for five years. Next the doctor does a residency, and then spends several more years preparing for a specialty in massage. And massage is not just a technique for loosening the muscles or relaxing stiff joints. Chinese massage is designed to release the flow of chi.*

EISENBERG: This is the massage unit. In this hospital, massage is taken very seriously. That's why there is a massage unit, just as we would have surgery or pediatrics.

MOYERS: What does massage have to do with medicine?

EISENBERG: Well, in Chinese medicine massage isn't just a rubdown but a way of treating some imbalance in the body. So these people have to know how to diagnose an illness, just as somebody does who works with acupuncture or herbs. Their treatment is through their hands instead of needles or herbs. But they look for the root of the problem. They don't just massage the point that is sore.

For example, these two women have what we in the West would call fibrocystic breast disease. They have pain in their breasts, but you see that the doctor is not touching their chests, but working on their backs.

MOYERS: Why is that?

EISENBERG: Why don't we ask him? Dr. Zang, why are you massaging this patient's back if her pain is in the chest?

ZANG: Because her breast problem is caused by obstructed chi in her liver. Following the line of the meridian, I am working on her inner organs in order to re-coordinate her chi and blood, thereby treating her disease. That is why she needs to be massaged not locally, but in areas far away.

MOYERS: How do you know that the chi is stuck in the liver?

ZANG: There are symptoms and physical signs. I can locate her sore points through her back and where her meridian is weak.

MOYERS: And massaging her back affects the liver, and the liver affects the breast?

ZANG: This is truly something special to Chinese medicine. The meridian is considered to connect the interior and the exterior of the body. Thus, our inner diseases can be treated through the exterior of the body. Once the chi of the meridian is opened up, the disease is cured.

EISENBERG: Dr. Zang has unbelievably gifted hands. What he is doing looks to you and me like massage, but he's worked on my body for months, and his hands are like radar. They can find spots you didn't know were sore. He can use a finger, or the ball of his hand, or his elbow. He makes it look easy, but it's remarkably difficult.

MOYERS: What did he teach you about using your hands?

EISENBERG: The first time he taught me, he brought in a bag of millet and threw it on the floor and said, "When you can use your hand to crush this to dust, then you have the beginning movements. But until you learn to crush it with your finger, you are not ready." It takes a lot of energy and skill to use your hand to crush millet into dust. That's the amount of force he can use, if he wants, on a single spot. Or he can use just the tip of his pinkie on one spot. He has to know many different manipulations—but more important, he has to know when and where to use them.

MOYERS: Dr. Zang, how long did you study this form of medicine?

ZANG: I spent six years studying medicine in college, and then a year later I was licensed to write prescriptions in the hospital. After that I practiced in the orthopedics unit for fifteen years. Then I began working on massages.

MOYERS: In the West, we think of massage as making the muscles feel better. But it's much more than that here.

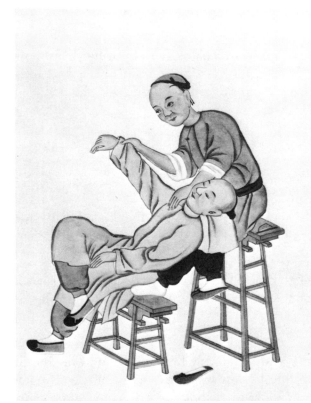

此中國剃頭棚放睡之圖也每日將頭剃完

筋骨疼痛者剃頭者坐于高橙之上其人躺

在剃頭膝上令其捶拿其快活無比

Patient Receiving Manipulative Treatment for Pain, 19th c.

ZANG: It is crucial to obtain an accurate diagnosis before one starts massage. Only when a diagnosis is reached can one begin to ponder the proper treatment. Muscular injuries should be attended to, but more important than that is the meridian. Through proper reconditioning of one's meridians, both exterior and interior diseases can be cured.

MOYERS: How do you recondition the meridians? Does the patient choose the treatment?

ZANG: No, the doctor decides what to do. We can choose from more than 160 different hand movements. These have been categorized into six main groups. Some involve turning, while others involve rubbing, pushing, striking, and vibrating. For example, in treating fibrocystic breast disease, we use the vibrating movement on the stomach. Eventually, the patient can't tell whether it's my hand or her stomach that is vibrating. After having been treated with the vibrating method, the stomach feels hot, and the sensation travels in her body, making her breast feel much better.

MOYERS: This is not just to make her comfortable.

ZANG: No, it's to cure her. She has an illness, and I am treating her illness. She has a lump which we are trying to get rid of. Her blood and energy circulation are obstructed. We are trying to open it up—then she will be cured. Her chi will no longer be obstructed.

MOYERS: Have you ever seen chi? Can you measure it or find it with a machine?

ZANG: Certain things cannot be detected by modern machinery. It's not merely physical force. Take this hand movement, for example. I am vibrating here, and she immediately feels a warm sensation. But she probably won't feel any warmth if I simply pat her.

MOYERS: You are using your chi to help heal her. But how did you locate your own chi?

ZANG: I practiced this particular hand movement from 1979 to 1986 before finally acquiring it—a total of seven years. It's not easy, not easy at all. You see, chi is more important than physical force. Only by practicing can you eventually acquire the ability to produce chi.

MOYERS: Why is chi more important than physical force?

ZANG: Because the patient suffers from obstruction of chi. Force alone is not going to do any good. Only my chi can help the circulation of her chi. For certain spots of the body we must wait for a while before the chi begins to circulate again. There is a saying in Chinese medicine: "Where there is an obstruction, there is pain." Once the obstruction is removed, the pain disappears. Take her breast pain, for example. Once her chi starts circulating, she will no longer feel the pain. In some cases, the problem is a matter of insufficient chi rather than an obstruction of chi.

MOYERS: I just don't see how it works. But why don't we ask the patient how she feels?

PATIENT: After having been massaged, my whole body feels hot, as if hot air is traveling in my arms and thighs. I feel particularly good after having been massaged, and I also feel the symptoms have subsided.

EISENBERG: How long have you had fibrocystic breast disease?

PATIENT: Eight years. I used to have cysts that multiplied rather rapidly. For a while the doctors even thought I might have breast cancer. But I feel basically well now, after only the seventh treatment.

EISENBERG: So you feel massage has helped?

PATIENT: Oh, yes. Over the years I tried all kinds of medication, both internal and external, but nothing really worked. So I came here, and after only the third treatment the lumps began to disappear and the pressure began to ease. The cysts can no longer be detected, either on mammogram or ultrasound machine.

EISENBERG: Dr. Zang, have you had many patients like her?

ZANG: Yes, I've had twenty-seven cases. Of these, I've cured eleven, healing them completely. In most other cases the size of the lumps was reduced. In two cases nothing worked.

MOYERS: How would you explain to a Western doctor how you healed this woman?

ZANG: Just as with a Western doctor, I needed the right diagnosis—but I got that diagnosis using Chinese methods. In this case I felt her pulse and looked at her tongue, and saw that her illness was caused by obstructed chi in her liver. So I adjusted the chi in her liver, not massaging anywhere near her breast, but instead, massaging her back, her stomach, and the acupuncture points along her arms and legs, and she was healed.

MOYERS: David, it must have been a stunning reversal for you to come here from a Western medical school and study with Dr. Zang. What would have been the treatment for this woman in the West?

EISENBERG: We don't have a satisfactory treatment for this disease. Most women who have severe fibrocystic breast disease are simply told to stop drinking wine or caffeinated drinks like coffee. But we don't have a good cure.

MOYERS: I still don't understand why the doctor deals with the liver by working on the feet.

EISENBERG: Well, he sees the body as a series of conduits through which chi flows. He is working on the liver, using this point down by the foot because the liver meridian flows down the feet.

MOYERS: You mean like the canals of Venice?

EISENBERG: This is the liver canal in the Chinese way of looking at the body.

MOYERS: And the energy allegedly is flowing through this canal, or meridian, to the liver.

EISENBERG: That's right. And unfortunately, in a certain area, according to Dr. Zang, the energy is stuck. So he's got to push it, move it, help it flow, and then, according to his way of thinking, the breast disease will become better.

MOYERS: Why? What happens when that chi is flowing?

EISENBERG: If I knew, I wouldn't have to keep coming back to China.

> *At Beijing Medical University, we meet a doctor who operates out of both frames of reference, East and West. Dr. Xie (pronounced "shee-yeah") never had any intention of learning traditional medicine, having been trained according to Western medical models. But in the fifties, Chairman Mao ordered many Western-trained doctors to study traditional Chinese medicine. Xie says he became profoundly interested and chose to make his life work the integration of both systems. Today he runs an entire department trained in both disciplines and consults on cases where Western medicine has met its limits. We talk to him about two cases of patients diagnosed as having ulcers. In one of these cases, Western doctors and Chinese doctors differed in their diagnosis.*

XIE: Now here's the case of a Mr. Lin, where the Western diagnosis, using X rays and an internal examination, is very precise: ulcers of the duodenum.

EISENBERG: Is that certain?

XIE: Completely certain. Look at the X ray.

EISENBERG: Yes, it's very clear. Here's the stomach, and this is the small intestine, and there's the duodenal ulcer right there.

MOYERS: I had one right there when I was a young man.

XIE: However, the Chinese doctors' diagnosis was totally different.

MOYERS: Same patient, different diagnosis?

XIE: Yes. Here's how a doctor using traditional Chinese medicine would diagnose the problem. First of all, we would look at the patient's tongue. Please take a look at Mr. Lin's tongue. On the front part of it is a white coat. The color of his tongue is a little bit pale. Pay particular attention to the sides of his tongue. There are indentations of the teeth. These are the particularities of Mr. Lin's tongue.

EISENBERG: Every student of Chinese medicine has to memorize more than one hundred tongue types. Students have to memorize the color, the texture, the coating, and whether there are indentations of the teeth. Every variation of the tongue is said to correspond to a specific problem of the individual internal organs.

MOYERS: So it's not just a matter of saying "ahh."

EISENBERG: There are very specific relationships between every tongue type and every internal organ. Tongues are different for different diseases. And every patient's tongue will change a little bit day by day, depending on the imbalance of chi.

MOYERS: So what does this tongue tell the doctor about the imbalance of his chi, his energy?

XIE: This tongue has particularities that indicate the patient has a spleen deficiency of energy, chi. The edge of the tongue is a little large and pale and has teeth indentations. These are all symptoms of spleen insufficiency. When this patient first checked in, the surface of his tongue was very white. Usually, a white surface indicates coldness, so we used a lot of warming medication as part of the treatment. After treatment, the color in the back of the tongue has turned light yellow.

MOYERS: You mean the ulcer is related to the spleen?

EISENBERG: From the Chinese standpoint, there's an ulcer in the stomach, but the root of the problem is an imbalance in the spleen. In this case you can see how different from the Western approach the Eastern approach to any particular problem can be.

MOYERS: So what comes after the tongue analysis?

EISENBERG: Usually, the doctor would then go on to pulse diagnosis.

MOYERS: The old lub dub lub dub.

EISENBERG: Not exactly. It's a lot more complicated. For the Chinese, there are probably at least forty common pulse types, twelve of which are found frequently in sick patients. Dr. Xie has to figure out which of these pulse variations are occurring at nine spots on each wrist. He puts his right hand on the patient's left wrist, and feels for three spots, each corresponding to a different organ. First he feels the pulse superficially, then moderately, and then by pushing down deeply.

MOYERS: And once he's found which of the forty pulse types any particular pulse is, what will that tell him?

EISENBERG: Again, using his line of reasoning, it will tell him more than just how fast the heart is beating, or whether this person has high or low blood pressure, or whether the pulse is regular. Those are things I can do. What he is feeling for is much more subtle. He will tell you whether a particular pulse indicates an insufficiency of heat or chi in the spleen, and he will tell you from this variation of touch that the spleen is the root of the problem. Even though this man has a bleeding ulcer, the pulse says the root of the problem is in the spleen. That's what always intrigued me when I studied this. Are these claims real? Could Western medicine verify that something was wrong with the spleen in this case? Do these associations between superficial pulses and internal disease really hold up?

Chinese pulse
chart, 1693

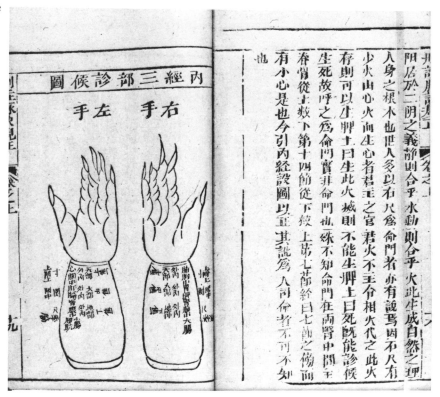

MOYERS: If the Chinese can diagnose that precisely by feeling the pulse, why can't we?

EISENBERG: We should test it. We have technology now that can measure the pulse in very sensitive ways. Why not take the best Chinese doctors and the most sensitive machines and see if claims about which pulse matches a particular organ hold up?

MOYERS: How long does it take Dr. Xie to analyze the pulse?

EISENBERG: He probably will do it for five minutes, in complete silence, just touching.

MOYERS: The last time I had my pulse taken, the procedure lasted about forty seconds.

EISENBERG: Yes, most doctors in the West are really just looking for the pulse rate and for whether the pulse is regular. Sometimes Chinese doctors will take the pulse for ten to twenty minutes, in silence. When you touch another human being for that long without saying anything, a lot is communicated nonverbally. You'll find out if the person is nervous or uncomfortable or seems unhappy or peaceful.

MOYERS: Is that connected with what I was reading in a book about Chinese medicine that describes the hands of the physician being able to discover something about the emotional state of the patient?

EISENBERG: That's right. Traditionally, each of these internal organ problems is connected with a particular emotional problem. For instance, in Chinese medicine, anger is said to be connected to the liver. So if the doctor touches somebody and feels this is a very angry person, he will pay special attention to the liver. If the liver is out of balance, he will try to tell whether this is a very angry person who is not in control of the anger.

MOYERS: We're making these kinds of connections, too, aren't we, in relation to stress and the heart?

EISENBERG: Yes. We are beginning to see possible relationships between certain personality styles and heart disease or cancer. But in Chinese medicine there is another reason for figuring this out through using the pulse. Doctors don't talk to patients about emotional issues. A Chinese proverb says the equivalent of "Don't wash your dirty linen in public"—don't turn your personal problem into a public disgrace. In other words, the patient does not share personal problems with the doctor, and the doctor does not ask these questions. So these kinds of feelings typically must be communicated without words. A lot of that happens when the doctor sits down with the patient and just touches him in silence for five or ten minutes.

MOYERS: So out of that old taboo came something positive. Did they try to teach you the forty pulses when you came here twelve years ago?

EISENBERG: Yes, but again, as with acupuncture, I wasn't very good. In fact, this was even harder than acupuncture. It probably takes five or ten years to be able to do it well. The analogy that I can make from my Western training is that when my cardiology professor gave me a stethoscope and said "Listen to this heart," I heard "thump, thump, thump." He would say, "This heart has a click and a murmur and then another murmur—do you hear it?" I would have to say, "No, I don't." But after a few hundred patients you begin to hear these subtle clicks and murmurs. If you have a good teacher, who guides you, you can learn the skill. It just takes a long time to be as skillful as Dr. Xie.

MOYERS: Dr. Xie, you were trained first in Western medicine, and you then took up the study of traditional Chinese medicine. Why did you change?

XIE: In my earlier practice I came across some problematic cases for which Western medicine did not offer any satisfactory cure. After I began to learn about Chinese medicine, I discovered that for these cases, Chinese medicine is more effective. That's when I really began to be interested in Chinese medicine. I then discovered that Chinese medicine had many advantages. For some acute diseases, such as viral infections, Western doctors and medication do not seem to provide a cure—but Chinese medicine offers some help.

MOYERS: Were you skeptical at first about Chinese traditional medicine?

XIE: Yes, I was, in part because I had begun my medical studies in Western medicine, and both the theory and practice of Chinese medicine are absolutely different from what I had learned of Western medicine. So I was very skeptical in the beginning. But after I tried the Chinese medicine and herbs, I found that they worked, so I began to change my mind.

MOYERS: What does Chinese medicine tell you about health and medicine that Western medicine can't?

XIE: In Chinese medicine the mind and emotions are closely related to health and disease. For example, disease can be caused by the intensification of any of the seven human emotions—joy, anger, melancholy, brooding, sorrow, fear, and shock. An excess of joy will do harm to the heart, anger will do harm to the liver, melancholy to the kidney, brooding and sorrow to the spleen, and fear and shock to the kidney.

MOYERS: And you could feel some of these emotions in the patients with ulcers simply by taking the pulse?

XIE: Partially, yes.

MOYERS: Since you practice Western medicine as well as Chinese medicine, would you ever use a drug like Tagamet for treating these patients' ulcers?

XIE: Yes, we use it very often here. Western medicine is effective in treating the ulcer, but a combination of both Western and Chinese medicine produces an even better effect. Take these two patients here for example: we gave them totally different Chinese medicine for their ulcers, and in both cases the medicine worked well.

MOYERS: So when you were diagnosing these patients, what did you learn from the pulse?

XIE: One patient doesn't have a special emotional problem—his ulcer had something to do with years of irregular diet. But the second patient is different. His pulse belongs to the "liver pulse," which has something to do with emotions. Habitual anger caused his ulcer, little by little.

MOYERS: And how does chi relate to that?

X I E :   These two cases are opposite. The first patient showed a lack of chi, while the second has excessive chi because of chi blockage in his liver. Chi can't pass through, causing his disease. But this chi excess doesn't mean there is too much chi in his body, just that the flow of chi stops in that particular area and is unable to travel farther.

M O Y E R S :   Is there anything in Western science comparable to chi?

X I E :   No, I don't think so. The concept of chi is hard to put into English. "Lack of chi" is often explained as a functional insufficiency, but "chi excess" is not equivalent to "hyperfunction." Sometimes it is, but at other times it means functional disorder.

M O Y E R S :   "Bad chi."

X I E :   Right, it's not good. We don't need this kind of chi.

M O Y E R S :   And the mind is closely related to chi.

X I E :   Yes. Take chi gong, for example, which is a method for adjusting and mobilizing chi with willpower and concentration. When you practice chi gong to a certain level, you might be able to mobilize all your body energy and focus it in one place. That's what we call "the phenomenon of chi gong." Chi is adjusted by the mind.

M O Y E R S :   Do you use your own chi when you are with your patients?

X I E :   No, I only suggest that patients use chi gong themselves to treat their illnesses. We do have some Chinese doctors here who can use their own chi to treat the patient, but I can't.

M O Y E R S :   Is it hard to integrate Western and Chinese medicine? Are they comparable in any way?

X I E :   We have to admit that the early period of integration for the two medicines was very hard. Gradually, we found that some aspects of Chinese medicine could be explained according to Western theory. For example, we noticed that certain herbs could strengthen chi, but we didn't know why. Then modern science showed us that some substances immunize people against disease. If a substance can do that, it can certainly strengthen chi, because "good chi" is the united power of body functions to resist diseases — and immunity is part of that.

M O Y E R S :   Your patients can choose either Western treatment or Chinese treatment. How do they make that choice?

X I E :   Many Chinese patients in fact know when to choose Western medicine and when to choose Chinese medicine. If they need an operation, they'll make sure to find a Western doctor, whereas for chronic diseases they'll prefer Chinese medicine.

MOYERS: But does Chinese medicine cure the illness, or does it just help the patient to live with it?

XIE: That depends on the disease. Some can be cured gradually and thoroughly, and some can't. But what I want to emphasize is that the application of Chinese medicine is fundamentally different from what is done in the West. In Chinese medicine, "disease" is defined as the struggle between human capability to resist disease and the pathogenic factors. Chinese medicine stresses the human capability to resist disease. Therefore, many treatments are designed to motivate this capability—once it is motivated, some diseases can be cured easily. That's the key point of Chinese treatment.

> *David and I keep talking about the mystery of chi. But to millions of Chinese, chi is no mystery at all. At dawn, in any Chinese park, you can see groups of men and women practicing what appears to me to be a ritual dance—but is actually an ancient exercise whose purpose is the movement of chi.*

MOYERS: This is an extraordinary sight. This park is absolutely full of people doing exercises.

EISENBERG: Yes, there are about three thousand people here. And every morning in every park, all over China, and all over the countryside, the same thing is happening. Some of these people are high-ranking government officials, and some are uneducated workers. Some are in fancy clothes, and some are poor. There are old and young.

MOYERS: So there's some democracy after all in Communist China.

EISENBERG: In terms of using Chinese medicine to maintain health, it's truly democratic.

MOYERS: What kind of exercise are they doing?

EISENBERG: Actually, this t'ai chi ch'uan exercise is twenty-three centuries old. They are trying to "move like the clouds, eternally transforming without the appearance of change." The exercise is supposed to be like nature, and the person exercising tries to connect with nature through movement. In Chinese medicine there's the idea that the body has to move, and that movement is as important as eating or sleeping or drinking. Centuries ago they started to make pictures about how people should move to keep the body healthy. So these people are moving, but it's more than that.

MOYERS: Is it like isometrics?

EISENBERG: No, they're moving all the joints, and using a lot more energy than it would appear. You can imagine how much energy it would take, for example, just

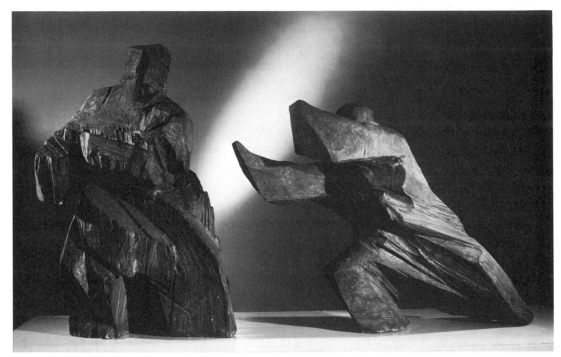

Ju Ming, *Tai Chi Boxing*, 1984

to stand with your knees bent for an hour. But in addition to physical strength, it also requires concentration. If you look at the faces of these people, you'll see that they're trying to do something more than just move their joints and strengthen their muscles. They're trying to focus their sense of the balance of energy, or chi. They're trying to feel where their energy starts from, and then to move it through their whole body. So although the exercise is physical, it's also very contemplative and meditative. To do this exercise, you have to be physically active, but you also have to direct your mind.

MOYERS: I'm astonished to see so many old people exercising here.

EISENBERG: A lot of these old people have probably been coming out here every day of their lives since childhood, when their grandparents taught them to do this.

MOYERS: Do they come in winter as well?

EISENBERG: Yes, and in northern China they come even when there is snow and ice. In Chinese medicine the body is a microcosm of the universe, a part of nature, so that as the seasons and temperatures change, people also experience these changes. It's part of living and dying.

Many of the old people here, who are in their seventies and eighties, can speak English because they grew up at a time when they went to high school where Americans taught them. Here comes a fellow I met yesterday, who introduced himself as we were walking around the park.

MOYERS: What is this? What are they doing here?

EISENBERG: This is another style of martial arts. To Westerners it looks a little like the kung-fu movies. It's called the "hard style." What we saw with the old people was the "soft style," where you're mainly trying to maximize your balance and feel where your energy center is. This harder style uses that as a prerequisite, and then it uses more speed and physical force, so it looks more martial, more aggressive. But the motions are the same, and the intent is the same: to center the energy and move it in order to maximize balance and health.

MOYERS: By martial, you don't mean aggressive, do you? They're not out to conquer or hurt anybody.

EISENBERG: We have a problem of language when we use the word "martial," because we think of being aggressive or striking somebody. But these exercises are really more like gymnastics, literally "push-pull" exercises—getting in touch with your energy so that you can push it, pull it, and move it to maintain health. If you speed up these exercises, they can look very aggressive. In the West we have this misconception that Chinese martial arts consists of kung-fu, or Japanese karate—but that's only one small portion of the spectrum. In the same way, we wrongly think of acupuncture as comprising most of Chinese medicine. It's only a tiny piece.

MOYERS: What do these exercises have to do with health?

EISENBERG: There is an ancient idea that if you don't move the body every day, it becomes stagnant. It's said that the body is like a hinge on a door: if it is not swung open, it rusts. So these people are moving their bodies, and because they're younger, they tend to want to do the more martial, aggressive forms of movement. They're still doing the ancient forms, the ones you saw their grandparents doing—but they're moving much faster, and they're less meditative in their approach. You don't see that look on their faces that you see on the faces of the ninety-year-olds—that they could be anywhere, in any park in the country. These young people want to be in a recognized group and wear flashy outfits and to be more aggressive in their style. But to perform well, you still have to know where your energy is and to move it appropriately. This man is doing another kind of ancient exercise: chi gong. His rhythmical, symmetrical movements enable him to feel where the energy in his body is and then begin to move it. Although it looks like he's just rocking back and forth, he's really trying to focus on where the energy in his body starts from. See, as he takes a deep

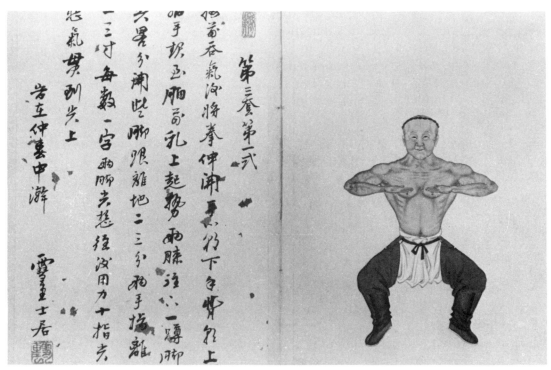

Chi gong exercise

breath, he's probably concentrating on feeling the energy in his body and moving it up or down through a limb. Everything we've seen is a way of learning how to move one's energy like this man is doing.

MOYERS: Do you believe that he really moves his energy in that way?

EISENBERG: I practiced t'ai chi for a year, and although I felt deeply relaxed and centered and balanced, I never felt this energy. If you ask this man, he'll say that he feels "heat" or "numbness," and that he can move this sensation anywhere in his body. Of the three thousand people here, I bet two thousand of them would tell you the same thing, and would also tell you that they've been feeling that energy for years. So either they are perpetuating a myth they all believe in, or they are feeling something they've been taught to feel which we don't understand.

MOYERS: If it's myth, it's superstition on a very large scale.

EISENBERG: Yes, and it's twenty-three centuries old.

MOYERS: Why do these people consider energy to be so important for health?

EISENBERG: All these people are trying to retain their proper place in nature because their notion of health is that the body has to reflect the balances in nature. So, as the seasons change, people are supposed to be outside in the seasons, and when they're outside, they're supposed to feel their energy. When they feel their energy, they can become balanced, but if they don't feel their energy, then they fall out of balance, and they get sick.

MOYERS: What do you mean by "balance"?

EISENBERG: Well, look at this man doing chi gong. He's probably creating an image of his feet going down three hundred yards into the ground, so that he is rooted like a tree. And in his mind his arms are probably moving like bird wings, very symmetrically, and very gracefully. That allows him to feel equal on the right and the left, up and down, and with that, he would tell you that he can feel balanced and centered. Then, he will tell you, he can begin to move his energy. All of these exercises have the same goal: to get that sense of balance and centering, so that you can feel your energy and move it. That, according to this tradition, is health.

MOYERS: When you were studying medicine here, did you do this?

EISENBERG: I did a variation of this, yes. I did t'ai chi ch'uan every day at dawn in a little courtyard in Beijing. That was really my favorite part of living in China, and it's what I miss most. There was something about being outside every day at dawn, even in the dead of winter, just moving, just feeling your body outside. We're not accustomed to that in the West.

MOYERS: Why did you give it up when you went back to the United States? You don't have to be in China to do t'ai chi.

EISENBERG: Because I became an intern at a big teaching hospital, and I had to be at work at six-thirty.

MOYERS: So your health was no longer as important as the health of other people?

EISENBERG: It was important, but I could no longer take care of it the same way. And that shows one of the differences between our culture and theirs. In China the patient is responsible for helping to prevent illness or maintain health. They resort to their traditional medicine—herbs and acupuncture and pressure points—only after they're no longer able to maintain their own health. If you take that point of view seriously, you'll get up every morning at dawn and go out into nature and do movement to keep your body limber and try to center yourself and feel balanced. In the West it's only relatively recently that doctors have recommended calisthenics and aerobics and said that physical stamina is essential in maintaining health or intervening in illness. The Chinese started on the other side, saying that this kind of exercise and centering is a prerequisite to health. You can't have health unless you maintain your body and use both physical exercise and mental discipline. One of my favorite things is seeing young people like these two women, who are so graceful and clearly so appreciative of their two-thousand-year-old art. They're not doing anything to challenge anybody, or to try to hurt anybody. They're just trying to figure out where their center is, what is a balanced form, where the right and left are. You might ask, what does that have to do with medicine? In the Chinese culture that defines health. If you can figure out where your center is and how to concentrate your mind, you're healthy, and once you lose that, you get sick.

MOYERS: What do you mean by finding your center? Are you talking about some kind of physical center?

EISENBERG: I'll put it in physical terms. This woman in white, who is so beautiful to watch—you could try to push her over, but if she's doing this form right, she won't budge, because at any moment she knows exactly where her center is, and she won't move from it. She's pretending that there is a rod running from her head down through her back into the ground. When people are taught this, teachers will actually try to push them off balance while they're doing a movement. If you can do everything that she's doing and never be pushed off balance, then you understand where your center is.

MOYERS: What does that have to do with health?

EISENBERG: If you don't know whether your body is out of balance, you can't know whether you're healthy or not. Where we would think in terms of being sick, they would say that their chi is too weak in one part, or too strong in another part.

MOYERS: Are they trying to get access to that chi, that energy, or are they trying to control it?

EISENBERG: Let me tell you the steps you have to go through. This woman has probably studied for ten years. She probably started learning very slow movements and was told to "move like the clouds, eternally transforming without the appearance of change." She had to learn every movement all these old people are doing. Then, after a few years of that, her teacher said, "Okay, now you're ready to feel where your energy is." As I said, I practiced this for a year and I never felt that energy. But many Chinese insist that after two or three years you can feel where your center of energy is in terms of physical warmth or heat or fullness. If you ask that woman, she will tell you she can actually feel that, and she can move it. Finally, she has to learn to move that energy while she's doing these fast actions. That's how she's taught this: to learn the balance, to meditate, to feel the energy, and then to move it at will.

MOYERS: It looks as if they are dancing.

EISENBERG: They are doing what's called "pushing hands." They're trying to use their balance to push the other off balance. It looks like a dance, but it's done with the intention of challenging your sense of balance. They're exercising not only their muscles, but also their sense of where their center of gravity is. It's hard to remain stationary when somebody is trying to push you off your feet. You have to know where your center of gravity is at all times. These women are probably in their sixties or seventies. Every day they come out to reexplore where their center of gravity is and to pay attention to it.

MOYERS: What about these people with swords? What are they doing?

EISENBERG: The swords are just ornamental, a kind of extension of where the body begins and ends. These people are not trying to strike anybody. They use swords to create postures as a way of experiencing balance. And like the other movements we've seen, these gestures have a two thousand-year-old history. I'm most fond of seeing the old people here in the corners of the park. They don't want the noise, and they don't want the big group. They are the ones who are trying to perfect the meditative side of their exercises, combining the mental as well as the physical. They're doing their best to meditate the whole time.

MOYERS: So is that part of what you mean by balance between the physical and the mental, and between action and contemplation?

EISENBERG: Right. The Chinese never separated them. In order to maintain health, you have to have physical movement, but also meditative balance. And you have to control not only your physical body, but also your will and intention and your thoughts. Without that mental overlay, the physical movements are just superficial calisthenics. In traditional Chinese medicine you don't just do calisthenics to get your heart rate up, and you can't just sit and meditate all day. One without the other is not enough. The combination is at the heart of Chinese medicine.

MOYERS: Somehow it seems more appropriate to be doing this in the woods.

EISENBERG: Yes, these people would much prefer to be in the woods, because their idea is that natural settings are the ones that allow you to be in touch with your energy. Traditionally, the Chinese did these exercises in places of natural beauty. We've been watching this woman for two or three minutes, and she's not moving at all. As I mentioned to you, all these exercises require both movement and meditation. She's concentrating on the meditative aspect. Just as an athlete needs to train in different ways—doing sprints as well as running long distances—you have to perfect different sides to do any of these exercises well. This woman is perfecting the meditative side.

MOYERS: What is she actually doing?

EISENBERG: If we interviewed her now, she would probably tell us that she is making her mind empty, and that she's trying to access the center of her body. Once she feels where it is, she'll tell you that she has a sensation of fullness or heat, and that she's trying to move that sensation up or down. As any thought comes to mind, she just lets it go and focuses on her breathing. This is similar to many other meditative traditions.

MOYERS: She looks as if she's about to fall asleep.

EISENBERG: I think she's quite awake. People who are meditating tend to be hyper-aware. I think she notices us, and she knows she is being filmed, and she is aware of everyone around her, but she's trying to let go of those thoughts. She would probably tell you that when her mind is emptied, these are the moments she feels most balanced, most physically in control, and most healthy.

MOYERS: This looks like an outdoor ballroom.

EISENBERG: Yes, this is ballroom dancing. You know, we're in the middle of Shanghai, and the people of Shanghai consider themselves to be the most Western in China. In the thirties and forties, Shanghai was the "place to be" for famous people the world over. Ballroom dancing was the thing to do in all the big hotels. Ballroom dancing has a hundred-year-old history, and chi gong has a twenty-three-hundred-year-old history—and they're both still going strong in Shanghai. Now this man is doing what's called "moving chi gong," or "walking chi gong." He's not just walking, he's also trying to meditate while he walks. He's walking with the intent of moving his energy with every step.

MOYERS: I wonder how long he will walk like that this morning.

EISENBERG: It would not surprise me if he walks for sixty or ninety minutes that way every morning, every day of the year.

MOYERS: What's happening to his body while he's doing this?

EISENBERG: Well, he's not getting the kind of cardiovascular workout he would get on a bike or a treadmill. But he's moving his limbs, and he's meditating, so he's probably relaxed.

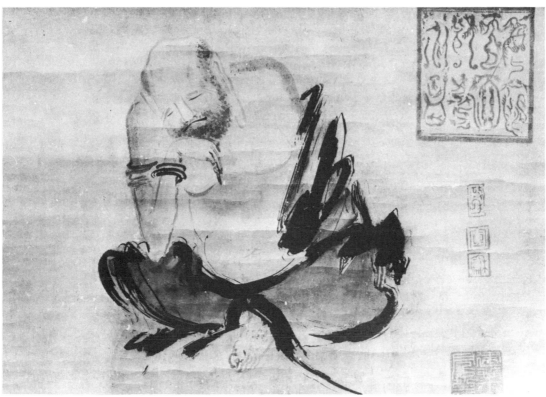

Honel-Ko in Meditation, Ming dynasty

But the big question is, do any of these martial arts change people enough to alter their disease, or make them live longer? If you ask the old people, they'll say, "This has kept me healthy." If you ask me, as a Western scientist, I'd say, "I don't know." But hundreds of millions of people have been out in the fresh air every day for twenty-four centuries in the belief that if they do these exercises, they'll maximize their health.

MOYERS: What do you mean by "maximize"?

EISENBERG: You know, some people are blessed with strong bodies and gorgeous facial features and powerful hearts, and other people have high cholesterol and high blood pressure and bad kidneys. The Chinese notion is that you're given a certain amount of bodily health, and then it's your job to maximize what you've got. And to do that, you've got to be out in nature every day, physically moving and meditating, or you won't be as healthy as you can be. You have the ultimate responsibility for your health.

Seeing hundreds of people exercising in the park—especially seeing the many older people—makes me wonder how t'ai chi and other mind/body exercises are learned. David takes me to the t'ai chi studio of Ma Yueh Liang, one of the greatest living practitioners of t'ai chi ch'uan, a Grand Master. He was trained in Western science and ran the clinical laboratories in a prominent Shanghai hospital. But at the same time, for more than seventy years, he has taught and practiced t'ai chi ch'uan. He is now ninety-one years old.

MOYERS: Did you learn t'ai chi while you were in medical school?

MA: Yes, when I was twenty, I began to study t'ai chi from a master. I became not just his student, but his disciple. A student is a learner on a regular basis, but a disciple is committed to the practice and teaching of t'ai chi.

MOYERS: Why did you begin the study of t'ai chi?

MA: As a student who studied bacteria, I would easily be infected by disease germs if I didn't keep myself healthy. That's why I learned t'ai chi—to keep fit. Practicing t'ai chi has many functions. One is that it makes you live longer. I'm ninety-one years old, and I can still take trips abroad by plane and teach t'ai chi to others. Even a young man cannot beat me in a t'ai chi martial arts competition.

Another function is to help heal chronic diseases. Yet another is to refresh. When you come home from work at the end of the day, if you calm down and practice t'ai chi, you will be refreshed, and your tiredness will disappear.

T'ai chi works for everybody. Practicing its slow movements is like taking a rest, except that there is movement in t'ai chi. It can also be used as a martial art, like boxing, but it is not designed to attack. Every movement of t'ai chi is designed for defense.

MOYERS: I'm a journalist, not a scientist. But journalists, like scientists, want evidence. They want to see something. In order to believe, I must see. How do you know that chi exists? You can't see it, and you can't measure it.

MA: I study bacteriology, which is a science. Science has to see something. If you say that something exists, but you can't find it, it's not science. But in China there are many things that are difficult to define in a scientific way. Take t'ai chi, for example. Chi is important in practicing t'ai chi. If you get chi perfect, you'll master t'ai chi.

MOYERS: But what is chi?

MA: I'll give you an example of chi. If you practice t'ai chi well, you will have the vitality of a child. The vitality of a child is strong, while the vitality of an old man is weak. As the old man gets older, his vitality gets weaker, and when there is no vitality left in his body, he dies.

MOYERS: Chi is life?

MA: There are two kinds of chi. "Yin" refers to the adequacy of vitality, while "yang" is the resistance against disease. Therefore, the Chinese terms "yin" and "yang" also explain "chi." You can't see it, but after practicing t'ai chi, you'll be able to direct the chi anywhere you want.

MOYERS: But what is chi? Is it energy? A life-force?

MA: Chi is the major energy of a person. You can see if a person has a strong chi. If the skin is not wrinkled, and there is no white hair, and the aging is slow, this indicates a strong chi or vitality. And this is the energy you just mentioned—the original energy of a person.

MOYERS: Where does this power or energy come from?

MA: When you are born, the chi is there as a natural thing. But as you grow up, the chi gets consumed, especially when you are sick or old or tired from excessive work. As far as I know, to practice t'ai chi helps to maintain vitality.

MOYERS: How long did it take you to discover your chi?

MA: It took me ten years to discover it. But it took me thirty years to learn how to use it.

MOYERS: That's very discouraging to most of us, who don't have the discipline to do it.

MA: This is where t'ai chi is most difficult. There are five aspects of practicing t'ai chi. First, you calm down. When you are about to practice, you think of nothing but t'ai chi. Second, you eliminate any exertion. To open your hand seems to be an exertion, but it's not—or it seems not to be an exertion, but it is. This is what we call "the state of t'ai chi." Third, you try to be consistent, neither fast nor slow, no intervals in between. As someone is practicing t'ai chi, he cannot be disturbed; otherwise he cannot do it well. You don't think of anything else but t'ai chi.

The fourth aspect has two principles: the first is to truly and precisely practice, and not in a slipshod way. The second principle is to study the proper movements of the body. In Chinese, the first three theories are referred to as "Quietly," "Lightly," and "Slowly." The fourth is represented by a Chinese character which has two meanings: to truly practice and to study. The word "study" here doesn't mean to study while practicing t'ai chi, but at the end of the practice, to try to recall what you have just done. Maybe you moved too high at some points or too low at some other points. Or maybe you violated correct form at a certain part. This is what we call study.

The fifth aspect is perseverance. When this word is applied to t'ai chi, it means to practice every day at the same time and for the same amount of time. If you have time in the morning, do it in the morning. If you feel noon is convenient, then do it at noon. If you have a chance only in the evening, then practice in the evening. Make sure when you practice, let's say one hour each time, you keep up with it. Don't practice more or less than you do normally. And if you practice the whole sequence only once a day, keep doing it once a day. If you practice the whole sequence twice a day, then you should always do it twice a day. Don't change.

MOYERS: You said it would take thirty years for me to discover my own chi.

MA: When I said it would take thirty years, I was referring to the highest stage of t'ai chi. A person who practices for just three months in order to get rid of an illness is like a person who has only graduated from high school and doesn't go on any further in education. But even if you practiced for only three months, you would see results. For example, if you were hypertensive, your blood pressure would go back to normal. I have taught many hypertensives whose blood pressure went back to normal in this way. But you don't stop practicing just because your body has regained its health. You still have to keep up with it, step by step, in order to obtain more of its advantages.

MOYERS: You're saying that this is not a matter of superstition, but that chi is a part of our body that we have to discover.

MA: Absolutely! There is no mystery in t'ai chi. The only difficult part is perseverance. To get any benefits, you have to practice it constantly. Once you see the benefits, you'll obtain an interest. When you have an interest, you will not want to stop. I have five students who are in their nineties. The oldest one is ninety-seven. I also have many students in their eighties.

MOYERS: Do you think Westerners can ever get this? We want our payoff now.

MA: If you want to practice t'ai chi, you must change your manner. If you try to take a shortcut, you will never develop the interest or understand the purpose of the five characters.

MOYERS: This morning, when I was watching you with your students, I saw you just lightly touch a young man, and he fell down. Was he just playing a game with you, or was something actually happening there?

MA: That was not playing a game. What I did this morning was just how I normally teach. It's not acting, it's a way of teaching. Chi can emanate from your body in this way.

MOYERS: You were pushing those men back with your chi?

MA: Yes. After practicing t'ai chi for a certain period, a person becomes more sensitive to chi. Therefore, when I was emitting my chi at him, he felt it and received it. He couldn't stand still, so he lost his center of gravity. That's why he fell down. For example, if a building is held up by four stable pillars, the center of gravity is maintained. But if one pillar is removed, the building will fall. My chi removed his center of gravity, and that's why he fell down.

I remember the chi gong exercises I saw in the park when David takes me to the chi gong unit of Xi Yuan Hospital. Here those same techniques are a part of standard medical treatment. Chinese doctors claim that chi can be sensed by anyone and harnessed to heal.

EISENBERG: This hospital is famous for the integration of Chinese and Western medicine. It has the usual Western medications and surgery as well as acupuncture, massage, and herbs. But it is especially renowned for this medical chi gong unit, where the doctor, as guide, teaches patients to use the mind to change their health. A Taoist proverb says, "When you have a disease, do not try to cure it. Find your center, and you will be healed."

MOYERS: This gets to the core of mind/body medicine, doesn't it? What illnesses are being treated here?

EISENBERG: The doctors told me that several of these people have chronic low-back pain or abdominal pain. Others have insomnia, or anxiety. Then some have chronic coronary artery disease with angina. In other words, the bread-and-butter problems of internal medicine are represented here.

The doctors are trying to train these patients to use their minds to decrease their symptoms. And in their way of thinking, this actually changes their disease and begins to cure them.

MOYERS: How do you explain chi gong?

EISENBERG: Chi gong can be translated in a number of ways: the manipulation of your chi, or energy; the ability to focus your mind on where the chi in your body comes from and then to move it at will, using conscious thought; or, "breathing skill," because chi means not only "vital energy," but also "breath." These people also use breathing techniques to move their energy.

MOYERS: Yes, this looks like a typical meditation class you might find in the States, with people doing breathing exercises.

EISENBERG: It's very similar to the Indian yoga techniques and to the Tibetan meditative practices. In fact, in almost every meditative tradition, the initial instructions are the same: "Sit quietly. Focus on your breath. As thoughts come to your mind, try to disregard them."

MOYERS: So what's different about this? I might do breathing exercises, but not for medical reasons.

EISENBERG: In Chinese theory, once you have learned to relax, to focus on your breathing, and to let go of all the thoughts, then you can actually find a spot in your body where your chi, your vital energy, begins. They call this the "Dan Tian point." It's a spot just below your navel. So when they say "Find this ball at the Dan Tian point," they are talking about a ball of energy which exists where chi begins in the human body. You concentrate on the ball of energy and learn to move it. That's the skill.

MOYERS: But what does that do for the woman with chronic arthritis, or for the man with back pain?

EISENBERG: After weeks or months of practicing this meditative tradition, their symptoms have decreased enormously—at least, that's what they say. But the question is, has it really done that? Is that just their subjective sense, or, more objectively, have their bodies physically changed so that the coronary artery disease or muscle spasms or the skin problems are helped. When you think about fifty or sixty million people in China who are doing this in response to medical conditions and who think that chi gong makes them better, you have to begin to wonder whether they really are better.

MOYERS: Unlike the acupuncturist, the herbalist, or the massage doctor, the chi gong doctor is not trying to do something for them. He is trying to guide them to do it for themselves.

EISENBERG: In this aspect of his work, that's right—he's a guide, a teacher. And traditionally, that's what a physician was, first and foremost—a guide to help patients maximize their health.

As you said, this is the core of mind/body medicine as the Chinese system understands it. This is using one's mind exclusively to alter one's body. It's a logical extension of the rest of the Chinese medical theory and practice.

MOYERS: You are a very rational man. I've learned that over the course of our time together here in China. But something keeps drawing you back to this.

EISENBERG: Well, you know, there comes a point when you meet a number of people with years and years of chronic back pain or migraine headache or duodenal ulcers, and they say, "I was miserable until I learned this, and now I'm much better. I feel better, I'm stronger, and I sleep better." Now that's anecdotal evidence that won't convince any of my skeptical colleagues. But if you interview dozens and dozens of people who seem very credible and realistic and practical, you have to wonder—are they all following some fantasy, or is there something here to be studied? That's why I keep coming back.

MOYERS: Given all these people you've interviewed, you must have yearned to submit chi gong to some kind of scientific proof.

EISENBERG: I would love nothing more than to help the doctors who are teaching these patients all over China, to create well-designed experiments in which one-third of the people do chi gong, one-third do not, and the last group thinks it's doing chi gong but has actually been given some kind of sham technique. A change in symptoms would translate into a new understanding of physiology, and that would be a big contribution to medical science.

As David and I talk, the patients begin to do the gentle exercises that I observed in the park.

EISENBERG: This is a moving form of chi gong, just like what we saw in the park, except that there, the people were doing chi gong to prevent illness, and here in the hospital, these people are trying to cure an illness that has already occurred. But they're using the same techniques of moving their chi around.

What has always interested me is that when you ask these people whether chi is something in their minds—imagery, perhaps, or the way they think about the body—they always say no. They'll tell you that chi is something physical that they can sense and, after months of practice, move around.

MOYERS: I tried biofeedback once and literally could feel the warmth in my body as I used my mind with the help of the biofeedback machine to lower my pulse rate. Is this comparable to the sensation of chi?

EISENBERG: I think they're doing similar exercises without the benefit of a machine to guide them. The teacher and their own sensations guide them. If all of these things do in fact lower blood pressure and pulse, and make people's symptoms go away, ultimately that has to translate into some physical, chemical change. If that's true, and if we could understand it, then we could translate this into the language of modern Western medicine.

MOYERS: But one of the patients said that you have to believe that it helps in order for it to help.

EISENBERG: If belief has the power to change the course of significant illness or disease, that would be fascinating, too, and would offer a wonderful opportunity to study the mechanism whereby beliefs and the mind induce physical change. And if it reproducibly shows that change, and you could "bottle" it or translate it into the chemistry that people in the West understand, that would be a major contribution to medical science.

MOYERS: The last few years of my father's life were so uncomfortable for him. He had chronic headache. I took him to several major medical centers in the United States, and nobody could help him. I watch these people and I keep thinking that there is something here that might have helped him by enabling him to deal with that pain.

EISENBERG: Then probably to you and to him, it wouldn't have mattered what the chemistry was as long as he felt it helped.

MOYERS: We tried, but he just wouldn't give this sort of method a chance. He thought it was superstition.

EISENBERG: So do a lot of people in the West, and so did I when I first came here. I was very skeptical and wanted to see if it really worked. Now I have a head full of amazing stories—but that's not enough.

Later David takes me to a doctor who was moving his hands in circles around a young man's skull, never touching a hair.

EISENBERG: This is the strangest and to me the most unbelievable form of traditional Chinese medicine. It's called "external chi gong." The notion here is that at an advanced level, people not only move chi in their own bodies but can emit it at will.

This idea grows directly out of the basic theory of the body—that the body is made up of channels through which the energy flows, and that this energy has to be in balance. If you can learn through physical and psychological exercises to control that energy, sooner or later you can learn to move it outside your body. That's what this doctor claims to be doing—performing external chi gong therapy on this patient, using his energy to help redirect the flow of the patient's energy. There are thousands of doctors all over this country who make the same claim and millions of patients who would claim to have been healed this way. This one is Dr. Lu, the director of the chi gong clinic.

MOYERS: And Dr. Lu is recognized as credible?

EISENBERG: He trained in traditional Chinese medicine for six years in Shanghai, and he also studied Western medicine. So he is trained in all the techniques we've talked about—acupuncture, herbs, massage, taking the pulse, looking at the tongue. But his specialty is training patients with every disease you can think of to use their minds to affect their conditions—and also using his own mind, or chi, to affect their condition.

Dr. Lu, what is this patient's illness?

LU: He is suffering from an inoperable brain tumor. I'm trying to increase his chi in order to activate his blood circulation and dissipate other obstructions.

MOYERS: Where does your chi come from, and where does it go?

LU: This chi is emitted from my body, but the key factor is the thought process. Generally speaking, when you emit chi, you shouldn't think about where it's coming from. If you do not focus on where the chi comes from, but think only of the need to cure the patient's disease and give him your chi, then the chi which is emitted will be complete and may even be greater than expected. The chi need not be forced out.

MOYERS: When you are treating him, does he need to do anything?

LU: No, absolutely nothing.

MOYERS: Because Westerners don't understand the emission of chi, could you please explain how you use your mind and thoughts in order to emit chi?

LU: It is very difficult to use language to express this process. It is also difficult to use language to explain chi gong to people who have never been in contact with it. The Chinese have a proverb which says, "There are some things that can be sensed but not explained in words." If you want to really understand the principles of chi gong, then you must practice it yourself. First "come inside," and then ask me questions. Don't ponder these principles when you are outside.

From another level it's a very simple matter to talk about chi gong, even though, in fact, it is a very complicated process. If I want to give him chi, then I just give him chi. That's all there is to it. The key is the mental process. According to Chinese medical chi gong, my chi will be wherever the object of my mental process is.

MOYERS: So for you, this chi is not merely a thought, it's a genuine phenomenon.

LU: Yes, that's true, you really do adjust your body. But that means you must focus only on your objective to give chi to the other person. You cannot use a false heart and a false mind to give chi.

MOYERS: How many years did you train in order to do this advanced chi gong?

LU: Our training was for six years, and we studied both Western and Chinese traditional medicine. After graduation I went to the Chi Gong Research Laboratory. At that time our work was different from what we're doing now. Our major task then was to train patients to do chi gong themselves. Ten years later, however, we began to use the external chi gong treatment.

MOYERS: Why did you change to that?

LU: There was an old doctor named Zhao Guang who was doing massage treatments. A woman patient with cardiorespiratory disease came to him for treatment, and he thought it was impolite to massage the breast of a woman, so he did an external chi gong treatment at her breast. The patient was very happy and said she felt much better, and she was no longer suffering from discomfort of the heart. Since then, we have been studying external chi gong treatment.

MOYERS: Were you skeptical of it at first?

LU: I didn't believe it at that time because I had been educated systematically in medicine. But we did a special clinical study, and external chi gong treatment proved to be effective, particularly with cardiovascular diseases, digestive diseases, and neurosis.

MOYERS: But isn't there a placebo effect going on here—the power of suggestion and the response of belief?

LU: This treatment, like any other medical measure, has its psychological effects. In human society, psychology cannot be eliminated from any branch of learning, so in this sense we say that chi gong is also under the influence of psychology. Psychological factors are especially important in the self-imposed exercises. However, our observations indicate that some effects cannot be totally explained by psychology.

But we should be cautious about external chi gong. Some people don't understand it and want to do away with it. I think we should study it, but at the same time not exaggerate its effects or overestimate its power. It's not a cure-all. We should place it in its proper position—not hold it too high or too low.

The next morning we visit Purple Bamboo Park, where a group of students is gathered around their chi gong teacher, Master Shi. Master Shi stands face-to-face with one of his students, barely touching, when the student doubles over as if a wave of electricity has passed through him. I ask the student what it feels like, and he replies, "Something is making me empty, like a void without structure or shape from the inside. It's like when you fill a plastic ball with water and then you extract the water. The ball collapses in on itself."

Master Shi tells his students, "Come here every morning at dawn for three years, and then I'll know you're serious." The students seem serious, and so does Master Shi—but the demonstration didn't look real to me.

MOYERS: It doesn't look as if Master Shi is actually using force.

EISENBERG: No, it's not physical force. He says his mind is directing the energy, or chi. And this is where it gets very confusing, because this is where Chinese medicine takes a wide turn away from what we understand and accept in the West. The people who claim to emit energy are the same people who master the herbs and who know the Taoist philosophy. So where do you draw the line? If you believe that they are empiricists, who know where to put the needles and which herbs help the body, then can you believe that they are also the ones who emit this fantastic force?

MOYERS: But if this is what it appears to be, it defies basic biophysical laws. It looks like a performance to me. The student is responding as he is expected to respond by jumping away.

EISENBERG: It looks that way, but they would say that this force is real, and that the student was "hit" by the chi of the master. They will say it's not just a learned behavior.

MOYERS: I can suspend belief for a moment while we're here, assuming that something is really going on. But I also have to confess that it reminds me a little of American wrestling.

EISENBERG: Yes, every time I see this, I have to ask myself: "Is this a learned behavior of the students from their teacher, or are they really feeling some energy that is physically hurting them, and making them jump away?"

You know, this alleged emission of energy is what a lot of the kung fu heroes exhibit. The martial art masters would emit energy, and it was that chi, not just their physical force, that defeated their opponent. So when you watch a Bruce Lee movie or a kung fu movie, that's what it is all about—the emission of energy by the master.

MOYERS: I know that something is there, but it also seems to be an insider's game. What do you think all this has to do with healing and the mind?

EISENBERG: It all has to do with the ability to use one's mental powers, one's thought, to change the body. In the West, we don't know if we can use our minds effectively to change disease. But the Chinese begin with the premise that the mind plays a critical role in maintaining health or curing disease. If you do t'ai chi exercises every day at dawn, you'll maximize your health and prevent disease.

MOYERS: Master Shi, do you think your good health is due to your practice of t'ai chi?

SHI: I have been doing these exercises here for more than a dozen years. Every day, without exception, I get up at four-thirty and walk for over an hour to reach here. On Sundays I stay here for half a day. I miss only one day a year, the first day of the lunar calendar. On that day I go to visit my mother to congratulate her on the new year.

MOYERS: Are there traditional Chinese doctors all over the city this morning, practicing t'ai chi so that they can be better doctors?

SHI: Yes, there are many.

MOYERS: How long would it take me to learn this?

SHI: It usually takes my students every day for three years to learn the basic techniques, depending on their capacity for understanding and the degree of their talent.

MOYERS: When did you begin learning t'ai chi?

SHI: When I was eight, my father began teaching me. Then I was taught by a master who was not well known because he rarely taught anybody. In the traditional Chinese culture, this is called "secret inheritance"—kept as a secret from the public.

EISENBERG: Do you think t'ai chi should be kept a secret?

SHI: No, it should be contributed to the whole human race. But the problem was that there were very few people who knew the art, so he didn't like to teach.

MOYERS: How is the practice of t'ai chi related to healing and the mind?

SHI: The purpose of practicing t'ai chi is not to attack people. A gun would be much better for that. The true purpose is to seek harmony with the world and with oneself, which is what Chinese medicine is really meant for. I use the force field of chi to balance the yin and yang.

MOYERS: But what is chi? If a man dies, and an autopsy is done, can you find evidence of any chi?

SHI: Chi cannot be detected by any instruments available. It is a kind of field effect. Everything has chi. No living being in the world is without the energy of chi. A tree grows because it has the energy for growing.

The state of t'ai chi is like the day at the point where it reaches its limit and becomes dark. Or it is like the dark at the point where it begins to turn into day. This is the transitional state, a point of emptiness. It is the primary source of the universe and also its final destination. Everything becomes its opposite through this transitional state. But chi itself is not a void or an emptiness. It can flow.

MOYERS: Christians might call this the spirit, the soul, the breath of life.

SHI: I have no knowledge of Christianity, but I believe there must be a reason for people to have faith in it, even though I don't know what that reason is. I believe in

Buddhism. I often say, "Buddha is in my heart." Other people say, "God is in my heart," or "The Madonna is in my heart." There is no great difference.

EISENBERG: Part of the difficulty in looking at Chinese medicine is that it's like going to medical school within the confines of a theological seminary. In the West, we separate religion and medicine. In Chinese medicine, the medical masters, the people who understood material things, were also the spiritual leaders. They never split the two. Imagine if Harvard Medical School were placed inside a large theological seminary, and classes were taught jointly. That's in large part what Chinese medicine is about.

MOYERS: Are you really talking about a spiritual discipline?

SHI: From its name in Chinese, Taoism sounds like a religion. But it's not a religion, it's a philosophy. Chinese culture has grown out of philosophical thinking: from two, there is bound to be three. Look, this is the index finger, and this next one is the middle finger. In between there is a space that is neither the index finger nor the middle finger. What is it? You cannot tell. That's why "You can talk about the Tao, but it is by no means simple." It is elusive when you want to define it. I can only say that it is a t'ai chi state, a state of harmony. The reason China is often called "the Middle Kingdom" is because it has found this truth of the Tao.

MOYERS: How do we learn chi?

SHI: By means of the basic training and by learning the way of thinking in the ancient Chinese culture. If you want to learn Chinese medicine, you have to read the *I Ching*, the book of Changes, which explains Chinese dialectical thinking. Over thousands of years, it has guided the development of Chinese civilization.

EISENBERG: So what you imply is that we foreigners can also learn chi.

SHI: Certainly. Chairman Mao used to say that Chinese medicine and Western medicine should be combined. China and the Western world should join together.

EISENBERG: This is to say that Chinese medicine and Western medicine combined is better than either of the two alone.

MOYERS: China is quite a laboratory.

EISENBERG: It's a big laboratory. Millions of people are doing t'ai chi. What if you took the people who did t'ai chi and compared them to people in their neighborhood who did not do t'ai chi but made the same amount of money and did the same work, and who were the same age and sex? If you studied both groups for ten years, would you find that people who practiced t'ai chi lived longer and got less cancer and had fewer colds? You know, China is a wonderful place to ask questions about mind and body.

I am interested in exploring healing and the mind—but David insists that healing is not separate from the rest of life in this culture—for instance, it is not separate from art, which uses the same philosophy of chi. We call on Master Wang, who was David's calligraphy teacher. In China, calligraphy is valued as highly as painting and considered an art in itself. A work of calligraphy reveals the spirit of its author—as they say in China, "the brush stroke is the man." After years of training, the master calligrapher can execute a complex Chinese character with a few splashes and lines that seem purely spontaneous.

All the while I talk with David, Master Wang demonstrates the "flow of chi" with beautiful, fluid brush strokes. Master Wang then ends our visit with a story.

MOYERS: What is Master Wang writing?

EISENBERG: He is writing the word for mountain, using a character that is four thousand years old. The character has something of the mountain in it because it was originally a pictograph—that is, the character looked like a mountain.

MOYERS: Master Wang, what is going on in your mind as you write this character?

WANG: When I write the character for mountain, I am feeling that I am a mountain. When I write the word for stone, I have to put more strength into it, and when I write "water," there is flowing, like practicing chi gong.

MOYERS: That's hard for me to understand: When I write the word "mountain," I don't think of myself as a mountain.

EISENBERG: He would also tell you that he can see a lot about a person by the way they write a single word. People in China who write for a living, or who are trained in calligraphy, put their whole personality into the written word. It's not just penmanship. There is emotion and expression in the way each character is written. So in the act of writing, he can express a different feeling in addition to what is expressed by the symbols.

MOYERS: You studied calligraphy under him when you were here, but you obviously learned more than calligraphy from him.

EISENBERG: Yes. Because Master Wang knows Taoism, he knows the philosophy of the whole culture. He would explain to me not only the meaning of the character, but the underlying notion of balance that is found throughout Chinese written words and ideas. We are born in a balanced state, but we fall out of balance. The physician's job is to figure out where the body and the mind are no longer in balance, where the yin or the yang are too much or too little.

MOYERS: And then to get the human being back into balance.

EISENBERG: Yes, both physically and spiritually. And that all comes from this very, very ancient notion of yin and yang, the two interdependent forces of nature in everything. Everything has its own opposite, and one cannot exist without the other. You can't know happiness without the idea of sorrow. So in everything in the universe—physical, moral, or spiritual—there are two sides. The body is also thought of in terms of yin and yang. Some of the organs are yang, and some are yin.

MOYERS: Somewhere along the way, we divided mind and body: they became opposites.

EISENBERG: But the Chinese never did that. There was no way to separate mind from body, because what we call the mind was part of the body. It was flowing in the body with the blood, and with the energy of the body. Also, in every yang is some yin, and in every yin there is yang. They cannot be completely separated.

MOYERS: So in every female there is male, and in every male, female. In every falsehood there is truth, and in every truth, falsehood.

EISENBERG: And to know strength, you have to have known some weakness. So in everything in Chinese philosophy and medicine, both forces are at work.

But these ideas of balance and chi are not easy to explain. For example, you can't just put chi into a bottle, or examine it in the laboratory. You can't speak it in words and totally describe it. That's impossible. It's like religious people in the West trying to describe what God is. So every time we ask somebody who understands Chinese theory or Chinese medicine or both, "Can you separate mind and body?" they give us the same blank stare you get when they try to tell you about chi.

MOYERS: So I'm trying too hard to grasp it intellectually, or rationally. It's spiritual.

EISENBERG: It is both physical and spiritual.

MOYERS: Both?

EISENBERG: Both. That's the point. The Chinese can't separate when it comes to chi.

MOYERS: So that might help to explain how is it that a calligrapher knows so much about traditional Chinese medicine.

EISENBERG: Well, Master Wang is very much what we would call a Renaissance man. In the old times in China it was not uncommon for learned people, the people who passed the examinations and became the ministers of this country, to have to master not only calligraphy, but also poetry, music, swordsmanship, the martial arts, and medicine. They studied all of these things to become a complete person: warrior, scholar, and spiritual being. Master Wang continues that tradition in a way. Most of Chinese medicine grew from the idea of balance to be found in Taoism, so he is also a scholar of Chinese medicine.

MOYERS: So as a calligrapher, Master Wang knows a lot about medicine. But what does calligraphy itself have to do with medicine and chi?

WANG: I approach calligraphy the same way I approach practicing chi gong. You need ultimate concentration and a quiet setting. Once you have obtained a sense of peacefulness, the chi in your body flows more smoothly and with less obstruction. If your thoughts or movements are in harmony with this chi, you will enjoy longevity, and a smoother flow of energy and blood inside your body. There is an old saying: "If one follows yin-yang and the four seasons, one will never suffer from diseases. Going against them, there comes catastrophe." In other words, we will enjoy true health if we follow the rules of nature, but will experience misfortunes if we fail to do so.

EISENBERG: So you incorporate a certain amount of chi while practicing calligraphy?

WANG: Yes, and this chi has to be controlled, just as if you were doing martial arts. But, as you know, it is difficult to comprehend chi, just as it is difficult to comprehend the birth of the universe. Some scientists believe that the universe was formed after an explosion. Before that explosion there was no time or space. What would that be like? This is as difficult to comprehend as the chi we've been discussing. In Chinese philosophy, before there was a universe, chi was already in existence. It is still around us, and however invisible and untouchable, it affects our bodies.

MOYERS: Physicists I've interviewed talk about the "primal energy" in the universe, the "big bang" that released an enormous force. And theologians I have studied with talk about the "breath of life." Is any of this related to the idea of chi?

WANG: They are all related. This chi that we breathe in and out also exists in the universe—but we don't understand it yet, even though Chinese doctors and Taoist philosophers have sought to understand it for many years.

The Chinese believe that before there was a heaven and an earth there was a chaos. This is also called the chaos of a light yellow tint. It was like the color of an egg yolk. Then it began to change, becoming left-right, bright-dark, up-down, male-female, yin-yang—the pairs of opposites. In every part of the universe there are these two opposing forces. They're interdependent—they can't exist without one another. You can't have one without the other. For instance, if you pick up a stone, the top is yang, or "male," and the bottom is yin. Even if you cut the stone in half, you still have a top and a bottom. So, according to this ancient philosophy, the universe is made of these two forces, and the struggle is in maintaining the balance between the two forces.

MOYERS: It's almost like the animals coming two by two in the Judeo-Christian tradition. But in the beginning, in Chinese as well as in other traditions, there was a void filled with chaos.

WANG: Yes. From the original chaos came the opposites. From one comes two. And from the two come three. Three is like the child coming from a father and a mother. By continuing this regeneration, we get the "ten thousand things." "Ten thousand" is metaphorical. In fact, the number is too great to be counted. This idea of origin is the most basic principle of Chinese medicine, from which all its methodology and knowledge are derived.

EISENBERG: Tell us more. What are the yins and yangs in the body?

WANG: Broadly speaking, male is yang, female is yin. In terms of having yin in the yang, take myself as an example: I am male, yang. My upper body is yang, my lower body is yin, my exterior is yang; however, my interior is yin.

EISENBERG: How do you explain illness with yin and yang?

WANG: I'll give you an example. Let's say I got sick, and my face was red, my lips were dry. At times I was constipated, and the color of my urine was yellow, or even with a slight redness. That would be a yang illness. On the contrary, if I felt chilly, didn't perspire, my face turned pale, my hands cold, I urinated a lot, and had loose stool, I would have a yin illness. So you see, the Chinese would divide the common cold into yin and yang. In the West, you would just say you had caught a cold virus. But here you could have an illness of too much heat or one of too much cold.

MOYERS: So this is a story, a way of seeing nature, including your nature and my nature, and the nature of the world.

EISENBERG: That's right. The key question is whether both the Chinese frame of reference and our frame of reference give us an accurate depiction of the universe and the body, even though these descriptions are totally different.

MOYERS: How does chi affect our health?

WANG: That question is both difficult and easy to answer. Let me start with the easy part. According to traditional Chinese theory, when chi is present in the heart, we call it happiness. When it is present in the stomach, we call it thoughtfulness. And when it is present in the liver, anger. We get angry sometimes not because we intend to or because we were provoked by someone else, but as a matter of tension.

Your neck gets stiff, your blood flows downward, your face turns red. Some people get so angry, they simply drop dead.

EISENBERG: There is a word in Chinese that means "to be angry to death." That happens when you have so much anger that your chi ends. And when you lose all your chi, then you die. This is an example of the Chinese way of thinking in which emotions and the body are inseparable. The emotions change the physical organs, and the organs change the emotions.

WANG: On this issue of the mind and health, many Chinese doctors have said the same thing: that our thoughts, our movements, our bodies, must agree with the force of the universe in order for us to have true health. The purpose of our living is not to become famous or to make a lot of money, or to struggle so hard to get something that eventually we lose our lives. In Greek mythology, Midas was the richest man in the world because he had so much gold—but he was also the poorest.

    According to a Chinese medical book, cosmic chi exists inside the body of someone who is always happy, not having much burden or desire. The vigor and vitality remain in the body, and when that is so, how could disease possibly invade?

    Tao is "the way," and it means to use nature as the rule, or paradigm. But now human activities are destroying nature. With our air polluted, and our water contaminated, it would be difficult for anyone, including me, to say "I am healthy."

MOYERS: Master Wang, what are the characters you've just written?

WANG: These are the characters for "lofty," "mountain," "flowing," and "water." As I write these four characters, I am reminded of an ancient tale whose title means, "I have someone who understands my melodies."

    Once upon a time, a musician was playing his instrument by the river, when a humble woodman began to listen to him. The musician asked, "Do you understand what I am playing?" The woodman replied, "You are playing about the lofty mountains." The musician was amazed and played him something else. The woodman said, "Now you're playing about the flowing water." The woodman proved himself to have understood everything the musician was playing, and they became very close friends.

EISENBERG: As we are, Master Wang.

WANG: A year later the musician returned to this place, hoping to visit his friend, not knowing that his friend had died. The musician went to the woodman's tomb to pay his last respects, then shattered his instrument against a rock: "I shall never play any music again. Never."

At this point in telling the story, Master Wang begins to weep, and then apologizes, saying that he has gotten carried away.

MOYERS: He said, "I am a mountain," "I'm water," and "There's someone standing beside me who understands me and is my friend." That's you, David. He's weeping because he's thinking of you.

EISENBERG: He's my teacher.

MOYERS: And you are his friend.

EISENBERG: There's a wonderful proverb in Chinese that says: "A teacher for one day is like a parent for a lifetime."

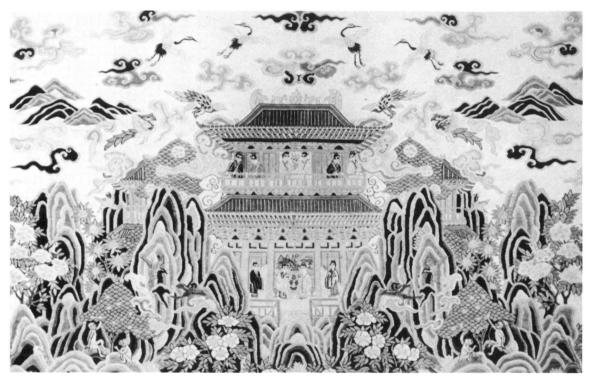

Immortals in the Mountain Palace, 1100

ANOTHER WAY
OF SEEING

David Eisenberg

DAVID EISENBERG, M.D., is an internist at Beth Israel Hospital in Boston and is on the staff at Harvard Medical School. In 1979 he was the first medical exchange student sent by the National Academy of Sciences to the People's Republic of China. Dr. Eisenberg speaks Chinese and is the Director of exchange activities involving Harvard Medical School, the Peking Union Medical College, and the Chinese Academy of Medical Sciences. A member of the Ad Hoc Advisory Panel, Office for the Study of Unconventional Medical Practices, National Institutes of Health, he is co-author of *Encounters with Qi: Exploring Chinese Medicine.*

EISENBERG: So, what do you make of all this?

MOYERS: I have lots of questions. The professional skeptic in me says that those herbs work because they have chemicals in them, as our drugs do, and that there's a placebo effect here—the power of suggestion. On the other hand, those patients we talked to were convinced and convincing, and the doctors were as credible as I've ever known sources to be. When I saw that doctor plunge an acupuncture needle into a woman, and she didn't wince, I had to say there's something there. So I have mixed feelings. I'm skeptical, but I'm also open, because I think that there's something here that might be useful to our society.

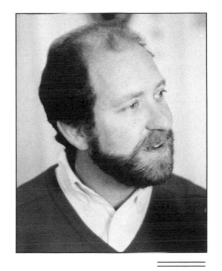

EISENBERG: When I first came here twelve years ago, I had exactly the same questions. But my main question was very simplistic: Does it work? And if it works, how does it work? How much of what's going on here has to do with the placebo effect? Is it just people's belief in traditional medicine that makes it work, or do the herbs and needles and massage really change the course of disease?

I think of the millions of people practicing chi gong and t'ai chi—they have the illnesses I commonly see in my patients in Boston: migraine headaches, abdominal pains, chronic pain, insomnia. The Chinese tell me that these contemplative practices help their symptoms, but I wonder. When I'm asked the question, "What do you think, Doc? Does it do the job?" I don't know the answer.

MOYERS: Is there anything here that might be useful to your patients back in Boston?

EISENBERG: You know, I wonder about whether herbs could help reduce side effects for patients getting chemotherapy for cancer, or lessen the effects of steroids for patients with ulcerative colitis? I wonder whether acupuncture could help people who have had strokes to regain some of their function? I wonder whether acupuncture and massage could help people in America with low-back pain get back to work and feel better?

But to answer any of these questions, there has to be a marriage of Chinese medicine and Western medicine. Some people would see that as a shotgun wedding. But the two sides have to come together because the Chinese doctors are not trained in science. They don't know about control groups, or randomization and statistics any more than Western-style physicians know about chi. But the two will have to come together and look at hundreds of patients, randomly assigned to different groups, in order to figure out whether these things work predictably, and, if so, how.

MOYERS: Every good marriage is trial and error over many years. So if we want to know whether Chinese medicine tells us anything about health that Western science can't, we have to scientifically test what the Chinese have done just as we would test any new drug before we brought it onto the market.

EISENBERG: Yes, if we apply what we know about designing controlled experiments, then someday we can answer that question. And if we don't, then I think the skeptics in the West have every right to say, "We don't believe this. There's not enough evidence."

MOYERS: Suppose these techniques did get scientifically tested and were proven to have validity for us. Do you think the American people are ready for this sort of thing?

EISENBERG: Oh, yes—millions of Americans are already using massage, med-

itation, acupuncture, and herbal remedies of all kinds, without their doctors'
recommendation.

MOYERS: I see plenty of evidence that
Americans are using these things to deal
with stress. You're saying it's more than
that.

EISENBERG: It's not just stress.
They're using these techniques for every
major problem you can think of: back
pain, heart disease, anxiety, inability to
sleep—the list is endless.

But the use of these techniques
points to something else as well. People
want to participate in the healing process. They don't want to be passive recipients of medicine, they want to be partners. My black bag can't be filled just
with pills and surgical scalpels, it also
has to be filled with advice about how to
prevent illness, how to screen your body
for illnesses that are at an early stage,
how to exercise, and how to use your
mind to deal with stress so that you can
maximize your health.

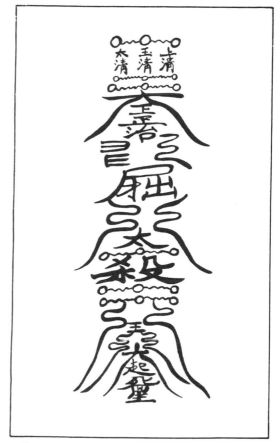

Taoist nostrum for curing all diseases

MOYERS: Do you think many Ameri-
cans are eager for another way of seeing health?

EISENBERG: I think they're eager for a more complete way of seeing health. It's
not "I'm a broken car, fix me," it's "I'm a human being with a lot of problems, and
a lot of fears—help me get better."

MOYERS: Are there legitimate, practical reasons why Western doctors don't recommend herbs and massage and acupuncture and these other techniques to their
patients?

EISENBERG: Physicians have many legitimate reasons for being cautious before
recommending these techniques. They don't understand them. They've not tested
them. They don't have enough evidence that these techniques help, or that they do
more help than harm, and that they're safe. And until physicians know that, they
can't in good conscience recommend these techniques to any of their patients.

MOYERS: And knowing that requires testing?

EISENBERG: Absolutely.

MOYERS: Chinese medicine is so much older than Western medicine—why did it get subordinated to Western medicine earlier in this century?

EISENBERG: That story is a bit of political history. In the last part of the nineteenth century, Americans and Europeans came to China with Western science and set up hospitals and universities. That's one reason we're welcome here. By the early part of this century, the leading class of China so favored Western science that they thought Chinese medicine should be outlawed. They tried to outlaw it, but that didn't work. Now traditional medicine exists side by side with Western medicine in many places.

MOYERS: Although traditional Chinese medicine feels alien to Westerners like me, I can see that it may have something to offer our practice of medicine. On the practical level it may give us treatments for certain diseases—herbs, or acupuncture therapy for stroke patients, for example. But at another level it also seems to offer a different view of health—that health is not just an absence of illness, it is a way of living.

EISENBERG: The whole Chinese medical system is based on the notion that the way you relate to other people, the way you think, and your emotions govern your health and illness—what kind of life you'll have and what kind of death you'll have.

MOYERS: Why do the Chinese grasp that in a way we don't? We don't look at our medical system that way. We want a cure.

EISENBERG: I think the entire Chinese culture is based on the notion that there is a correct way to live, and that how you live ultimately influences your health. It's not just diet or exercise, it's also a spiritual or emotional balance that comes from the way you treat other people and the way you treat yourself. That has always been the highest goal of living in all the Taoist and Confucian traditions. And since that's the basis of their culture, it spills over into their medicine.

MOYERS: So there is an ethical foundation to Chinese medicine.

EISENBERG: Yes, the Chinese medical system is based primarily on Taoism, which claims that it's not just your physical well-being that determines your health, but also your behavior toward others. The doctor was part priest, part martial artist, part scholar, and part empirical scientist. But most of all, he was a teacher. And he not only taught you about diet and exercise, but also guided you psychologically and spiritually to become a better person, because that would shape your health. The doctor tried to teach people the best way to live their lives.

MOYERS: Is that ideal still alive today?

EISENBERG: You know, we are talking about an ideal that developed two thousand years ago and reached its pinnacle probably four or five hundred years ago. Today physicians in Chinese hospitals spend most of their time with the practical applications of Chinese medicine: the herbs, the needles, and the pressure points. So some of the religious objectives are no longer discussed as much.

MOYERS: Did the ancient doctors think that living in this way would contribute to longevity?

EISENBERG: The ultimate objective of Taoism was immortality. Much of Chinese medicine is based

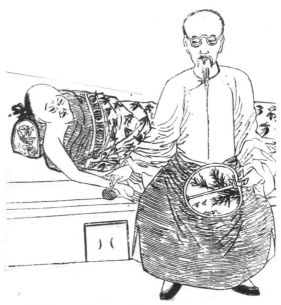

Chinese Doctor Feeling Patient's Pulse, 19th c.

on the notion of obtaining immortality—the wise doctor was said to help you live for one hundred years. Chinese classics written twenty-four centuries ago say that "in the old days, people lived to be one hundred, but now"—that is 400 B.C.E.—"they are not in control of their spirits, their emotions, or their thoughts. They do not know how to find contentment within. For this reason, when they reach fifty, they begin to deteriorate."

From its very beginning two thousand years ago, Chinese medicine said that what goes on in our minds influences our health. To us this is merely a hypothesis.

MOYERS: You know, I think millions of Americans are ahead of your profession in the practice of mind/body medicine. They often go off into the superficial aspects of it, the pop psychology and all of that. But they're searching for something, and they seem to know that the mind has something to do with health.

EISENBERG: Yes, I think people in the West are beginning to pay much more attention to the way they live, the way they eat, and the way they think. Science often lags behind popular experience.

MOYERS: But we are beginning to admit the possibility of a mind/body connection in our own Western medicine.

EISENBERG: I think in the last fifty years we have begun to accept the notion that thinking in harmful ways—being chronically anxious or depressed, for example—may lead to illness or increase your risk of heart disease. But what about the other side? What about the notion that if you become kinder, more thoughtful, or more relaxed, you can change your body positively?

In Chinese medicine, the idea is that your "will" governs your chi, so that what you decide to do governs the energy in your body. Two thousand years ago, one of the most famous Taoists, Mencius, said, "Where the will goes, the chi will follow." Whatever you decide to do, the way you live your life, your convictions—these will change your physical being and the organs in your body.

MOYERS: My goals in life, my intention.

EISENBERG: Right, and your desire or lack of desire. The Taoists believe that desiring too much or too little will harm you physically as well as mentally, emotionally, and morally. It's all a matter of balance.

MOYERS: And that affects your body?

EISENBERG: I think it's one of the most interesting questions the West could ask: Does your morality and intention really matter to your health? The Chinese, however, would not be interested in this question because to them, health was not limited just to one's physical health, but also included one's moral health. So, if you were physically strong but morally weak, you could not be considered "healthy." To us, this approach is a combination of religion and medicine. But to them, the way you lived your life and your physical health were inseparable.

MOYERS: You're saying these people still see human beings as we were before Western knowledge broke us up into compartments, and separated the study of health into medicine and psychology and religion.

EISENBERG: Yes, we invented the notion that "biology" and "physics" and "psychology" and "psychiatry" are separate. But if we want to deal with health, and we're looking only at the chemistry or the emotional state, we have an imperfect glimpse. The patient sitting before me brings with him or her not only chemistry, but also family, relationships, emotions, and character. The distinctions we bring to a hospital in terms of mind and body are abstractions that we make. The patient is still a whole person, and to help him or her get better, ideally we would deal with all of these aspects—the balance of a person's life.

If you put the focus on health instead of disease, you can begin to understand the Taoist approach. In the West, most medicine is defined from the point that somebody gets sick. Somebody has symptoms, or we find an abnormal laboratory test. We start looking at what's wrong, what's the pathology, what's the disease. We're dealing with a sick person.

To the Chinese, health was viewed as a continuum. Even if somebody didn't have physical symptoms, the doctor would look at him and say, "You could become healthier if you did the following." The doctor might recommend herbs or massage or acupuncture or diet or t'ai chi or chi gong simply in order that the patient might go from a disease-free state to even greater health. The doctor's job was not simply to cure you when you were ill, but to help you reach your maximum health by helping you lead a more balanced life, thereby increasing your vital energy, or chi.

MOYERS: I wonder if that chi—which no one has ever seen, or measured, or put in a vial, or held under a microscope to examine—is anything like adrenaline?

EISENBERG: I think the Chinese would say it's much more than that. It goes beyond any one chemical. Chi is governed by the way you live and think. Your mind governs your energy. The question is, how do you translate that into Western scientific terms? How do you make people back home open to the possibility that the way you think alters you physically to the point that it can affect disease? And how do we use our modern scientific tools to test this possibility?

MOYERS: I admire the Chinese way of seeing us as whole human beings, but I have to say that the logic behind Chinese medicine is so complex as to make it inaccessible to Americans.

EISENBERG: I think you're right, but Chinese patients don't understand all the theory either. For example, it took a long time for me to learn about chi. In fact, it wasn't until I had been in the Chinese medical college for months that my teacher finally drove it home that the whole system is based on chi energy, and on the balances of yin and yang.

MOYERS: We see that notion of balance in Chinese architecture. The spheres and circles and roofs of the temples come down in a balanced, symmetrical way. They even have names like "The Temple of Perfect Harmony."

EISENBERG: The temple is symmetric, and it's supposed to fit into nature perfectly.

MOYERS: Their architecture is based on philosophy and geometry, but is their medicine based on anything more than philosophy? Is it scientific?

EISENBERG: Chinese medicine is scientific up to a point. I guess you could say that the basis is a kind of "early" protoscience. To do science, you have to watch something, see a pattern, and then experiment with it. We call that empirical science. An observation leads you to a theory, and you test the theory over and over again. I think for the last thousand years Chinese doctors have done that. They have tried herbs, needles, and pressure points and have observed that in some instances those things helped individuals with particular illnesses. They've noticed patterns and used them, and that's empirical science. But that's not science of our standards today. In the last hundred years we've gone from that to a lot more sophisticated science. To satisfy my colleagues back home, you need more than just a few anecdotal case histories. You need to control an experiment. You need to give one group the right medicine and another group sugar pills and see if the medicine worked and the sugar pills didn't. You need to follow hundreds of people over time and use statistics to be certain you're not observing just a chance event.

MOYERS: How did they come up with this particular geography of the body we saw them using in the hospital? They have meridians and channels of energy. We have nerves and arteries and all of that. Why the difference?

EISENBERG: The simplest answer is that they didn't do any anatomical dissections. They never opened up the body. You see, in Chinese culture the body was viewed as the gift of one's parents and, ultimately, the gift of one's ancestors. To open the body through surgery or autopsy would be to deface the gift of one's ancestors. So their knowledge of anatomy never developed as ours did in the West.

MOYERS: Do you have to leave something behind when you come here as a Western doctor?

EISENBERG: Yes, it's another world—a wonderful world, but very different.

MOYERS: When you first came here, what did you find most fetching about this culture?

EISENBERG: The people are incredibly warm and caring and funny once you get past the habit of trying to figure out what they're thinking.

MOYERS: Why do you keep coming?

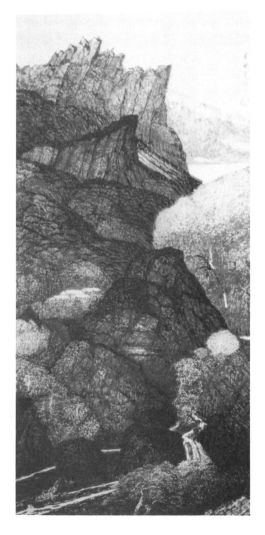

Yu Chengyao,
Landscape, 1987

EISENBERG: Because I think some of these practical things—like the herbs, the acupuncture, the massage, the mental disciplines—do work. Some probably work through belief, and some work through mechanisms that can teach us a lot about the body. Some of those herbs have active chemical ingredients in them. Some of the work with needles can teach us a lot about the nervous system in the way we sense pain. Some of the meditative techniques can teach us about how the mind influences hormones, our endocrine system. That's fascinating to me.

All of these things may teach us something biologically. But I'm at least as interested in those techniques that work through the power of placebo—those that work because patients believe they are working. I think that's even more precious than any of the active ingredients in herbs. If we could predict the degree to which an individual patient's belief in a treatment leads to a decrease in symptoms and a change in body chemistry, and if we could understand that change in body chemistry, we would have a revolution in biology.

MOYERS: We would then know something about how the mind shapes our physical response.

EISENBERG: Exactly. Chinese medicine and the millions of people practicing these ancient arts offer a wonderful opportunity to study how the mind changes the body.

MOYERS: So in China it's not just a matter of what we know about the immune system through science, but how our thoughts, our philosophy of life, and even our friendships have consequences on our bodies.

EISENBERG: Yes—and that way of thinking is rather new in the West. Does what you think and feel and believe matter to your health? Does it really make a difference? I wondered that twenty years ago.

MOYERS: Is that why you first came to China?

EISENBERG: Well, the rational answer is that twenty years ago I read James Reston's column in the *New York Times* about how he had an emergency appendectomy in China, and his pain was controlled by needles. It was the first time I had ever read about acupuncture anesthesia. Reston called the column an "obituary" to his appendix. I read it and thought, "This is very strange."

About six months later I entered college, and I asked my biology teachers if I could do a study of acupuncture anesthesia, and they said, "Sure." Unfortunately, they didn't know, and I didn't know, that in all the libraries at Harvard College, there wasn't a word in English about acupuncture anesthesia. All I could find were translations of two thousand-year-old Chinese medical texts. My favorite was *The Yellow Emperor's Canon of Internal Medicine,* which is still the book they use in the hospital

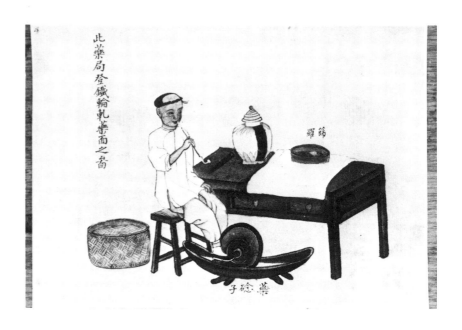

Apothecary (grinding medicinal ingredients for pills), ca. 1800

此藥局登鐵輪乳藥而之畜

羅篩

藥碾子

we just visited. I thought it was so interesting that I decided to learn the language and study Chinese medicine as well as Western medicine. When you're seventeen, you can think such grand thoughts.

MOYERS: Well, I read that Reston column, too, and I was interested—but what caused you to make such an enormous personal investment in this?

EISENBERG: I don't think I was aware of it at the time, but looking back, I can see that it had to do with a personal tragedy when I was a boy. When I was ten, three of my grandparents passed away of unrelated illnesses, and that same year, I lost my father, who died at thirty-nine of a heart attack. It was hard to understand why all that happened, and nobody talked very much to a young boy. I always wondered whether there was more of a reason than just fate. Why do people live longer or shorter lives? Does it matter how you live, or think, or feel?

MOYERS: Have you found anything in traditional Chinese medicine that's valuable to you in trying to answer these questions?

EISENBERG: No, but a lot of things here have helped me understand the limitations of medicine. I have fewer hopes of being able to cure everybody, and a deeper appreciation of the possibility that maybe the endpoint of life is not how long you live, but the way you live. I think that drives me professionally and personally in everything I do.

China also taught me that we in the West don't have a monopoly on understanding the human body or the relationship between the mind and the body. I am more and more convinced that to understand health, I can't limit my study just to the physical body. I also have to understand the mind and spirit.

V

WOUNDED HEALERS

"Nothing so concentrates experience and clarifies the central conditions of living as serious illness."
— ARTHUR KLEINMAN

I watch from a distance. Although they have welcomed me here and generously shared their thoughts and emotions, I am, as a visitor, an outsider to this moment.

They are saying goodbye after a week together. As they shake hands, embrace, mug for one another's cameras, make small talk, and joke, it is hard for me to imagine them as they were a week ago: strangers, arriving here tense and fearful. They were strangers to one another but not to the afflictions of illness that rack the mind when the mind knows there may be no cure. A week ago their only bond was a knowledge so personal it can hardly be spoken to oneself, much less to others: *I have cancer.*

Throughout the week they have learned to say it aloud, even to laugh together about it, and go on to more important things. They have learned from one another that the most important thing is healing, coming to terms with a life they may soon be leaving.

Most of us, brought up in the tradition of Western medical science, tend to regard illness as a kind of mechanical breakdown of our bodies, requiring a mechanic under the hood to replace the parts and rewire the connections. Standing in a dimly lit service station on a lonely road late at night, waiting for the attendant to diagnosis the sputtering engine, or pacing the waiting room while a surgeon sets my son's fractured arm, I have uttered a thousand hosannas for just such skills, and for the people who possess them.

But here at Commonweal, a retreat for people with cancer, north of San Francisco, healing is a matter of meaning, not mechanics — a moral response, if you will, that seeks to understand the experience of illness as part and parcel of life. Here it is not the patient who is healed but the person.

The distinction is greater than a play of words. Before coming here, I read the recent meditations of Arthur W. Frank, a medical sociologist in Canada, who was stricken at age thirty-nine by a heart attack and a year later by cancer. *At the Will of the Body: Reflections on Illness* describes how Frank and his wife came to see that their struggle was not against cancer but with the nature of life, to preserve the wonder of it against the shambles illness would make of it. "When a person becomes a patient and learns to talk disease talk, her body is spoken of as a place that is elsewhere, a 'site' where the disease is happening," Frank writes. "Illness is the experience of living through the disease. . . . Illness begins where medicine leaves off, where I recognize that what is happening to my body is not some set of measures. What happens to my body happens to my life . . . to *me*. Not *it*, but *me*."

The danger is that "taking pain entirely into my own body, making it too much my own, carries the danger of becoming isolated in that body." Isolation, he discovers, is the beginning of incoherence, the loss of "future and past, of place and innocence," and above all the loss of connections to other human beings. People suffering from illness "need most a sense that many others, more than you can think of, care deeply that you live." To Frank, "caregivers" are people "who are willing to listen to ill persons and to respond to their individual experiences. Caring has nothing to do with categories; it shows the person that her life is valued because it recognizes what makes her experience particular. . . . Care is inseparable from understanding, and like understanding, it must be symmetrical. Listening to another, we hear ourselves. Caring for another, we either care for ourselves as well, or we end in burnout and frustration."

Commonweal is about care, receiving and giving it. Overlooking the Pacific Ocean, on the edge of the Point Reyes National Seashore, the retreat grew from the experience of Michael Lerner, its founder, and Rachel Naomi Remen. Lerner is a former political scientist who, when his father, Max, was diagnosed with cancer ten years ago, decided to devote his life to working with people confronting illness and death. Remen, trained in pediatrics, suffers from Crohn's disease, a serious chronic condition that has required her to undergo major surgery seven times. She is Commonweal's medical director.

With a small staff, they operate a program where usually eight people at a time learn to navigate the life passage called cancer. Each day begins with quiet exercises—yoga, deep breathing, meditation, and relaxation. After breakfast the participants meet for two hours, telling their stories and listening to the stories of others. Then comes lunch. In the afternoon they go for individual counseling, for massage, or for walks on the beach. At five there are more yoga exercises, and after dinner they attend a class in cancer care or poetry. Before bed they gather in a circle to pray for everyone there.

The routine is simple, the environment quiet. When I arrive, I know it will not be easy to capture on film what Lerner and Remen have told me occurs here—the bonding between strangers whose experience is so personal that journalism is at a disadvantage and risks altering the process it is trying to observe. But our cameras are not outsiders after all. They capture the rhythmically repeated yoga classes and breathing exercises, the poetry readings which evoke both tears and laughter, the walks, the quiet conversations, and the camaraderie of mealtimes. The participants invite us to watch them work on sand trays, shallow wooden boxes filled with slightly moistened sand, pleasant to the touch, which they will sculpt into a representation of some yearning, hope, or fear.

I am struck especially by the participants' response to massage. For most people with cancer, touch is largely confined to having doctors probe their bodies in a painful search for disease. Now, massaging one another with healing intent, these people welcome touch and the relaxation it brings their bodies. Watching, I remember those studies demonstrating that human touch increases the chances of survival among premature babies; remember how, in the last days of his life, my father finally allowed me to rub his head and shoulders, sighing deeply as my hands gently pressed his temples; remember, too, that the laying on of hands is one of the oldest of the healing traditions.

"We are all healers of each other," says Rachel Naomi Remen. "Look at David Spiegel's fascinating study of putting people together in a support group and seeing that some people in it live twice as long as other people who are not in a support group. I asked David what went on in those groups and he said that people just cared about each other. Nothing big, no deep psychological stuff—people just cared about each other. The reality is that healing happens between people. The wound in me evokes the healer in you, and the wound in you evokes the healer in me, and then the two healers collaborate." Everyone here is wounded, she says, "and they can't cover it up the way the rest of us can. Because they can't cover up their woundedness now that they have cancer, they can trust each other."

During the week, says Michael Lerner, "the group bonds profoundly. They often become closer to each other than they've felt to almost anyone in many years. In the course of this quieting and turning inward, issues that they may have carried within themselves for years tend to bubble to the surface. They listen to each other." One of the patients writes a poem about this. She calls it "Mother Knows Best":

> Don't talk about your troubles.
> No one loves a sad face.
> Oh, Mom, the truth is
> Cheer isolates,
> Humor defends,
> Competence intimidates,
> Control separates,
> And sadness,
> Sadness opens us each to the other.

Sharing sorrow makes us "wounded healers," as C. G. Jung described people whose knowledge of inner healing came from experience with their own wounds. Professionals give advice; pilgrims share wisdom.

Consider this conversation between Howard, seventy-four, a retired professor with Hodgkin's lymphoma, and Dyanna, forty-six, a real estate agent. Howard's situation at home is shaky; he thinks he is becoming a burden. "Everyone wants me to be the way I've always been," he says, "regardless of how sick I am, so my daughter has let me know that she has two little girls to raise and she has just so much energy to handle, and of course, I don't blame her for that—"

"Listen, Howard," Dyanna interrupts. "I don't know you. I don't know your daughter, certainly, and yet I feel a sadness and anger that you're very complacent and so accepting that she's so busy she's not available for you. I don't think there is such a thing as busy-ness. I mean, such an opportunity in her life to have a moment with you, and you're offering it. Why, I'd be so grateful."

"Well, I don't want that much, you know. All I want is just to be there, but I think it's her thing that she has to do something heavy for Dad. And that's not what I want. I just want to be welcome there."

"And have you had this conversation with her, as simply as this?"

The suggestion emboldens him. "Not quite. But it has to, it should come soon."

"Yes."

"I have a very special affection for my daughter, and I think she has a very special affection for me, and I love—"

"That's great."

There is a silence between them. They look at each other knowingly, strangers no more.

"Thank you," he says. "Thank you."

When I mention the exchange to Remen, she describes it as the core of what happens here. "What we begin with is the first and most powerful technique of healing, which is simply listening, just listening. One of the greatest gifts you can give another person is your attention."

I ask about the danger of romanticizing illness. "There is nothing romantic about illness," Remen answers, and even as she speaks, I remember that this woman has had major surgery seven times. "Illness is brutal, cruel, lonely, terrifying. You have to understand that anything positive that emerges out of a real illness experience is not a function or characteristic of the nature of illness but of human nature. People have the natural capacity to affirm and embrace life in the most difficult of circumstances, and to help each other despite their circumstances."

I watch from a distance. The participants have gathered on the front steps for a last snapshot, joshing one another, asking silly questions, teasing, playing the clown. Then—almost in slow motion, it seems to me—they form a group, their arms around one another. They smile, and the camera clicks.

Back in my room, I start to pack. Arthur Frank's book is on the table. I pick it up and turn to his interpretation of the Old Testament story of Jacob. Influenced by a Chagall print hanging in his living room, Frank has chosen Jacob's story as part of his personal mythology of illness. "Stories we tell ourselves about what is happening to us are dangerous because they are powerful," he has written. "We have to choose carefully which stories to live with, which to use to answer the question of what is happening to us."

In Genesis, Jacob wrestles with a stranger, whom Frank imagines to be Jacob's own nature, his divided self. "Jacob has to decide which side of him will prevail, the servant of God or his dark twin, the trickster." In the struggle "Jacob wins not by defeating his darker side, but by realizing that the other he is contesting shares the face of God. Jacob does not overcome his opponent; instead he finds divinity in him." The struggle ends as "the sun rose upon him, and he halted upon his thigh." This is the end of the struggle, but not the end of the story. "Wounded, Jacob becomes whole. Whole, he is renamed." For Arthur, "this is what it is to be ill: to wrestle through the long night, injured, and if you prevail until the sun rises, to receive a blessing."

I close the book and think of those people who have just bid farewell to one another and are now making their way back into the world beyond Commonweal. Strangers a week ago, they are now linked by something far more powerful than the shared knowledge of cancer. They have blessed each other: the ultimate gift, the deepest healing.

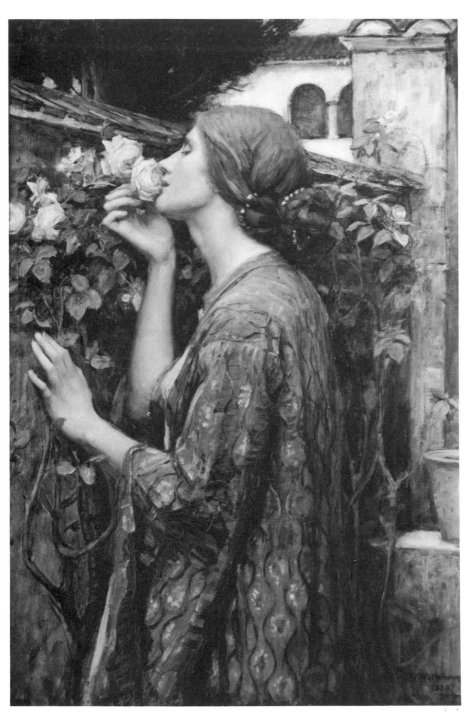

John William Waterhouse, *My Sweet Rose*, 1880

HEALING

Michael Lerner

MICHAEL LERNER, Ph.D., is founder and President of Commonweal, a health and environmental research center in Bolinas, California, and is cofounder of the Commonweal Cancer Help Program. Awarded a MacArthur Prize Fellowship in 1983, Dr. Lerner is a Fellow of the Fetzer Institute and a Policy Fellow of the Institute of Health Policy Studies at the School of Medicine, University of California, San Francisco. He served as Special Consultant to the Office of Technology Assessment of the U.S. Congress for the 1991 report *Unconventional Cancer Treatments*.

MOYERS: When people come to Commonweal, have they given up on traditional medicine?

LERNER: No, we work only with people who are under the care of an oncologist or other qualified physician. Some of the people, of course, have been told by mainstream medicine that there's nothing more that can be done to help them. So they come to Commonweal to find out what they can possibly do for themselves at this very difficult point in their lives. This Cancer Help program is not a therapy, it's an educational program. Most of the people who come here are under some form of active treatment, even if it's a fairly advanced cancer.

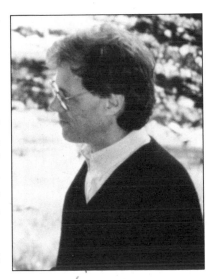

MOYERS: Realistically, don't you think they're hoping to be "fixed"?

LERNER: Sure—everyone with cancer who wants to live, hopes to be cured in some sense. But one of the most fundamental distinctions we start with is the distinction between curing and healing. Curing is what allopathic mainstream medicine has to offer, when it can, and that's what the physician brings to you. Healing is what you bring to the encounter with cancer and with mainstream medicine. Healing comes from inner resources. We make very clear from the beginning that this program is focused not on curing, but on healing.

MOYERS: When I was growing up, I knew that when my uncle was healed of his broken leg, his leg was good again. Or when a neighbor was healed of an infection, she was cured. So the distinction here between curing and healing requires us to think differently about healing.

LERNER: Well, it's a very important distinction. Take your uncle, for instance. The doctor may have set the broken leg, but the doctor didn't make it heal. The healing took place from within. The reintegration of the bone was an internal healing process. For a cure to work in mainstream medicine, the biological and psycho-biological healing response of the individual has to be functioning. Some people, for example, are too sick for an antibiotic to cure an infection, or have too few inner biological resources for a bone to heal, or even for a wound to heal. The body has to participate in healing. Mainstream medicine creates certain conditions under which healing becomes possible again. You set the bone so that it can heal, or you sew up the wound so that it can heal. But the healing process is an internal one.

There are different levels of healing. There's a biological level, an emotional level, a mental level, and, depending on what language you use, a spiritual level. But the point is that at the very simple biological level, mainstream medicine does not make a wound heal. It creates the conditions under which the tissue can knit back together. What we bring to the encounter with any life-threatening illness is our healing resources, our healing potential.

MOYERS: But doesn't it follow that the healing that takes place here would help the individual to overcome the biology of cancer?

LERNER: That's a very interesting question, to which we don't know the answer.

MOYERS: If my uncle's internal healing process has brought his leg back to normal, the parallel assumption would be that the healing process you focus on here would help the body dispose of cancer.

LERNER: There's more to it than that. First, cancer is a very difficult illness to reverse. I've spent over ten years studying the whole field of cancer treatment. While few people with cancer have truly life-threatening cancers, when the cancer has metastasized, or spread to different parts of the body, the person is likely to die of that cancer. People in this situation may have long lives, but they are likely eventually to die of that cancer. It's very difficult under any circumstances to completely reverse that. Mainstream medicine does not have cures for metastatic cancer. And, also, the internal healing processes seem to have a tremendously difficult time with metastatic cancer. So we should start with the fact that if we look at all the people using all the different alternative healing methods with cancer, we find relatively few well-documented cases where people have fully reversed a cancer, and it has never returned.

MOYERS: No cure, so to speak.

LERNER: There aren't a lot of cures. Documented, spontaneous remissions from cancer are reported in the medical literature, and these cases are a very important field of research. There are hundreds of articles describing probably thousands of cases in the world medical literature, but if you look at the individual level, and study the likelihood that someone with a metastatic breast cancer or a lung cancer or a pancreatic cancer will, by his or her own inner resources, be able to reverse this cancer and have it go away forever—well, that's a very steep slope. So the more interesting question to ask is not "Is this cancer going to disappear completely?" but "Is more than an improved quality of life going to take place as a result of healing interventions?" The answer to that is, we really don't know. We don't have a lot of good research out there with controlled clinical trials in which people have been randomized to two treatment groups, and one has received mainstream medicine and healing interventions, and the other has received just mainstream medicine. That's important work to do. But at this point no one really knows the answer to that question.

MOYERS: So, knowing that there's no documented evidence for a cure based on the healing you focus on here, why do people come? Exactly what are they looking for, Michael?

LERNER: Different people come for very different reasons. This program has no ideology. We don't want everybody to leave here at the end of the week doing imagery, or eating a vegetarian diet, or doing yoga, or anything else. We have no agenda. Our essential message to people is that if you come here, we will provide you with a variety of opportunities to explore. Some of these will be cognitive, mental explorations, and some of them will be more experiential, psychological explorations. And we hope that you will find something of benefit to you.

MOYERS: And by benefit, you mean . . .

LERNER: By benefit we mean something that they will feel is useful. By the end of the week people have found things that make a profound difference in their quality of life. That's the most fundamental thing they've found. The words "quality of life" are not adequate to describe the shifts that many people experience here in terms of their relationship with the cancer. You talked about how difficult it was to

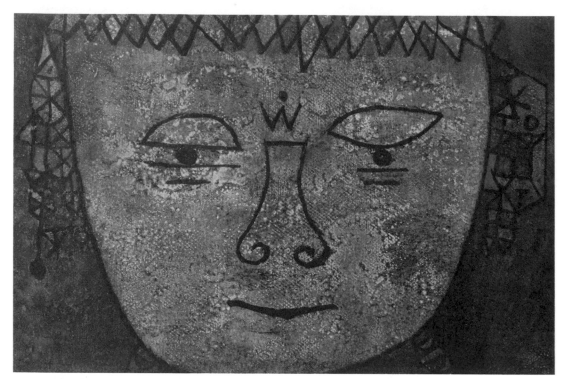

Paul Klee, *Child Consecrated to Suffering,* 1935

understand the distinction between curing and healing. Another important distinction is that between disease and illness. The disease is defined biomedically. But the illness is the human experience of the disease. There's a similar distinction between pain, which is the physiological phenomenon, and suffering, which is the human experience of pain. And, as we said, there's an important distinction between curing, which is the scientific effort to change what's happening in the body, and healing, which is the human experience of the effort to recover. All of these distinctions can be listed under the difference between biomedicine, which is the scientific effort to cure, and what's called "biopsychosocial medicine," or patient-centered medicine. Patient-centered medicine is based on the knowledge that it's not enough just to focus on the scientific facts. You also want to focus on the human experience of the disease, because the human experience may feed back into the biology of the disease in ways that we don't understand yet. That's why this is such an exciting field.

MOYERS: If I hear you, you're suggesting that there is a difference between the person's experience of illness and the physician's attention to that illness. What's the importance of that difference?

LERNER: It's the difference between how you feel going through this experience of cancer and what the biopsy slide looks like to the physician. Now you may have a thousand women, each with an absolutely identical breast cancer biopsy, so that the disease is essentially identical for each one, but there may be a thousand different illnesses, a thousand different human experiences of what that's like, a thousand different relationships to that disease. Biomedicine intervenes entirely on the biological disease that it's making an effort to treat—but it doesn't address the individual illness. I should say, by the way, that my brother's an oncologist, and that my father's life was saved by a great oncologist. I have enormous respect for biomedicine, and I see it as the great contribution of modern science to the treatment of disease. But what has been lost in that is the human experience of illness, which the ancient traditions of medicine addressed.

MOYERS: But Americans are so accustomed to end-oriented goals—you do this, and that happens—that it is very hard to get us to think of recovery as something other than simply being fixed medically.

LERNER: I would not encourage anyone to think of recovery as something other than being fixed medically, because to me, recovery does mean a cure. But the process of living with cancer, of seeking to do what you can physically, mentally, emotionally, and spiritually to change your quality of life and your relationship to your illness—this process can be useful. Of course, for many people this is simply not appropriate. In other words, this is not something I'm on a crusade about. We offer it to those people who come looking for it. But there are many people who are not interested in self-exploration. They simply want a doctor to make an effort to fix them, and if the doctor can't fix them, they really don't want to do anything else. I respect that greatly. I don't see that as a lesser approach.

MOYERS: Then why did you start Commonweal?

LERNER: I started Commonweal because I was interested in the conditions under which healing can take place. I was interested in what conditions allow people to explore—physically, mentally, emotionally, and spiritually—what they can do to recover from life-threatening illnesses.

MOYERS: Tell me about some of the techniques you've used here over the past ten years—meditation, for example.

LERNER: Perhaps the best way to respond to that is to tell you the first words I would use to describe the Cancer Help program: stress reduction, health promotion, and group support. Stress reduction involves things like meditation, progressive deep relaxation, and stretching exercises, all techniques that are fairly well known in the culture as a whole right now. In other words, we use meditation as a technique for stress reduction. Herb Benson calls it "the relaxation response." There's a very large literature showing the benefits of meditation, or the relaxation response, on a whole series of physiological parameters.

MOYERS: In layman's language, what does meditation do for you?

LERNER: Meditation quiets your mind. It is a way of simply sitting quietly and allowing your mind to empty of all content, either by focusing on something, such as a sound, or your breathing, or an idea, or else by just emptying the mind and allowing things to come in and go back out again. There are a variety of meditation techniques.

MOYERS: It's hard to do this, though, because the mind is constantly full of chatter. It's like monkeys up in trees, chattering back and forth. If you quiet the monkeys in this tree, the monkeys in that tree begin to sound off.

LERNER: The mind is well recognized as being a monkey. We all have a monkey mind. In meditation you give that monkey something to do. For example, one traditional image is to tell the monkey to stand a hair on end. An equivalent of that is giving the monkey a sound to repeat, or telling the monkey to focus on his breathing so that you can get beyond the conscious mind to a place where there's some quiet. This is a very old tradition. Every spiritual tradition I know of has had a meditation tradition.

MOYERS: It's hard for me to imagine stilling the monkey mind if I had cancer. My mind is constantly full of the chatter of the mundane world. How much more vociferous that chatter would be if an invader like cancer entered my body. I'd be wanting to think about that all the time.

LERNER: Meditation is not for everybody. It's just an approach. Some people may be better off playing tennis, or shooting pool, or listening to Bach.

MOYERS: The people who come here are taught yoga. What's the purpose of yoga?

LERNER: There's nothing magical about yoga. It's just a useful package of effective stress-reduction practices such as gentle stretching exercises, deep-breathing exercises, meditation, and progressive deep relaxation.

MOYERS: What do they have to do with the mind and the body?

LERNER: They help quiet both the mind and the body. Doing progressive deep relaxation, tensing the muscles and then sequentially relaxing them, focusing on the breathing, and breathing deeply, watching the breathing, meditating—those things tend to have a deeply relaxing effect. It doesn't have to be yoga. There are other exercises you could do as well. If you do gentle stretches, or progressive deep relaxation, or if you sit quietly and look inward, that's the equivalent of yoga. Yoga's just a word for a packaging of those things that came together and were refined thousands of years ago in India. Many health-promotion programs use it as a basic framework because it's an efficient way of accomplishing stress reduction. But sometimes the language gets in the way. People hear "yoga," and they think of some

Moritz von Schwind, *Forest Chapel*, 1850

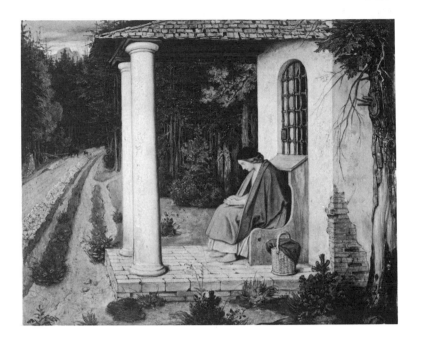

strange foreign practice. But if the word gets in the way, it should be thrown out and replaced by some other package of ways of relaxing the mind and the body.

MOYERS: What do you think the ancients knew about the body that brought yoga into use as a healing instrument?

LERNER: I don't know, but I think what is clearly true is that because they didn't have all the technologies, they paid attention to what they had. And what they had was their bodies, the natural world around them, diet, herbs, caring for people, imagery, and belief in God. It's interesting that shamanism, which is the old tradition of healing that comes out of all the great cultures around the world, is remarkably similar in many different parts of the world. Some researchers have suggested that shamanism touched some bedrock of human experience and that the reason it's so similar in different places is that people came to the same conclusions about what was helpful. In all those places you find some combination of ways of quieting the mind, and of going inward. The native healer will try to come into contact with the part of the self that the person is not aware of, and to elicit it, so that there's some possibility of consciousness and growth leading to a new perspective that might help with the illness.

MOYERS: As I understand it, the native healers—shamans—had experienced suffering, illness, and pain themselves, and they shared with others what they had learned in those experiences.

LERNER: That's right. They were "men of sorrows and acquainted with grief," in the words of the Christian tradition. Almost without exception, the shamans were people who had gone through a life-threatening illness and recovered. It was in that recovery that they found their mission of helping others. And by the way, it's very common for cancer patients to say to themselves, "If I recover from this cancer, I want to devote the rest of my life to helping other people."

MOYERS: What about the value of massage? It was obvious in watching the people here that massage was a part of the healing process.

LERNER: Massage goes back to the very ancient reality of touch. If a child gets hurt, what does the mother do? The mother says, let me kiss it or touch it or rub it and make it better. A lot of people with cancer have been touched only with medical intent for a very long time. Every touch has been a touch for a procedure. And also, very often, their bodies have changed. They've lost breasts or other parts of their bodies. So to receive loving touch, supportive, caring touch as well as the kind of touch that works out all the kinks in the muscles and just relaxes you—well, again, it's just common sense. You're tense, and you haven't been touched in a caring way for a long time. Most cancer patients just melt at the idea of getting a massage. The massage is nourishing. It reduces the stress of cancer and reinforces that even the scarred body can be touched in a caring way.

MOYERS: But the legacy of Puritan America has been hard to overcome. So many Americans think of touch as sex, and they think of sex as taboo, and then the mind begins to raise barriers to this form of nourishment.

LERNER: Absolutely.

MOYERS: What have you learned about the inner mechanism of healing from using meditation, and yoga, and touch? What insights have you gleaned about the connections between the mind and the body?

LERNER: Well, there are two pieces to that. One has to do with the science of it, and the other has to do with the experience. Let me speak to the experience first, because that's what we work with here. At the experiential level we take eight people from very varied backgrounds who share in common only that they believe that if they came here for a week, they would benefit from it. We have found that if we do this combination of things intensively for a week, it characteristically produces very important and lasting shifts in people's experience of their illness. They will often say things like "This is the most important thing that's happened to me since I had the diagnosis," or "This is one of the most important weeks in my life." Simply caring for people like that in a very intense way for a week, and providing a safe place for them to get together and share with each other the experience of cancer creates experientially transformative effects.

As to science, we've gleaned nothing about that because we're not doing the science here. But the people who are doing the science have found that many of the pieces that we use here have generally beneficial physiological effects on people, whether they're sick or healthy. From the scientific point of view, the question is whether these stress-reducing activities have any effect beyond quality of life. Do they extend life? Nobody knows the answer to that yet, because that hasn't been adequately studied.

You've been at Stanford with David Spiegel and his group of women with metastatic, or recurrent, breast cancer. You know about the discovery of a difference in the average length of life for women who had a support group in addition to their treatment, versus women who simply got mainstream medicine. To his astonishment, the average length of life for the women who participated in the support group was double that of the women who got only mainstream medicine. That is an extraordinary finding. Of course, it needs to be replicated, and many people are attempting to do that now. But if a new chemotherapy for metastatic breast cancer had doubled survival time, it would be headline news. There would be a massive effort to find out if that was, in fact, the case. When a psychological intervention that costs almost nothing suggests in a carefully done controlled clinical trial that this may, in fact, happen, there's a replication effort, but because of our scientific orientation, nowhere near the same level of resources are committed to the effort. I'm not judging that; I'm just noticing the difference in our response in terms of the resources that we bring to the evaluation of different modalities. But the point for us is that Spiegel has found that group support, which is one of the things that we do here, appeared to double survival in metastatic breast cancer.

Many of the women who come to us have metastatic breast cancer. We don't take a position on whether group support extends survival or not. We simply say, "Here's this study. It may be of interest." There were shortcomings to the study, and we need to see what others who are replicating the study say. But people of common sense may decide that getting together to share the experience of cancer certainly increases their quality of life. And maybe it does some of the things David Spiegel talks about, as well.

MOYERS: You encourage people here to be very open and honest, to be frank about their feelings, their angers, their fears, their loneliness, or their desires. Why do you do that?

LERNER: We do that because we see it as part of the process of discovering who you are at this point in your life, and how you want to live. We believe that moving away from old patterns which may no longer fit you, and toward ways of living that feel authentic to you is very beneficial for everyone, whether you have cancer or not. But in the crisis of cancer, where so many people feel that old values and things that they once thought were important are no longer important, and where other things become important, there's an intensive opportunity to explore what has emerged as important in your life. So the emphasis on expressing what is going on for you has to do with the exploration of what the new authenticity for you is, now that you have this diagnosis.

MOYERS: But in practical terms, what does expressing my pain, or expressing my feelings, do for me as a cancer patient?

LERNER: There's a very interesting scientific study by Lydia Temoshek, who looked at patients with malignant melanoma, which is a serious cancer. Temoshek looked at the difference between patients who expressed their feelings and those who didn't, and discovered that the ones who expressed their feelings had more immune activity at the site of their lesions. They also had thinner lesions than the people who did not express their feelings. Now again, that's only one study, so I don't want to make too much of it. But it suggests that expressing one's feelings and saying how one really is in the world may have a stimulating effect. That's the scientific side. But if we go back to the quality-of-life side, experientially, we all know that to sit on how we're feeling, and to not be able to be who we are in the world, is intrinsically less satisfying than being who we are. In this culture we are trained to suppress a lot of who we are in terms of our work, or our families, or whatever else we do, so that the opportunity to explore who we are is a very important aspect of authenticity.

MOYERS: What do you mean, "who we are"?

LERNER: Well, there's a wonderful line from Goethe that goes something like, "Whoever said that we have only two beings wrestling within us underestimated the number by a considerable amount." We all have many, many facets that are jostling about inside us. The process of really coming to grips with all those different aspects of our personalities and beginning to integrate them and bring them forth is a lifelong task.

MOYERS: So if I feel deep and unrelieved fear over the diagnosis of cancer, that's who I am, and I need to express that fear. But if I don't express it, although I feel it, I'm pretending to be something other than what I am.

LERNER: I see what you're saying. If you feel deep fear with the diagnosis of cancer, which is absolutely natural, one of the things you can learn is that you may feel the fear, and it may be an aspect of you, but it is not your core self. But expressing the feeling or emotion that's going on for you right now clears the way for what may be next. You may have noticed how much laughter there is here. There's a lot of lightness and a lot of joy. And the laughter and the joy come mixed in with very intense emotions of pain and sorrow and anger. When you're able to express the fear

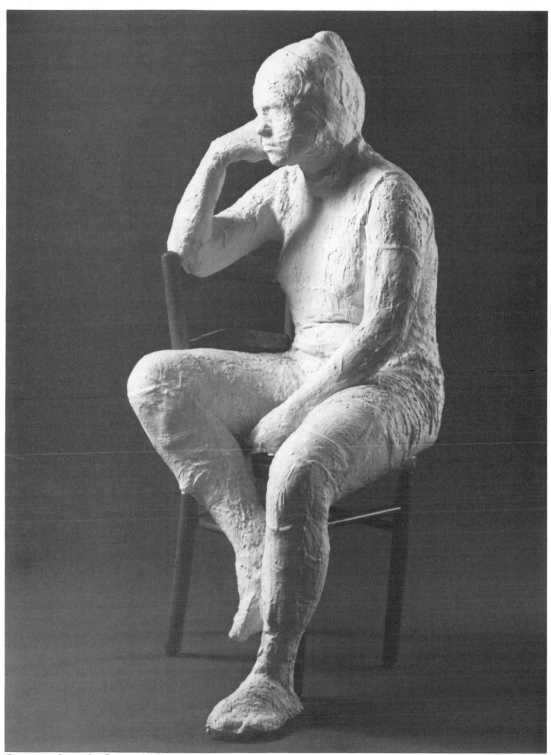

George Segal, *Seated Woman*, 1967

and the pain and the sorrow and the anger, then there's room for the lightness and the joy as well.

MOYERS: As they are revealing and sharing their feelings, what's happening to healing?

LERNER: At the emotional level of healing, expressing the feeling gives you an opportunity to look at it. You've put it out there in a safe and supportive context, and now you can look at it. And as you look, the experience of the feeling begins to turn, and you begin to be able to step back from it, and to experience that you have a self separate from this terror or anxiety. The capacity to identify and disidentify with different aspects of oneself is one of the processes of individual evolution that appears in many traditions.

MOYERS: What do you mean?

LERNER: For example, feeling that I am a father when I'm in the father role, but I'm not only the father, I'm more than that. I am a worker in this factory, or whatever, but I'm not only a worker. I am a wife, but I'm not only a wife. These are different roles. I am angry, I am afraid, but I am not only angry and afraid. What this does is take you back to a core self, the self from which we observe the world. When that self is not identified with one of these feelings or roles, it is actually in a peaceful place. So when you put the feeling out there and express it, there's a release, and the relaxation that goes with that release, and a sense of relief. You have a chance to step back from it and say, "Ah, yes, I have that feeling, but that is not me. I'm beyond that." So expressing your feelings is part of that movement inward, toward a core self where one can find some peace.

Now when people get a diagnosis of cancer, their whole world turns over. Some of them become acutely anxious.

MOYERS: The very word "cancer" brings a kind of terror with it.

LERNER: Yes, but not everybody reacts that way. Some people experience a sense of recognition, as if they expected this to happen. They may get very peaceful. They may say, "This has come to my attention." There are many, many human responses to cancer. Not everybody has a response of anxiety. But the point is that whatever one's response, it opens up an opportunity to look at life anew.

MOYERS: Do we have to get cancer to come to this realization?

LERNER: No, but it's a very common theme. People will sit around the room together and say, "It's crazy that I had to get cancer to learn this stuff." But you know, there's that saying that illness is the Western form of meditation.

MOYERS: Yes?

LERNER: In theory, at least, in the East, people used to think deeply on these subjects before they became ill. But in the West, with our less contemplative tradition, it is often only when we become ill that we begin this journey of inner exploration that we might not have undertaken under any other circumstances.

MOYERS: I prefer our times to those ancient days, but I do think there is a kind of wisdom we have lost in our information and technology.

LERNER: The essence of much that we do here is to recover that wisdom and put it in a very commonsense, modern language that is completely accessible to people in our time, so that it can be integrated with first-rate mainstream medicine, which I would not give up for a quarter of a second. We need to bring that old wisdom together with mainstream medicine so that mainstream medicine can become humane and compassionate in the application of its technologies. I think one of the truly great tasks of our time is to make these technologies compassionate. As almost every American knows, sometimes the technologies of mainstream medicine are applied with enormous compassion, and at other times the technologies drive what's happening in a way that forgets what the integrity of the human being is. When that happens, the process is tremendously destructive. So the recovery of that wisdom and compassion, both on the part of the physician or the healer and on the part of the person with the illness, is one of the most important things we can do in medicine.

MOYERS: Yet you're very emphatic that this kind of healing is not to be pursued at the expense of traditional medicine, and that traditional medicine has done some wonderful things in curing disease and extending life and relieving pain, so you don't give it up for this healing process.

LERNER: I'm profoundly emphatic about that. In fact, I will often find myself suggesting to cancer patients who have overlooked what mainstream medicine has to offer that they're not going to find in these healing approaches the curative potential that exists for many cancers in mainstream medicine. Sometimes I will have an idealistic person who believes that he is going to cure himself as well as heal himself just through diet and imagery and meditation and so forth, without using the mainstream medicine. And I will say to him, "I've looked for ten years, and if I thought there was a cure for cancer among the adjunctive, complementary approaches, I'd be the first to say so. But I have not seen a cure for cancer there." Now that does not mean there aren't case histories of spontaneous remissions. But it does mean that the complementary or the adjunctive or healing approaches, which may support quality of life, and, potentially, extend life for some people, are not curative in any systematic way. In mainstream medicine you find a series of modalities that are demonstrated to be absolutely curative for some cancers. So to avoid those curative potentials is a very great mistake. I see the two as fitting together.

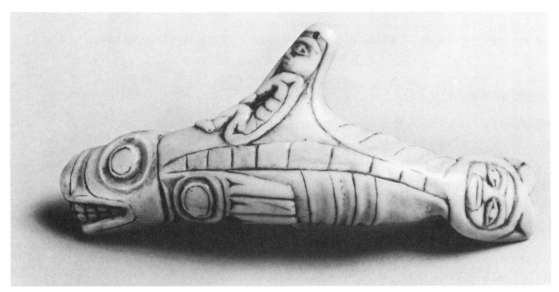

Amulet, Tlingit, 19th c.

MOYERS: Does it frustrate you that you can help people feel better while they're here but that they still don't leave physically cured?

LERNER: I don't know that it frustrates me. I know that very often I would give anything to help someone recover physically from cancer. I feel acutely the pain that they have and what it means for them to die and leave small children or whatever it is. It's just very painful. But my response is not one of frustration. My response is of knowing that from the beginning of time this has been the human condition, and that the wisdom is in coming to have a different perspective on it. It's a perspective that includes all the pain and all the anger and the sorrow. But there is also the possibility of opening up to something besides pain and sorrow. Are there other lessons, other meanings of life? Is there anything worthwhile in this very difficult experience you've been given? When people gather here, they discover with each other that there's a great deal that's worthwhile.

MOYERS: What happens to them when they leave? Do they crash?

LERNER: Sometimes they do. After an intensive week like this, people often leave on a psychological and physical high. But they also leave having learned deep inner lessons, their own individual lessons. The physical high often crashes three or four days out, but the lessons remain. We've talked to people who have been out of the program for years and asked them what remains of use, so we have a good sense of the deep things that last. After they go back out into their lives, what they have learned here may appear to dissipate—but then they return to it as something that they've found for themselves. It's as if they've glimpsed a new territory while they were here, and then they come back later to explore it.

MOYERS: What have you learned about emotions here? Are there emotions that make us ill and emotions that help us recover?

LERNER: That's a very complicated issue. I think it's possible to get stuck in emotions, over long periods of time, that may contribute to changes in health. For example, I don't imagine that it's good for someone to be caught in a severe depression over a long period of time. On the other hand, if you're talking about active emotions like anger, sorrow, grief, and joy, I'm not sure that any of those emotions are bad for you at all. They're natural. If they're processed or expressed in some way, I don't think they're bad for us.

Now, when you ask what I have learned, I have to respond experientially to your question, not scientifically. The experience and the expression of authentic human emotions, the whole range of them, is natural and human and healthy. But sometimes we get caught in an emotion because we can't express it or work it out.

MOYERS: So if I'm stuck in the anger I feel about my cancer, it may actually accelerate my condition.

LERNER: There we have to be very careful again, because that's a scientific question to which I don't know the answer. But if you tell me you're stuck in your feelings of anger about your cancer, and you're unable to express them, I would say that in terms of the quality of your life, you're certainly going to regret being caught in that situation. If I were to hazard a guess, I would bet that if the research is ever done, it will turn out that sitting on unexpressed emotions is not a good thing. But, on the other hand, I've looked at cancer therapies in Japan, where the expression of emotion is not necessarily a positive thing. So I think that large elements of culture enter into what is a healthy response to these situations.

MOYERS: Do you find that people often blame themselves for their cancer?

LERNER: Yes, and I think that's very unfortunate. One of the illnesses of the "new age" is the view, "I caused my cancer, I should be able to reverse it." That's an incredibly simplistic and unfortunate attitude. We live in an age where cancer is essentially an epidemic illness, for reasons that have nothing to do with individual personalities. It may be that psychological factors in an individual life contributed to the multifactorial mix that caused the emergence of a cancer, but to say that you caused your illness because of some set of events or some way that you related to the world ignores all the other things over which you had absolutely no control.

MOYERS: I asked one of the women at lunch yesterday, "What kind of week has it been for you?" And she said, "Well, it's been a very good week. I came guilt-ridden, and I've rid myself of that guilt this week." And I said, "Guilty about what?" "About my cancer," she said. That's what you're talking about.

LERNER: Yes.

MOYERS: What helps people realize that they're not responsible for this sudden bolt out of the blue?

LERNER: Sometimes just an educational process in which you learn about cancer as an epidemic condition in this country. If you're blaming yourself for having brought this upon yourself single-handedly, you're just overlooking some very fundamental facts of life.

MOYERS: Back to the influence of touch. The laying on of hands, as it's called, is a very old religious tradition. I've long been curious about the phenomenon of the healing touch—massage is somehow connected to the same notion.

LERNER: In just the way massage is comforting, to put your hands on another person with healing intent is tremendously comforting. It's a way of expressing and receiving caring. That much we know. Then the question is, well, what may be happening beyond that? First of all, on the experimental level, we know there's a literature on a technique of laying on of hands, which is called therapeutic touch. It's used in many hospitals and involves the nurse entering a state of quiet meditation and holding the hands above the patient, not on the skin, and then feeling healing energy coming through her. Some interesting studies suggest that this induces physiological changes in the patient such as a change in blood chemistry. There's even one very exciting study, which controlled for the placebo effect, where wounds healed faster in the people who received therapeutic touch than in the people who didn't. So there's apparently some still-unknown physiological energy coming through when one does laying on of hands that has that effect.

But then, beyond that controllable energy there may be forces or factors we may never understand, which are beyond human rationality. That's part of the Christian tradition and, in fact, of every great tradition. I allow for the possibility of grace. And I believe in the potential efficacy of prayer. I didn't come to that because somebody told me to believe in that; it's just that in my life experience, prayer and caring seem to have important effects on people that I don't begin to understand. I've found that when people pray, positive things sometimes happen. And because all these great traditions support that, I'm willing to make that part of my life.

MOYERS: Even as we talk here, your father, Max Lerner, whom I know, is critically ill.* Can you talk about what's going on in regard to his illness and you?

_____

*Editor's note: Max Lerner died June 5, 1992.

LERNER: I got into the cancer work because my dad developed cancer, and I wanted to see if there was something out there other than what mainstream medicine had to offer. Little did I know that this was going to be a very large piece of my life. When my dad first got ill with cancer, people didn't expect him to live for more than a couple of years. And he's lived ten years. One of the things I like most is that he never used any of the adjunctive approaches that I've explored. He stuck entirely with mainstream medicine, and with his own instincts. The one thing he got from the work that I'd done was that if he could find the way to live that was truly vital for him, that might be helpful. He really incorporated that in his own life. And to me, that's the real truth of the situation. Diet and imagery and relaxation and meditation and all those other things that one can do may be helpful to some people. They have certain intrinsically beneficial effects. But the deep question is, how do you want to live? How do you want to be in this period of your life? And my dad wanted to immerse himself in his writing. As a result, he got ten good years, after a very serious cancer diagnosis. Now at the age of eighty-eight, he's back in the hospital with a third cancer, and it's very serious. He is fighting to recover and be able to get out of the hospital and get some more time. I have almost never met anyone who loves life as much as my father does. It's just a visceral thing for him, how much he loves life.

MOYERS: The will to live?

LERNER: Oh, I'm sure there's a will to live.

MOYERS: What is it?

LERNER: I think it's just a deep, deep instinct that varies in intensity from person to person. And by the way, there's nothing wrong with deciding that you've had enough. Dying is okay. That's one of the real toxicities of our culture: that it makes dying not okay. It's such a fundamental and natural act. One of the things that happens here is that people come to grips with the fact that it is okay for them to die. You know, there is no shame in it. They don't have to fight and do diets and all those things. They can accept the fact that they might die. At a certain point, for many people, the will to live becomes less intense. My father happens to be one of those people who would happily live to be 180 and who has a list of books a yard long to complete. His will to live is as ferocious today as it was fifty years ago.

MOYERS: Dying may be okay, but nonetheless, you will feel a deep, permanent loss when he's gone.

LERNER: Oh, yes. I will.

MOYERS: So what does that say about dying being okay?

LERNER: I simply mean that it's very personal, and different for different people. For some people it's never okay to die. They want to go out fighting, and that's how they go out. But other people want to come to terms with death and perhaps see it as a process that might be interesting to experience. That's the way Aldous Huxley died—very interested in his own dying. And, of course, before modern medicine, there was the great tradition of the deathbed scene, where your death was the culmination of your life. In many cultures, people are aware of when they were going to die, and so death is integrated with life in a very different way.

But you're asking me about my father's death. When my father dies, I will be sad about two things. First of all, I will be sad that he didn't get the chance to keep living, just because he wanted to so much. And the other thing is that he has such an extraordinary mind, and I will miss talking with him.

MOYERS: After our lunch yesterday, I stood apart for a while and watched the people leaving. And I thought, some of them may not be here very long. Some will not be around for one of your reunions. It was hard to imagine those physical beings I was seeing not being any longer. And then I realized I might not be around any longer than they are. And it was hard for me to imagine myself not being.

LERNER: Yes, it's a very hard thing to imagine.

MOYERS: Do you think about your own death at all?

LERNER: I do. Doing this work, you can't help thinking about your own death.

MOYERS: What do you think about it?

LERNER: I want to live to be at least 108. I love life with a passion. And I very much hope that when I die, I can die in the way that some of my friends who have come through the Cancer Help program have approached their death, which is with courage and with curiosity. I hope to die conscious and actively curious about what's happening. I don't know what happens after death, but it is a mystery worth contemplating. And I will be very interested to see whether I find some friends on the other side of it, or whether that's all there is.

MOYERS: What's been your own personal experience with illness?

LERNER: I've been remarkably fortunate in my own health. I have something called benign essential tremor, so my hands shake. And I went through a period where I was diagnosed with a heart condition, and they didn't know whether it was serious, and whether I might have a heart attack. They wanted to do an invasive procedure that involved pumping radioactive dye into my heart, to determine whether I really had heart disease or not. And I said to my doctor, who's a wonderful man, "Thank you, but I'm just going to do good health practices for six months and see if I can deal with this pain in my chest myself." So I went through six months of not knowing for sure whether I had a serious heart condition, but not wanting to put radioactive dye in my heart. But one morning I woke up and realized that the fear I

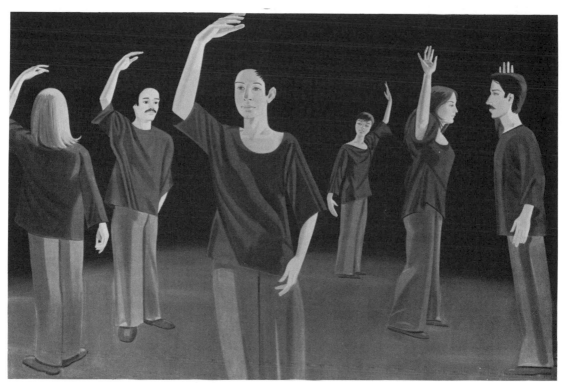

Alex Katz, *Song, Laura Dean Dance Company,* 1977

was living with as a result of not having the diagnostic test done was more harmful to me than the radioactive dye was going to be. So I had the radioactive dye pumped through me, and it turned out that my heart was okay. But for that six months I really lived in the place that people with cancer live in when they come here, which is really not knowing whether I was going to live or die. It was a very deep learning experience for me.

MOYERS: How would you sum up what that experience was for you?

LERNER: I experienced that life was incredibly precious to me, and that the things that mattered most to me were my son and my wife. Driving down a highway at night, just looking at the fog—moment by moment, life was precious. I had that experience that so many people come here with, that the whole world has shifted and that they're seeing the world in a new way. It's an unfortunate fact that human beings learn through pain and suffering. If you ask yourself, have you learned most from the parts of your life that were easy, or the parts of your life that were painful, I imagine that like the rest of us, you've learned most from the parts of your life that were painful. Well, cancer is an enormous pain. And like every other pain, it has opportunity in it as well as suffering.

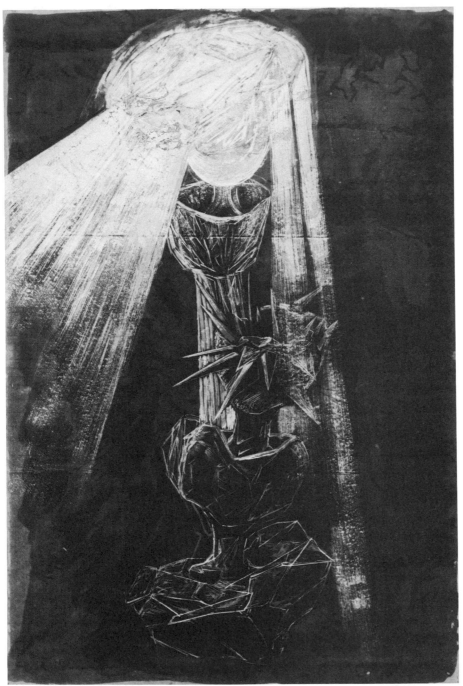

Morris Graves, *Hold Fast to What You Have Already and I Will Give You the Morning Star,* 1943

WHOLENESS

Rachel Naomi Remen

RACHEL NAOMI REMEN, M.D., is founder and Director of the Institute for the Study of Health and Illness at Commonweal and the cofounder and Medical Director of the Commonweal Cancer Help Program in Bolinas, California. Dr. Remen maintains a private practice in behavioral medicine, specializing in the care of individuals and families with life-threatening illnesses. She has served on the faculty of the Stanford Medical School and on the clinical faculty of the School of Health Sciences, University of California, Berkeley, and the School of Medicine, University of California, San Francisco. Dr. Remen is author of *The Human Patient*.

MOYERS: Who are these people? Where do they come from?

REMEN: They're just ordinary people who happen to have had cancer. In this particular retreat we have people from the East Coast to California. We have many people from Canada and some from as far away as Europe. Just people.

MOYERS: What brings them here?

REMEN: The search for healing is what brings them here. How they get here is really interesting because we have no publicity or public relations. We don't even have a brochure. They get here just by word of mouth—one person with cancer telling another person with cancer.

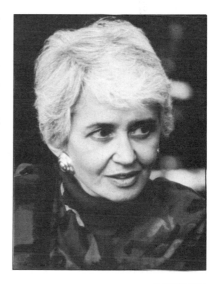

MOYERS: Will most of them eventually die of cancer?

REMEN: Some of them will. I don't know if most of them will, because cancer doesn't mean death anymore, even though that's what people sometimes think when they get the diagnosis. Cancer often means life under altered circumstances. But yes, some of them will die.

MOYERS: I asked Chris, one of the women who's just completed a week here, "How are you?" And she said, "I'm terminal—but I can say that now without that stroke of fear that used to stab me like a knife."

REMEN: You know, in medical school I was taught the attitude that if somebody dies, that's my failure and that when I do my work right, nobody dies, ever. But there is a way that people can die, which is a healing. People can heal and live, and people can heal and die.

MOYERS: When I arrived here, that was an oxymoron to me. A healing, dying patient.

REMEN: Healing is different from curing, you know. Healing is a process we're all involved in all the time. It's very close to the process of education. "*Educare*," the root of "education," means "leading forth, wholeness, or integrity." Healing is also the leading forth of wholeness in people. Sometimes people heal physically, and they don't heal emotionally, or mentally, or spiritually. And sometimes people heal emotionally, and they don't heal physically.

MOYERS: Are you tempted to try to "cure" them of cancer?

REMEN: No, that was the goal of my old life as a pediatrician. You know, the people in this group taught each other a lot about healing. This morning, as they said good-bye, they each talked about what they had gotten here. And they weren't talking only about what they had gotten from the staff, but about what they had given each other. People have been healing each other long before there were doctors.

MOYERS: It's clear to me that that's taking place here.

REMEN: Yes, they've always been able to do it. Part of it is seeing and listening to each other and not offering solutions. Nobody offers anybody solutions here. My sense is that this thing works because everybody here is wounded. All people are wounded, but the people who come here can't cover it up the way the rest of us do, thinking we're the only wounded people in the world, right? Everybody has pain, everybody is wounded. And because the participants can't cover up their woundedness, now that they have cancer, they can trust each other. You see, it's our woundedness that allows us to trust each other. I can trust another person only if I can sense that they, too, have woundedness, have pain, have fear. Out of that trust we can begin to pay attention to our own wounds and to each other's wounds — and to heal and be healed.

MOYERS: I've seen that. But despite what happens here, they leave with the same cancer they had when they came.

REMEN: It doesn't take the cancer away. It takes the fear away. And when the fear is taken away, people are empowered to deal with whatever they need to deal with and to seek and find meaning in the events of their lives. Being here opens up opportunities for people to be listened to, and heard, and validated. They're not stuck anymore. If you ask, "How does that happen?" I have to say that I'm not sure — but it does, and I trust that. I think the greatest thing you can ever give someone else is your attention — not with judgment, but just listening.

MOYERS: But you know, if I had come to you in your life as a medical doctor, and you had told me I had cancer, I think the greatest gift you could have given me would have been to cure me.

REMEN: It's not always possible, Bill. We don't know how to do that with everybody. For example, for thirty-six years I have had Crohn's disease, which is an autoimmune disease of the intestine and the joints. I was fifteen when I first became ill — and after several operations, I don't have most of my intestine anymore. I think I would fairly say that without the doctors and nurses who helped me, I would have died. And I'm grateful for that. But if I had had only the surgery and the medications, I would have been an invalid. As a matter of fact, when I was first diagnosed, I was told that I would have multiple surgeries, that there was no cure for this disease, and that I would be dead by the time I was forty.

MOYERS: Do you remember the feelings you had when you learned at the age of fifteen that you had Crohn's disease?

REMEN: Yes, I do — and they're very much the same feelings that many of the people who come here feel. You feel separated from the whole human race. You feel as though you're looking at the world through plate glass. You can see other people, but you feel as if you can't touch them or be with them, because you are different.

MOYERS: That's loneliness.

REMEN: Yes. And that's what most people who come here talk about. They say that the sense of isolation, of being separated from people who are well, is as painful as chemotherapy, as cancer itself. They feel that other people don't want to listen and don't understand. I think it weakens people to feel isolated.

MOYERS: How did you get rid of your loneliness as a fifteen-year-old girl hearing that you had a devastating disease?

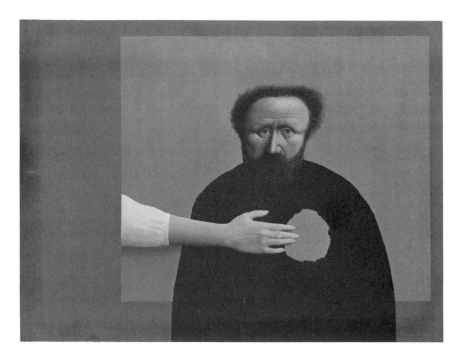

Alfredo
Castañeda,
Consideration,
1986

REMEN: I'm not sure I have gotten rid of my loneliness. I've just invited a lot of people into it, to be there with me. I think, ultimately, being a human being is a very lonely thing. But powerful things happen in the midst of that loneliness. It's not what we do that makes a difference, but what we allow to happen. There is a natural process that moves towards wholeness in me and in every human being. Chris, the woman you were talking to, said that cancer has ultimately healed her sense of loneliness. I think what she means is that the process of being deeply wounded in this way has made her able to open herself to the love that is around her and that was always around her. This disease, in showing her her deep vulnerability, has given her the gift of humanness.

MOYERS: But isn't the best thing a doctor can do for people who are ill is fix them?

REMEN: If it's possible, yes. We all want somebody to take away our pain. But there are limits to what technology can do. And not everything is fixable.

MOYERS: But what about your own experience? The surgery fixed you.

REMEN: No, it just gave me another set of problems to live with. We don't fix the people who come here, we simply offer them an experience which allows them to explore who they are as human beings and get in touch with strengths they didn't know they had, and to see themselves and their lives differently.

MOYERS: Let's talk about some of those techniques. You use imagery a great deal. Why do you ask people to imagine, to visualize?

REMEN: Well, you know, the visual is only one way in which we imagine. We usually trust one of our ways of perceiving and processing the world more than others. Some of us are visual, some auditory, some kinesthetic. For example, I'm not a visual person. My experience of you is not what I see but what I hear or sense about you. And forty percent of people are like me in not being primarily visual. These are the people who come to Commonweal and think they "can't do imagery" because they can't visualize. And yet imagery, like healing, is part of everybody's birthright as a human being. We all do imagery—but in our own way. Even worry is a form of imagery.

MOYERS: You mean when we worry, we are imagining?

REMEN: Absolutely. Once a man came to my office who had the same disease I have. I asked him, "How many times have you had surgery?"

He said, "Oh, ninety-three times."

"Ninety-three times!"

"Yes," he responded, "but only three of them actually happened."

You see, that's more than just a joke. What we imagine, we experience, and what we imagine affects us. It affects our immune system, and our strength, and our optimism. So we need to take control of our imagination and use it for our well-being.

MOYERS: And that's what imagery helps us to do.

REMEN: It can. Imagery is the way the mind and body talk to each other. That's why Olympic athletes often have imagery coaches to help them to imagine their optimal performance and thus improve their actual performance.

MOYERS: What happens in this mind/body conversation? For example, why does the body of that old man react with stress when he imagines a surgery that he hasn't actually had?

REMEN: I really don't know why, I just know the way things happen. We all know the power of imagination to affect the body. For example, I might say to you, "Bill, increase your heartbeat by ten percent." While some people can do this, most of us can't. But if I started telling you a scary story, especially one that has feelings and images attached to it, your heartbeat would naturally go up. Images are the primal language. Maybe the first way we experience the world is through images. And images bring back the old memories and feelings. There was a very beautiful moment on this retreat where one of the men broke down and cried because I asked him to imagine eating the oatmeal that he ate as a child. As he imagined swallowing it, all of the deep love he felt from his mother as a child came back to him, and he felt safe.

MOYERS: Even though he had cancer.

REMEN: Yes, because being safe is about being seen and heard and allowed to be who you are and to speak your truth.

MOYERS: And who you are in this case is somebody with cancer who is in deep need and having difficulty finding others who accept you.

REMEN: Who you are is not somebody with cancer. Who you are is somebody. Somebody who matters. People here come to appreciate that they're each unique — and that's not about being perfect, that's being as you are. I think we all look for acceptance of ourselves from others, and when we are accepted as we are, we are empowered in some way.

MOYERS: That's what the poetry writing is about — expressing uniqueness?

REMEN: Yes. You know, it's ironic that I should have introduced poetry to the program, because I don't like poetry, basically. I hated it in school. It always seemed to me to be pretentious, with references to the Greeks and that sort of thing. I never understood it. And then I came across a certain kind of poetry that was different — the poetry of Wendell Berry, for example, who is basically a farmer. A lot of his images are from his daily experiences, and they're very powerful. His images are of common, personal experience — things that are true for him. So we started writing that sort of poetry here as a way of helping people listen to the part of themselves that knows what's true for them and speak that in a simple and real way.

And when we started writing poetry together as a group, people's first response was that they didn't know what was true for them. What they really meant was, they don't know what was right. Everybody knows what's true. What's true is whatever is happening right now. It comes directly out of our experience of life: it's "I'm confused," or "I'm scared," or "There's nothing happening inside." We do a little relaxation to help people catch a poem. "Close your eyes, and with each breath in, just begin to move closer inside, to the part of yourself that knows what's true for you, and just listen. And let yourself know something that is true for you about illness or life or death or love, or whatever. Write it down as simply as you can, and then we'll read it to each other."

My sense is that creativity and healing are very close to each other, in some way that I really could not say too much more about. At first most people don't believe they can write poetry. They'll say, "I can't do this," or, "I'm not good at this." There's some way that our culture has caused us to become alienated from the intuitive and creative in us, perhaps by calling up in us some habit of judgment. We're supposed to produce something perfect or professional. But we help people reclaim this healing, creative part of themselves by having them write poetry. And you know, we've never had anybody who couldn't write it.

MOYERS: So what do you think is happening to them when they're writing poetry? Are they getting out what they really feel inside is true?

REMEN: Maybe what they *know* inside is true. And when people speak their truth in this way, it's highly personal, but it will be true for everybody. It's from the place where we all connect, our common humanity.

I was thinking about what was for me the absolute high point of this retreat, and I think it is in the many moments in which people show themselves in the beauty of their own humanity. One day, while your crew was filming here, we were reading our poetry to each other, and the cameraman couldn't go on. He put down the camera, and he started to cry. That was a wonderful moment of great healing for everybody because it made clear that there really is only one group. He was as human and as touched and as vulnerable as anybody there. He tried to cover it over, but one of the participants wouldn't let him. She said to him, "Wait a minute, what happened for you?" She invited him to tell his story, and he started to cry again, and said he just felt very intensely how fragile life was and how precious. He was thinking about his wife and his children and how he loved them.

MOYERS: That was an image.

REMEN: Yes, perhaps an image, but also more than that, it was a reality for him. You see, in a way imagery is reality because it helps connect us to what's most real in us. People are using imagery now in relation to cancer—imagining white cells eating the cancer cells up, for example. I think these uses of imagery need to be investigated, but that kind of imagery is different from what I'm interested in. The kind of imagery that is important to me is what is evoked spontaneously from people. Each person's imagery is unique and has a life of its own. Even if two people have the same image, like the image of a wolf, that wolf has a totally different meaning for one person than for another. As you evoke these images, it's almost as if a movement towards wholeness is also being evoked. That movement is there in everybody, sometimes weak and sometimes strong, but it's there. It's like the will to live. And it will clothe itself in images so that it can be seen by anyone who happens to be in the room.

MOYERS: But it's a very private movie, one that I am showing myself.

REMEN: It's the one that is yourself. While we were doing imagery, one man said he experienced a sensation in his chest that was unfamiliar to him. It was as if he had always lived from his gut, and suddenly his energy, or life, had moved up into

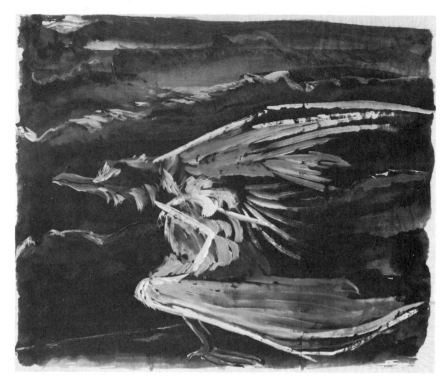

Morris Graves,
Wounded Gull,
1943

his chest. It was a very powerful experience which ended with the spontaneous image of a hawk riding, balanced, on the updraft. I asked him how he felt about that, and he said the hawk was precarious and alive, and it could see a long, long way. And then he said, "You know, the experiencing of opening your heart is precarious and alive, and you can see a long, long way." And then there was a long pause, and he said, "It's the only thing worth doing." I wasn't telling him anything, I was simply directing his attention inward, and something within him spoke to him. That is his healer, not me.

MOYERS: But you don't want to give the impression that people should stop going to doctors and come here.

REMEN: No, people don't need to come here. Anyplace where human beings meet together they can do this work, because it's part of what's natural between human beings. It's not about doctors. People have been healing themselves and each other since the beginning. It's as if we've given some of that power away. Doctors contribute the expertise that is required for curing, but the healing happens with each other all the time.

In my practice I see at least thirty people with cancer each week, and I spend one week a month here at Commonweal. People sometimes say to me, "How do you stand this? How come you're not eaten alive?" But I'm not eaten alive at all. As a matter of fact, at the end of the week I feel fed and strengthened. Healing is natural. It's not something I do to you, but something that is mutual, that comes out of the integrity of the relationship between us. So both of us will be healed in that process. I have been healed by every one of these retreats, and so has the rest of the staff. You know, because of the events in my life, it's been very hard for me to trust life. But every time I go through a retreat like this, I trust life.

MOYERS: What do you mean, you trust life?

REMEN: I mean that we're not in danger, and that I trust the ability of each one of us to deal with our own pain, fear, and loneliness, and to become in touch with who, essentially, we are.

MOYERS: But when you say we're not in danger, I could argue that we are in danger—we're in danger of disease and pain and death and being alone. Life is dangerous. Zorba the Greek said, "Life is trouble. Only death is no trouble."

REMEN: That's one way of looking at it. But my sense is that the worst thing that happens in life is not death. The worst thing would be to miss it. A friend of mine, Angeles Arien, says all spiritual paths have four steps: show up, pay attention, tell the truth, and don't be attached to the results. I think the great danger in life is not showing up.

MOYERS: Sometimes you're pushed onstage when you don't want to be. No one has asked to be here. Every one of us comes into this experience by somebody else's action. Nobody asked me if I wanted to be born.

REMEN: I don't know, maybe somebody did ask you to be born. Maybe that wasn't the total accident that you seem to be making it to be.

MOYERS: Coincidence, at least.

REMEN: Yes, maybe. Before the retreat I called one of the participants, who had a very powerful sense that she recognized my voice. I didn't recognize hers, but when I walked in at the beginning of the week, I remembered her as the nurse who had taken care of me ten years ago, when I was in the hospital with a tube in my heart to keep me alive. And now she's here with cancer, in this program I'm involved in.

MOYERS: Coincidence.

REMEN: Maybe. You know, every one of us is wounded, and every one of us has healing power. I heal you, and you heal me. That's how it goes in life. Several times a day we may switch those positions. It's not about expertise, it's about something much more natural. We're all wounded healers.

MOYERS: In a sense, did you put expertise behind you when you left the traditional role of the physician to take on this work?

REMEN: I wonder sometimes. Maybe it's a different kind of expertise. But it's not as if I know something other people don't know. I trust something other people may not trust, and I help them to trust it, too—the natural power of growth in people.

MOYERS: Is what happens here a kind of encounter group therapy?

REMEN: No, I'm not a psychologist or a psychiatrist, I'm a pediatrician, so I know a bit about growth and about the fact that many of us still have our child alive in us. No, that's not what happens here—unless any two people sitting anywhere talking is an encounter group, or a therapy session. Of course, maybe it is. Maybe we always have the opportunity of healing each other. As someone talks, other people feel very deeply what's being said in the room. We don't fix things or offer solutions, we just listen.

As one of the women in the group was listening, she was crying and feeling very touched and also feeling her own pain. The next morning, lying in yoga class, she had a vision. Sometimes on retreat someone will have a spontaneous vision, which is probably a vision for the whole group. Suddenly, this woman saw a city of gold, very vividly, with the light shining off the buildings. She said that although nobody was visible, she felt that it was filled with people, and there was a great sense of peace in seeing it. It was a very powerful experience for her. It kept fading out, and she kept saying to herself, "Oh, please come back," and it would come back and fade out and come back again. And the third time it faded out and came back, Ashoka, who leads the yoga class, spontaneously began saying the words of "Amazing Grace": "Through many dangers, toils and snares, I have already come; 'Tis grace hath brought me safe thus far, and grace will lead me home." Where that image of the golden city came from, I don't know.

MOYERS: Well, it's a traditional image from the Christian scriptures.

REMEN: At that moment in her life the image was just hers—it just happened. These things are part of ordinary life. They're part of what's available to us as people.

MOYERS: Is this kind of work with the imagination related to what I saw people doing with sand trays? They were placing small figures in the sand, almost like children playing with toy figures on a beach. What do the sand trays have to do with healing?

REMEN: They're just another way of putting people in touch with the fact that not everything they know is in their conscious mind. There is an unconscious part of the mind that has great power and strength, and, indeed, wisdom and truth. The sand-tray work is like a waking dream. Many dreams are healing, even dreams that are frightening. I once read a dissertation about the dreams of pregnant women. Many of the dreams were terrible nightmares filled with anxiety and fear and loss. But the study showed that the women who had the worst nightmares had the easiest deliveries. Maybe in feeling their anxiety, even if only in a dream, they were released from it so that when their time came, they could give birth in an easier way. In the sand-tray work that deep intelligence that is in every human being, and that knows what is needed for healing, can tell its own story.

MOYERS: So what is going on when Chris brings an image of her own burial out of the sand?

REMEN: It may be about her story. It may also be symbolic, because as we start something new—a new attitude, a new belief, a new way of life—something else ends. There should be a word that means beginning/end because nothing begins without something dying.

I have sometimes done sand trays with people here. One of the most powerful was with a man who died two weeks after the retreat ended. He hadn't wanted to do the sand tray, because it seemed silly to him. And yet when he came into the room,

which has all these tiny objects everywhere, he very purposefully went to a large crystal paperweight and said, "This is mine." And he took it, and put it in the sand, and buried it, right in the middle of the tray. Then he put twelve very long, thin candles around the buried diamond, and lit them, and then began singing "Happy Birthday."

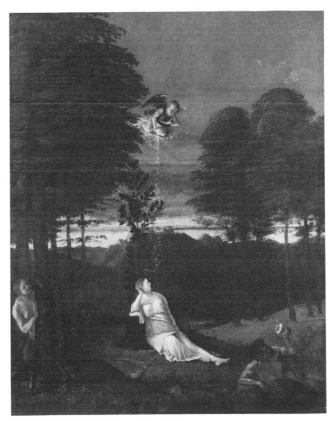

MOYERS: So what do you make of that?

REMEN: I think it was telling him something about his death or about death in general. But you don't have to make something of it. Just the expression of

Lorenzo Lotto, *A Maiden's Dream,* ca. 1505

what's true, just being able to say it in the form of a sand tray, and have it heard and accepted by someone releases something. It is healing just to do these things. I never interpreted that tray, I just witnessed it. After he did the sand tray, a lot of fear left him, and throughout the rest of the retreat he seemed very deeply at peace. I have no idea why, but I do know that receiving the truth of another human being is enormously empowering to both.

MOYERS: You're asking us to think of healing as wholly different from how most of us were raised to think of it.

REMEN: Healing may not be so much about getting better as about letting go of everything that isn't you—all of the expectations, all of the beliefs—and becoming who you are. Not a better you, but a realer you.

MOYERS: But my expectations, my fears, and my beliefs are all part of me. They are as much me as my hands.

REMEN: Not true. You were born with your hands. You weren't born with your beliefs. Some of your beliefs may help you to live, and some of them may not. And you need to be able to sort them out, because only the ones that are true, only the ones that can help you to live, are the ones you want to keep.

Let me give you an image. I bought a little falling-down cabin on the top of a mountain. It was so bad that when Michael Lerner came to see it, he said, "Oh, Rachel, you bought this?" But with two carpenters, an electrician, and a plumber, in three years we have remodeled the whole thing. We started by just throwing things away—bathtubs, light fixtures, windows. I kept hearing my father's voice saying, "That's a perfectly good light fixture, why are you throwing it away?" We kept throwing away more and more things, and with everything we threw away, the building became more whole. It had more integrity. Finally, we had thrown away everything that didn't belong. You know, we may think we need to be more in order to be whole. But in some ways we need to be less. We need to let go, to throw away everything that isn't us in order to be more whole.

MOYERS: I understand you, but at the same time I don't want to throw away more years. If I have an illness that you can treat, I expect you as a doctor to extend my life.

REMEN: And if I'm lucky, I'm going to be able to do that, too. All doctors feel a very great satisfaction in being able to do that. But you know, extending life isn't the highest goal, because people can live miserable lives for long, long periods of time.

MOYERS: It's true that extending life is not always the highest goal, but there is this will to live. I want to live, and I want to live as long as I can.

REMEN: I think that's too low a goal. Of course you want to live as long as you can, but don't you want to live well?

MOYERS: Yes, of course.

REMEN: It's interesting that many of the people here this week have survived a terrible childhood. Now all of us have done certain things in order to survive, and survival is about living longer, right? But I think what has to happen for people at some point in their lives, and what certainly is happening for all the people who were here, is that many of the things we've done in order to survive are different from the things we need to do in order to live and to live well. For example, perhaps my childhood taught me that in order to survive I had to become voiceless and invisible so that my alcoholic mother never noticed me. But in order to live, I need to re-own my own voice and its validity. Or, in order to survive, I had to trust no one. But in order to live, I need to trust enough to love and be touched by other people.

You know, touching is a very old way of healing. We don't touch each other in this culture, and touching is often misunderstood or even sexualized. As a physician, I was taught that you touch people only to diagnose them, and if you touch them in any other way, even in a comforting way, they may misunderstand. And yet, touch is the oldest way of healing. Touch is deeply reassuring and nurturing. It's the first way a mother and child connect with each other. Many people with cancer will tell us that they're often touched as if they were a piece of meat. One woman said, "Sometimes when I go for my chemotherapy, they touch me as if they don't know anybody's inside this body." And so we try to touch people with the tenderness of a mother touching a child, because what a mother is saying to her child with that touch is "Live."

MOYERS: And "I care about you."

REMEN: Yes—"Your life matters to me." That is enormously important. The opposite of love is not hate, but indifference. Many people tell us that they experience being touched with indifference when they go to hospitals. I don't think it's really indifference, by the way. A certain percent of the people in my practice are doctors who are burned out. They've seen so much suffering and pain they can't fix, they can't feel anymore. They are numb. And if I'm your doctor, and I feel numb, you may experience me as indifferent. But I've become numb because I care too much. We have to learn how to train people so that they can do this work with their hearts wide open. That's a real challenge.

But let me go back to the touching issue for a minute. Years ago, when I was associate director of the pediatric clinics at the Stanford Medical School, one of my colleagues, Marshall Klaus, did a study which at the time was extremely innovative. He was chief of the intensive care nursery, where all the babies were these tiny little people you could hold in your hand. Each incubator was surrounded by shifts of people and millions of dollars worth of equipment. Everything was very high-tech. Of course, we didn't touch these infants because we'd get germs on them. But Klaus decided to do an experiment in which half the babies in the nursery would be treated as usual, and the other half would be touched for fifteen minutes every few hours. You'd take your pinky finger and rub it down the little baby's back. And we discovered that the babies that were touched survived better. No one knows why. Maybe there's something about touching that strengthens the will to live. Maybe isolation weakens us.

MOYERS: Do you really believe there is a will to live?

REMEN: Yes, I do.

MOYERS: Can it be evoked?

REMEN: That's the question. I think that's what healing is—evoking the will to live. And it's evoked not by doing something, but by receiving another person, by letting another person know that their pain and their suffering and their fear matters. By not being indifferent. You know, the will to live is a kind of a mystical concept. Some people live despite everything, and others die for no apparent reason. Brendan O'Regan, at the Institute of Noetic Science, did a study of people, most of them with cancer, who had been sent home to die, and for unknown reasons the cancer went away. These stories, with all the lab values and X rays and so forth, are usually "fillers" in medical journals. O'Regan began to collect these stories and discovered that there are thousands of these case histories of spontaneous remission. In our drive for expertise and mastery, we look past the mystery, which is right there for us to wonder about. I don't know why people get well. I have no idea.

MOYERS: How did you get well when you were suffering for so long from Crohn's disease?

REMEN: I don't really know, and I still suffer. As we're sitting here, I can't see you very well because I have cataracts in my eyes from the cortisone that was given to me years ago. You know, these drugs were given to me in very high doses, because it wasn't expected that I would live. No one expected me to be here to not see you. But I don't think life is about avoiding suffering. And I don't think health is just about the physical.

MOYERS: But lots of people suffer who don't emerge healthy, as you did.

REMEN: But I'm not healthy.

MOYERS: When you say you're not healthy, you're refuting everything you're about, because you're surviving, and you're surviving with meaning. Isn't that healthy?

REMEN: I'm not healthy in the way that most people use that word—physically sound. I probably couldn't run down the beach with you this afternoon. My body won't do that. So I'm not healthy—but I'm whole. You see, we start moving into paradoxes here. Sometimes illness evokes health in people. Many of the people on this retreat seem very healthy, very alive—and yet, like me, they're not physically healthy. And some of the most boring people are those who are jogging and eating health food as if the physical health of the body is their goal in life. Health is not a goal, it's a means to doing what is purposeful or meaningful in life. You can often do that more easily if you're physically healthy. But you can do it anyway, even when you're not physically healthy.

MOYERS: People want to feel good. Are we talking about emotions and not actual physical fitness?

REMEN: You know, some of the most important times of my life have been those in which I haven't felt well. During those times I have had a much deeper sense of the integrity in myself, even though I wasn't feeling very well physically.

MOYERS: What do you mean, "integrity"?

REMEN: That I am what I am. And that there's no need for me to find your approval or to seek it. And that wounds and all, there is an essence and a uniqueness and a beauty—like all other people have, too. I make sense exactly as I am. People talk about self-approval, but self-approval is just another form of judgment. Self-acceptance is closer to what it's about.

MOYERS: Is part of this finding the right emotion, or finding the good emotion that takes the place of the bad emotion?

REMEN: You know, it would be nice to reduce life to some simple formula, but I don't think we can. I don't think there's such a thing as a bad emotion. The only bad emotion is a stuck emotion.

MOYERS: What do you mean?

REMEN: I think of people who are angry for years, or who feel they always must be cheerful. When I became ill, I was angry for years. I was fifteen years old, and it looked as if my whole life was being taken away from me. My response to that was to be furious and to hate all the well people. I did that for a long time, until eventually I realized that my anger was my will to live, expressed negatively. I realized that life was important, that it was valuable and precious to me, and that I didn't need to be angry in order to know that. My anger was useful—it got me through—but if I hadn't eventually come out of that mode, I would have lost much of what is precious in my life.

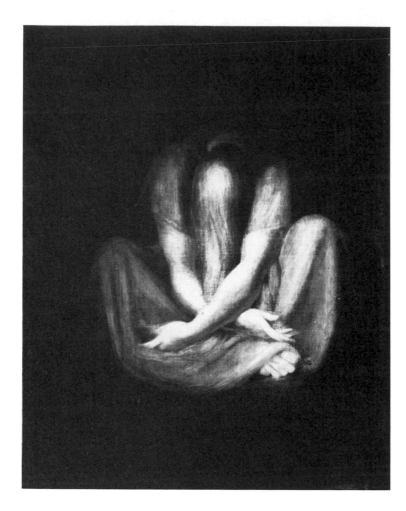

Johann Heinrich
Füssli, *The Silence,*
1799

I really worry about people who get cancer and don't get angry, because I feel
that somehow they're not holding to life, they're not engaged with life, or they're not
passionate enough about life. When I was working in hospitals, they used to send
me around to visit people with ileostomies, because I have an ileostomy, and it helps
people to meet somebody else who is living with an ileostomy, when they've just had
this surgery. I'd walk into these rooms, and I would feel whether or not the person
was angry. And if they were not angry, I would be concerned that somehow they had
become resigned too much, in a strange kind of way. Anger is a demand for change.
Many people initially experience their strength through anger—just as I did.

MOYERS: We know of many angry people who live and many cheerful people
who die.

REMEN: Yes, and the reverse is also true. There's no formula. I don't believe in
positive emotions. I think all emotions can be positive.

MOYERS: I don't understand that.

REMEN: Perhaps positive thinking is not the same as positive emotions. You know, when people first get a diagnosis of cancer, they often run out and buy a hundred dollars worth of books about what you need to do in order to live and what you mustn't do or you won't live. People talk about how love and cheerfulness and optimism are positive emotions, and sadness, fear, and anger are negative emotions, and negative emotions are dangerous. But my experience is that all emotions, to the extent that they engage you with life, are positive. For example, the person who feels sadness at the thought of losing her breast—well, life is precious to that person. I'm very suspicious of people who say, "Oh, well, you know, what's a breast?" That doesn't feel real to me. There's almost a tyranny of the emotions now where people are afraid to feel their feelings because they think that if they feel certain "negative" emotions, their cancer will get worse. People are called upon to edit themselves.

MOYERS: Have you learned anything from your experience, or your own illness, or from the retreat, about who gets sick and who doesn't?

REMEN: It's an absolute mystery—which is very frustrating for those of us who would like to be in control. You know, once a year we invite professionals who work with cancer to come to Commonweal for a little R&R. While they're here, they often talk with each other about the things they really don't understand, even though they've spent years working in this field. What often comes up is that there isn't a simple formula. There's a lot that is mysterious here. People who intensely want to live sometimes don't, while people who seem to be very negative, will. As we do retreat after retreat, we discover that all our cherished beliefs get taken from us by the experience itself.

MOYERS: When I was a boy, I would use my glasses to start fires on dry leaves by focusing the sun's rays through them, causing a combustion from the intensity of the focus. And doesn't being told you have cancer do that to you? Doesn't it so focus your thoughts on yourself that your feelings and fears are heightened? And isn't this retreat, therefore, an experience out of the ordinary, in which the healing that occurs here couldn't be understood by people out there?

REMEN: I don't think so, really. The people who come here have known they've had cancer for some time. And my sense is that everybody has pain. You know, if it isn't cancer, it's something else. There's no way to be alive and avoid pain and loss and suffering. It's all part of life. Most serious diseases call into question the way you live and what's important. There is a whole reshifting of values. Someone once described it to me as a "wake-up call." I sometimes think of that poem by e. e. cummings:

i thank You God for most this amazing
day: for the leaping greenly spirits of trees
and a blue true dream of sky; and for everything
which is natural which is infinite which is yes

(i who have died am alive again today,
and this is the sun's birthday; this is the birth
day of life and of love and wings: and of the gay
great happening illimitably earth)

how should tasting touching hearing seeing
breathing any—lifted from the no
of all nothing—human merely being
doubt unimaginable You?

(now the ears of my ears awake and
now the eyes of my eyes are opened)

I think that's what cancer does to people: "The ears of my ears awake and the eyes of my eyes are opened. . . ." But you don't have to have cancer to experience that. It can happen to anyone, anywhere. We suddenly realize that very little is random or trivial, and that life is full of opportunities to love and connect and grow in wisdom. We're not a special group of people here, we're just human beings, frightened, lonely, hurting, and able to grow in response to crisis. That's what's available if you're willing to allow yourself to be human.

MOYERS: Cummings also said that if we want to help people, we have to start with the minute particulars of life. I suppose that healing is part of the discovery of life in the minute particular.

REMEN: That's right.

MOYERS: But when they left down that road today, they still had cancer.

REMEN: Yes, they still had cancer. But they had a bigger piece of themselves than when they came. Some people are going to heal, and some people are going to die, but they may do it better than before they came here. There's something important about the healing power of a community of human beings. Even if it's only for a week, you know there's a place where you can belong, even if you haven't got a breast, even if you haven't got an intestine, even if there is a big mass growing in your lung. There's a place where you can be accepted and loved and see reflected back to you that you matter. Knowing that heals the isolation and helps you return to the human race.

MOYERS: Do you have to come here for that?

REMEN: No, we do that for each other all the time.

MOYERS: Ideally, but not really.

REMEN: What are families about, then?

MOYERS: Well, some of the most wounded of society are in families. Families can create casualties—abused children, for example. We romanticize the family and community, don't you think?

REMEN: Yes, but there is real community. Real community is about a sense of belonging, just the way you are.

MOYERS: Essentially, what you have done is to help them accept their cancer, and to live with the inevitable.

REMEN: No, actually when people leave here, they're able to fight better, to do whatever they need to do. But this point about acceptance is very, very complex. My sense is that all power comes out of the ability to accept what is. Acceptance is what allows change. Accepting that one has cancer is the first step to healing yourself.

MOYERS: Yes, but they haven't defeated the cancer, so some people will ask, "What's the good of acceptance?" As Zorba said, "What good are all those books if they don't tell you the answers to these questions?"

REMEN: Maybe you won't be cured of cancer, but you won't lose your life—and it's easy to lose your life these days. Seeking physical healing is important, but it may not be the ultimately important thing, at least not for me.

MOYERS: What is?

REMEN: Being alive, which is not a matter of length, but of moment to moment. Being alive is being aware, being able to be touched and moved and changed, being able to respond rather than to react, being able to see and hear. Several of my patients have had near-death experiences. In one case, the woman told me that she came away from that experience with an awareness that the purpose of life was not about being a doctor or a mother or creative or smart or rich, but to grow in wisdom and to learn to love better. And that's all.

MOYERS: So what does all of this have to do with the mind?

REMEN: I'm not sure that the mind is the highest human function. I think of it as the storehouse of knowledge. I think it has to do with the soul rather than the mind. It's the difference between perfection—a mental construct—and wholeness. I wrote a poem that goes something like this: "O Body, for thirty-six years, one thou-

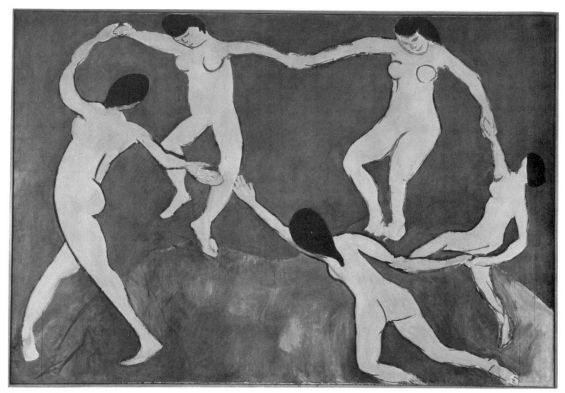

Henri Matisse, *Dance,* 1909

sand three hundred and seventy-four experts with a combined fourteen hundred years of training have failed to cure your wounds. Deep inside, I am whole." There is something in every one of us that is invulnerable to loss, suffering, and decay, that just shines on. We don't usually talk about these things with each other. We're a little ashamed of them, so we hide them as if they were weaknesses, when they're really our strengths. Here is an opportunity for people to share their fears, their darkness, their strengths, their light—who they are. Here is an opportunity to be whole. And that is a healing experience for people.

MOYERS: So what have you learned from this about death?

REMEN: Well, what I've learned about death is that it's an unknown, but by fearing it, we tend to deal with it as if it were a known. Here we are, meeting where the United States begins, the very edge between the land we know and the ocean, which is the great unknown. We're having a meeting on the very edge—and cancer can take you to the very edge of what is known about life. I have no idea about what death is, but because I have been in association with it so intimately, I have a much greater sense of the value of life and of what life can be.

MOYERS: Doesn't that make you sad about leaving it one day?

REMEN: Not really. We talk about death a lot here. What people say is something like, it's an unknown, and the unknown gives me a sense of adventure. I would be very sad about leaving behind certain things. But I don't know what it is I'm going towards.

MOYERS: I'm not afraid of death, but I can't imagine not being. Can you?

REMEN: Well, that's what Freud said—that we are such egos that we cannot imagine our own "not being." And maybe that's right. Maybe there's a reason why we can't imagine our own "not being," Bill. Maybe there is no such thing as "not being." Maybe in some way we do go on. I don't know, but I wonder about it constantly.

MOYERS: Do you think that all the great religions and spiritual traditions of the world have at the core something irreducible that is common to all times and places?

REMEN: Yes. I don't know what it is, but I know it's there. I think that healing happens only in the context of our imminent awareness of something larger than ourselves, however we conceive that. When Sylvia got that image of the city of gold, everyone in the room recognized that it was like a promise. This is not something that can be proved to anyone, but it's something one can experience. Thank God that for twelve years I've been talking to people with life-threatening illness and that I've done forty-five retreats with cancer patients, because otherwise I'd sound like Pollyanna even to myself. I can only share what my experience has been. That's all I have—my experience. And I don't believe that we're alone. We are such a gift, each of us to each other, we human beings.

FAMILY

His Holiness said,
"I hope these words I've spoken today
have been worthwhile—
but if not . . . it doesn't matter. . . ."
I cling to the string on my neck
that he left,
and I wonder.

Tears hang behind my eyes
like fog hangs off the beach
spilling forward . . . just . . .
as I imagine myself out of range,
they wash loose the grief and the dust
of the corners and soften
all the edges of pain.

In the dark here
I remember your loving hugs,
urging me on.
I can still see you gathered
—such an unlikely family—
and I know I can find
my way home.

CHRISTINE SAXTON
b. November 17, 1945–d. November 29, 1991

INDEX

PICTURE CREDITS